Neural Fate Decision:
Understanding Cells and their Signals

Neural Fate Decision: Understanding Cells and their Signals

Edited by **Cheryl Chang**

FOSTER ACADEMICS

New Jersey

Published by Foster Academics,
61 Van Reypen Street,
Jersey City, NJ 07306, USA
www.fosteracademics.com

Neural Fate Decision: Understanding Cells and their Signals
Edited by Cheryl Chang

International Standard Book Number: 978-1-63242-286-6 (Hardback)

Printed in China.

Contents

Preface

This book presents an insight into the understanding of neural stem cell fate decisions. Over the past few decades, several studies on regenerative medicine and stem cells have emphasized on novel therapeutic techniques for treatment of many neurological disorders. It has been observed that the present optimism over potential stem cell therapies has propagated from novel comprehensions of stem cell biology leading to particular cell fate decision. This book aims at providing a basic understanding of signaling pathways underlying the ability of differentiation of various types of stem cells into neurons at the time of development; elucidating progress in cellular therapy that could be employed to recover central nervous system dysfunction in pathological conditions; and helping readers to comprehend the changes in signaling pathways under pathological conditions.

After months of intensive research and writing, this book is the end result of all who devoted their time and efforts in the initiation and progress of this book. It will surely be a source of reference in enhancing the required knowledge of the new developments in the area. During the course of developing this book, certain measures such as accuracy, authenticity and research focused analytical studies were given preference in order to produce a comprehensive book in the area of study.

This book would not have been possible without the efforts of the authors and the publisher. I extend my sincere thanks to them. Secondly, I express my gratitude to my family and well-wishers. And most importantly, I thank my students for constantly expressing their willingness and curiosity in enhancing their knowledge in the field, which encourages me to take up further research projects for the advancement of the area.

Editor

Section 1

TGF-Beta Signaling and Neuronal Fate Decision

Chapter 1

Insulin/IGF-Signalling in Embryonic and Adult Neural Proliferation and Differentiation in the Mammalian Central Nervous System

Tanja Vogel

Additional information is available at the end of the chapter

1. Introduction

1.1. General overview of insulin/IGF-signalling

The IIS cascades are initiated by binding of Insulin or Insulin-like growth factors (IGF-1 and -2) to their receptors, the Insulin receptor (IR), and the two Insulin-like growth factor receptor 1 (IGF-1r) and 2 (IGF-2r) (Fig. 1). While high affinity binding occurs between the cognate ligand-receptor pairs, each ligand binds to the other receptors with lower affinity [2]. IR, IGF-1r and -2r are dimers that occur as homo- but also as heterodimers, the latter of which are studied in various cancer cells [3]. Such hybrid receptors are also found in the central nervous system, however a clear function for them has not emerged as yet [4] although activation of different signalling cascades followed by a different biological effect is a likely scenario [2]. IR, IGF-1r and -2r are tyrosine receptor kinases that phosphorylate themself as well as downstream adaptor proteins like the insulin receptor substrate proteins (IRS-1-4) [5]. Through phosphorylation, IRS proteins bind to SRC-homology-2 (SH-2) domain-containing proteins like SRC, SRC homology2-B (SH2-B), protein phosphatases like Tyrosine-protein phosphatase non-receptor type 1 (PTPN1), or the p85 subunit of phosphatidyl inositol 3-kinase (PI3K).

Two major signalling pathways are activated through IIS: the PI3K- and/or the RAS/Mitogen-activated protein kinase- (MAPK) pathways that are implicated in the regulation of a plethora of different cellular processes.

PI3K belongs to a family of lipid kinases that are grouped into three classes. Class IA PI3K are heterodimers of a p110 catalytic and a p85 or p55 regulatory subunit [6]. Binding of PI3K is followed by activation of the p110 catalytic subunit of the kinase, which catalyses the increase of phosphatidylinositol-3,4,5-triphosphate (PtdIns{3,4,5}P3) lipids. PtdIns{3,4,5}P3 induce phosphorylation of phosphoinositide-dependent protein kinase 1 (PDK-1), and the AGC kinase AKT. In mammals, AKT has three different isoforms, AKT-1,-2, and -3. Each of them has two critical sites in their activation domain, Thr308 and Ser473 that need to be phosphorylated both to achieve full kinase activation. Inactive AKT is localised in the cytosol, but it is recruited to the plasma membrane together with PDK-1 through association with phosphatidylinositol-4,5- diphosphosphate (PtdIns{4,5}P2) and PtdIns{3,4,5}P3. As a result, PDK-1 and AKT colocalise at the plasma membrane, which allows PDK-1 to induce phosphorylation of AKT at Thr308. AKT phosphorylation at Ser473 occurs by integrin-linked kinase (ILK) as well as mTORC-2 that are therefore PDK-2s for AKT [7]. Substrates of AKT are numerous, including pro-apoptotic proteins like BAD or anti-apoptotic proteins like BCL-2, NF- κB, and MCL-1, Forkheadbox transcription factors of the FOXO family as well as GSK-3β. AKT also phosphorylates and inhibits the dimer tuberous sclerosis complex-1/-2 (TSC-1/TSC-2), which acts as inhibitory GTPase-activating protein for RHEB. The GTPase RHEB can activate mTORC-1, which has several substrates like p70 ribosomal protein S6 kinase (p70S6K), the translation initiation regulator 4E binding protein (4E-BP), and the proline-rich AKT substrate PRAS40. Through this signalling cascade, IIS activates mTORC-1 to promote cellular growth, translation, transcription, and autophagy. mTORC-1 activation initiates a negative feed back loop through active p70S6K that phosphorylates and inhibits IRS, thereby preventing activation of PI3K in response to IIS. As indicated above, mTORC-2 also influences upstream IIS by phosphorylating AKT as PDK-2 and is involved in spatial growth by regulating the actin cytoskeleton. However, little is known about mTORC-2 activation through IIS. Recent data suggest that mTORC-2 activation through IIS relies on a putative PI3K that is insensitive to the negative feed back loop that controls activation of mTORC-1 [8].

IIS triggering the RAS/MAPK pathways can lead to activation of a subset of three downstream kinases, ERK, JNK, and p38 [9] (Fig. 2). Activation of ERK is dependent on the RAS/MAPK pathway, in which IIS results in phosphorylated IRS or SHC that recruit growth factor receptor-bound protein 2 (GRB-2). GRB-2 associates with the protein son of sevenless (SOS), which is a guanine nucleotide exchange factor. SOS acts by binding RAS-GTPase and forcing it to release bound GDP and to bind GTP instead, which results in an activated state. Activated RAS phosphorylates RAF, which in turn phosphorylates MEK that is responsible to activate the MAPK ERK-1/-2. Jun aminoterminal kinases (JNK-1/-2) are further members of the MAPK pathway that are as well activated through IIS. JNK activation is dependent on PI3K, whose catalytic subunit does not bind to p85 but to the small RHO-family GTPase CDC42 [10]. This complex activates MKK-4 (or MAP2K-4 (mitogen-activated protein kinase kinase 4), which finally phosphorylates JNK-1/-2. The mechanism of p38 activation via IIS is so far unclear [9].

PI3K- and RAS/MAPK-pathways also converge on some downstream molecules like FOXO proteins. Phosphorylation of FOXO through AKT leads to nuclear exclusion and interference with target gene expression. Several other sites are phosphorylated through ERK and p38 MAPK. Interference with these posttranslational modifications leads to decreased promoter binding together with ETS-1 transcription factor (TF) [11].

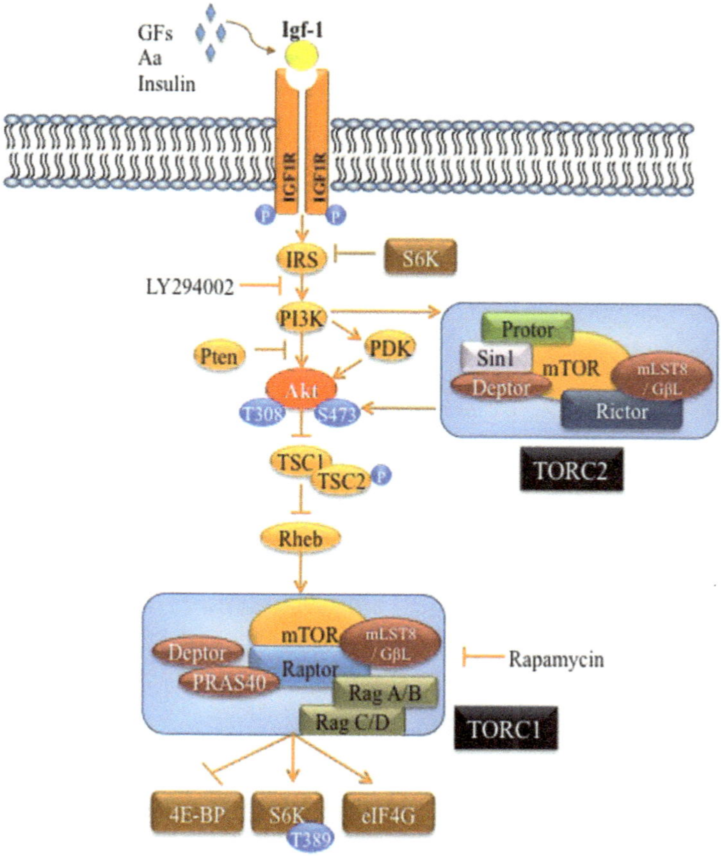

Figure 1. General overview of PI3K-dependent and mTor-driven IIS cascade and points of interference of serveral inhibitors commony used to study downstream IIS.

2. Insulin/IGF-expression in the central nervous system

Insulin, Igf-1 and -2 as well as the three corresponding receptors are widely expressed in the developing and mature central nervous system (CNS) (for a recent review refer to [1]). Expression of Insulin and Igfs is in part under the control of Growth hormone (GH), but action of several tissue- and developmental-specific transcription factors are also involved in Insulin/ Igf expression as is the nutritional status (our own unpublished observations and [12-14]). Coordination and regulation of the biological activity of Igf-1 and -2, but not Insulin, is not only achieved by transcriptional or translational control but also through a set of proteins that have the ability to bind these ligands, namely the Igf-binding proteins (Igfbp). Upto date there

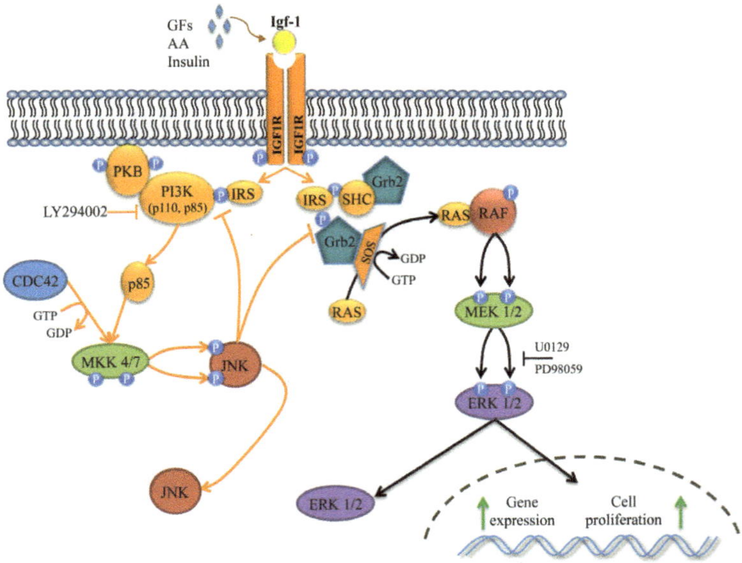

Figure 2. General overview of IIS activating ERK in RAS/MAPK-dependent and JNK in CDC42-dependent manner.

are several Igf-1 and -2 binding proteins as well as Igfbp-related (or -like) proteins that bind to the ligands with varying affinities. Igfbps serve different functions, such as stabilisation and regulation of the concentration of diffusible Igfs, as well as facilitating receptor binding and modulation of Igf-bioavailability in the extracellular space [12]. Altogether, the various subtypes of Igfbps bind 99% of circulating Igf-1 and -2. Within this fraction, 75% are bound to Igfbp-3. Only 1% of Igf-1 and -2 is freely available in the extracellular space [15].

Igf-1 and -2 as well as the Igfbps are widely expressed in the brain [16,17]. Their expression patterns have been described in multiple studies, mainly based on mRNA-detection methods (summarised in [12]). Accordingly, Igf-1 is strongly expressed in the spinal cord, midbrain, cerebral cortex, hippocampus and olfactory bulb (OB) during development. Igf-1 transcription decreases postnatally as cell maturation advances to reach low levels in the adult central nervous system. In the OB, Igf-1 expression persists at high levels in cells that are constantly renewed even in the adult organism [18]. Igf-2 is also expressed in various brain regions and also declines over development. However, it is considered to be the most abundantly expressed Igf in the adult brain.

Igfbp-1 seems generally not to be present in sufficient amounts for detection in the central nervous system [1,19]. Expression of Igfbp-2 is found over all gross neuroanatomical structures of the rat brain, increasing from E15 until adulthood [20]. In preneurogenic stages (E10], rat Igfbp-2 is strongly expressed in neuroectodermal structures of the neural tube and the neuroepithelium [21]. In the postnatal brain it is mainly confined to astroglia as well as to the choroid plexus and leptomeninges [22]. Accordingly, IGFBP-2 is found closely associated with human astroglial tumors. In this research field, it serves not only as a staging marker for glioblastoma but is exploited for therapeutic intervention [23]. IGFBP-2 as well as bound IGF-2 are overexpressed in high-grade astrocytomas. MMP-9-mediated proteolysis of IGFBP-2 leads to increased IGF-2 levels in these tumours. This accounts for increased aggressiveness of the tumours through growth- and motility-promoting effects [24]. Expression of Igfbp-3 in the brain is apparently not studied in great detail. However, Igfbp-3 expression increases after brain insults and it has been shown to be upregulated in Alzheimer's disease brains [25]. Igfbp-3 interacts with retinoic acid and might therefore also be implicated in cell differentiation [26]. Igfbp-4 expression is also detected in most brain regions with declining levels over development [20], being highly expressed in the hippocampus and cerebral cortex in adult stages [27]. A function apart from regulation of Igf action has not been described yet. However, Igfbp-4 expression is decreased in the cerebral cortex, hippocampus and the cerebellum in an *in vivo* model for amyotrophic lateral sclerosis (ALS) [28]. Igfbp-5 is expressed mainly within thalamic nuclei, leptomeninges and the perivascular sheaths in adult rats [27]. Igfbp-6 seems to be expressed in differentiated but not in proliferating cells. Embryonic expression of Igfbp-6 in the CNS seems restricted to the trigeminal ganglia. Igfpb-6 transcription increases postnatally after approx. 21 days in the forebrain and cerebellum, primarily in GABAergic interneurons. Higher levels are found in the hindbrain, spinal cord and dorsal root ganglia [29]. According to this strong association of Igfbp-6 expression with the cerebellar sensorimotor system, overexpression of Igfbp-6 results in a reduced size of the cerebellum [30]. Igfbp-7 is produced in the adult hippocampus, e.g. in the dentate gyrus (DG) [31]. In the postnatal hippocampus, all components of the extracellular Insulin/Igf-signalling molecules were detected apart from Igfbp-1. Variable amounts of individual components were detectable over two developmental time points studied, as well as in different cellular sources, which comprise neurons as well as glial and endothelial cells, albeit Igf-familiy member expression in the latter two cell types were not studied in comprehensive detail.

In rodents, the Insulin-receptor (Ir) is expressed in the olfactory bulb (OB), cerebral cortex, hippocampus, hypothalamus, pituitary, cerebellum, and the choroid plexus [32]. Expression is high in early stages of development and declines in the adult, and is also more enriched in neurons compared to glia. Within mature neurons, enrichment is observed within the postsynaptic density [4,33]. Accordingly, Ir-signalling including downstream mediators like Ras/MAPK and PI3K/Akt/mTor are implicated in synaptic connectivity and dendritic structure [4]. Igf-1r has a similar expression pattern with high expression in the developing cerebellum, midbrain, OB, and hindbrain [12]. However, although expression of Ir and Igf-1r is observed in hippocampus, there are local differences in their distriubtion: Ir is enriched in the CA1 region and Igf-1r is more prominent in the CA3 region. Levels of expression of the Igf-1r are higher during development and decline to adult levels shortly after birth in the brain parenchyma, while it stays relatively high in the choroid plexus, meninges and vascular sheaths.

Igf-2 receptor (Igf-2r) is also known as the mannose-6-phosphate (M6P) receptor, which has a role in lysosomal enzyme trafficking. Accordingly, the main function described so far is to internalise the Igf-2 ligand through endocytosis and to mediate degradation of Igf-2. However, recent studies reveal that Igf-2r is also implicated in specific signal transduction, e.g. in the context of memory enhancement or fear extinction [13,31]. Igf-2r is also expressed in all major neuroanatomical structures, with high expressions in the hippocampus, OB, retina, pituitary, brain stem, and spinal chord. Further it is detected in the choroid plexus, ependymal as well as endothelial cells [12].

Detailed analyses of expression of the upstream Igf-signalling members has been reported for the mouse late embryonic and postnatal cerebellum [34]. Igf-1r is ubiquitously expressed, whereas Igf-1 is detected in a subset of Purkinje cells (PC) at E17.5 and in postnatal stages. Igf-2 is confined to the meninges and blood vessels. Both ligands are not detectable in dividing cerebellar granule precursor cells (CGP). Igfbp-1 is not detected, but Igfbp-2 is expressed wide spread in the meninges, PC, internal as well as external granule layer, and choroid plexus. Igfbp-3 is restricted to PC, Igfbp-4 to meninges and choroid plexus, and Igfbp-5 to Calbindin-negative cells of the PC layer. Igfbp-6 is only detected in later stages in a subset of PC.

According to the widespread expression of members of the upstream IIS, their developmental dynamics and cell type specificity, it is conceivable that this signalling pathway exerts important function for development, maintenance as well as function of the various parts of the central nervous system. Some of these functions that are mainly attributable to neuronal development and fate decision will be highlighted in the following sections.

3. Biological effects associated with Insulin/IGF-signalling in neural development

3.1. Insulin/IGF-signalling in ESC

Insulin and IGF are important factors to keep human ESCs in a proliferative state and to promote self-renewal, where upon IGF-1R has been identified as essential component [35]. Blocking of IGF-signalling results in differentiation, but it is unclear whether a certain cell fate is favoured under such condition. Downstream signalling of Insulin and IGF has also been studied in this context and revealed that blocking of this pathway at various points induced differentiation. In this study, blocking is achieved on the level of PI3K through LY294002, of AKT-1, and of mTOR-1 through Rapamycin. Treatment of human ESC with LY294002 results in loss of phosphorylation of the downstream molecules AKT, p70S6K, S6 as well as GSK-3β [35-38].

Together with stromal cell-derived factor 1 (SDF-1/CXCL-12), pleiotrophin (PTN), and ephrin-B1 (EFNB1) IGF-2 induces differentiation of human ESC into TH-positive dopaminergic neurons [39].

Interestingly, retinol/vitamin A also induces Nanog transcription and the signal is transduced over the IGF-1R, IRS-1, AKT and both mTOR complexes, mTORC-1 and mTORC-2 [40]. Expression of Nanog is a hallmark of proliferating, pluripotent stem cells. However, Insulin has differentiating capacity into the neuroectodermal lineage when human ESCs are cocultured with endodermal derived cells. This effect is dependent on PI3K/AKT signalling [41]. Together, these results reflect context-dependent IIS, and possibly cross-talk with other signalling pathways activated e.g. *in vivo* through development or *in vitro* through cocultures.

3.2. Insulin/IGF effects in embryonic neural precursors

The Insulin-receptor (Ir) is expressed in distinct regions of the CNS, including the olfactory bulb (OB), hypothalamus and the pituitary. Accordingly, a Nestin-cre mediated conditional, CNS-specific knock-out of the Ir early during development results in increased Luteinising hormone (LH) release from the hypothalamic-pituitary axis that leads to a deregulation of energy homeostasis and endocrinology of the reproductive system [42].

Neurospheres generated from embryonic striatal precursors in the presence of Egf respond to Igf-1 treatment with increased neuronal differentiation, presumably over an Igf-1r dependent signalling cascade. However, this has not been addressed comprehensively through receptor inhibition but was deduced from lower differentiation upon Igf-2 and Insulin stimuli [16,17,43]. Igf-1 treatment in this setting is not accompanied by increased cell proliferation, but cotreatment with Insulin increases the fraction of dividing cells. It might be that this effect is specific to this combined treatment.

In the cerebral cortex, increased Igf-1 expression after Growth hormone (GH) treatment of rat embryonal neural precursors is involved in increased proliferation of early (E14) and late (E17) progenitors and is accompanied by increased neuronal differentiation at both time points. In addition to neuronal differentiation, astrogenesis is also increased but only when late progenitors are exposed to GH. This effect is also blocked in the presence of an Igf-1-blocking antibody and thus illustrates that IIS is transducing GH-induced effects [42,44].

Increased proliferation of E14 rat cortical progenitor upon Igf-1 is observed *in vitro* after treatment of cultured cells, and *in vivo* after intrauterine Igf-1 injection [45].

Igf-1 function in the brain is highly context-dependent and cell-type specific. This interpretation is corroborated by the finding that Igf-1 treatment of E19 rat embryonal hippocampal progenitors does influence survival of these cells [46].

In another setting, Igf-1 treatment evokes cell survival of mouse E10 neuroepithelial cells [47] and it is mitogenic for sympathetic neuroblasts [48], showing that progenitor subtypes respond differently to IIS. It is so far ill defined what kind of signalling events, including cross-talks to other pathways, are associated with this differential outcome of Igf-1 stimulation. Interaction with Egf- as well as Fgf-2-signalling and Igf-1 has been studied in striatal-derived neural progenitor cells (NPCs). In this setting, highest numbers of formed spheres are obtained in the presence of Igf-1 and Egf or Igf-1 and Fgf-2. Sphere formation in this context is highly dependent on presence of Igf-1, since no spheres were observed in the absence of IIS [49]. These data show that Igf-1 is also affecting NPC proliferation in cooperation with other signalling molecules, emphasising the pleiotrophic nature of IIS.

Igf-1-signalling seems to increase the effects of Fgf-2 on NPC proliferation as has been shown in various stem cell populations, like rat adult SVZ neurospheres [50], neurospheres from mouse E13.5 forebrains [51], mouse embryonic OBSC [52], and mouse embryonic striatal NPC [49]. Although not shown in all stem cells investigated so far, it is likely that in one scenario Igf-1 promotes survival and proliferating competence of stem cells but that other mitogens such as Erk-activators are needed to increase proliferation. However, other stem cell populations might proliferate upon IIS without further mitogenic instructions as has been observed by Fgf-2-independent Igf-1-mediated proliferation in rat embryonic NPCs from the cerebral cortex and the hippocampus [45,46].

NPCs from neonatal rat forebrain undergo neuronal differentiation upon Insulin-treatment [53]. The content of GFAP-positive cells in the neurosphere-based assay is unchanged, thus suggesting a preference for neuronal differentiation in this cellular model.

Embryonal stem cells from the olfactory bulb (OBSC) are strongly dependent on IIS as shown *in vitro* as well as *in vivo*. Igf-1 increases OBSC proliferation as well as differentiation without strong lineage restriction, thus affecting neuronal as well as glial differentiation [54]. OBSC proliferation however does not depend strictly on Igf-1, Insulin or pro-Insulin, they rather potentiate the proliferating effect of Fgf-2 and Egf [52]. This study also showed that Igf-1 induces differentiation into the neuronal and astroglial lineages, but oligodendrocyte differentiation clearly depends on presence of other growth factors.

Several data support the finding that Igf-1 and -2 increase cerebellar granule cell precursor (CGP) proliferation as well as survival of the same [34,55]. Different effects were linked to different concentrations of the cytokine, where lower concentrations favoured survival and higher proliferation [56]. IIS is supporting Sonic hedgehog (Shh) action that is a potent mitogen for CGPs. Blocking of signal transduction through the Igf-1r diminishes Shh-mediated cell proliferation, as well as endogenous supply of Igfbp-5. However, other Igfbps do not interfere with Shh-mediated proliferation, but decrease Igf-1-dependent cell division [34].

Igf-2 treatment of CGP also results in proliferation. However it is unclear whether this occurs over the Igf-1r or 2r [57] but it indicates also important function for Igf-2 in the context of development of the central nervous system.

Igf-1 prevents cell death in primary rat embryonic hippocampal cultures after exposure to glucocorticoids. While increased levels of corticosterone reduce Akt-phosphorylation and lead to cell death, Igf-1 rescues cells from dying by increasing pAkt-levels in a PI3K-dependent manner [58]. The same effect is observed by applying Insulin instead of Igf-1 [59].

Signalling of Insulin/Igf affects NPC proliferation, survival as well as differentiation *in vitro* and this finding is corroborated *in vivo* by studies of knock-out and transgenic mouse models. Transgene-mediated overexpression of Igf-1, driven by the Nestin-promoter, supports *in vitro* finding that Igf-1 influences NPC proliferation as well as neuronal differentiation during development. Cumulative BrdU-labelling shows that Igf-1 decreases the total length of the cell cycle through acceleration of the G1-phase. This higher proliferating activity is paired with a higher rate of cell-cycle re-entry. The overall increased number of progenitors provides a larger pool of NPCs for neuronal differentiation and thus increases numbers of neurons residing in the postnatal cortical plate of Igf-1-overexpressing mice [60]. *In vivo*, Igf-1 also exhibits survival function since apoptosis is reduced upon its overexpression [61,62] which further contributes to increased numbers of neurons in the cortical plate. Igf-1 signalling does not affect all neuronal populations in a similar manner but shows regional differences. The neuronal composition of the motor cortex is more increased than the somatosensory cortex of Igf-1-overexpressing mice, which is however also increased compared to wildtype animals. Neurons in the cortical plate are also differently affected. Layer 1 neurons comprise the most increased neuronal fraction in Igf-1-transgenic brains, layer 6 neurons show the smallest increase [63]. It is thus likely that NPC are more sensitive to IIS during early developmental events of the cerebral cortex in which neurogenesis of frontal precedes that of caudal regions and layer 1 is preceding generation of layer 6.

In line with *in vivo* overexpression studies, complete loss of Igf-1 in mice leads to the opposite effect of decreased numbers of specific neuronal populations in the cerebral cortex, e.g. hippocampal granule cells and striatal parvalbumin-positive interneurons. Dopaminergic neurons of the midbrain, basal forebrain cholinergic neurons, as well as motoneurons in the spinal cord do not depend on Igf-1 presence [64]. Further analysis of this Igf-1-deficient mouse revealed Igf-1-dependence of axonal growth and myelination that are strongly impaired. Overall, Igf-1-deficient mice have a decreased number of myelinated axons. This observation goes in line with studies of human IGF-I overexpression driven by a mouse metallothionein promoter, that revealed increased myelin production by an unchanged number of oligodendrocytes in adult brains [65].

Overexpression of Igf-1 driven by the Igf-2 promoter results in general brain overgrowth. The greatest effect is seen in the cerebellum, although Igf-1 deletion does not lead to an observable phenotype in this part of the brain, maybe because of compensatory effects from Igf-2 [55,64].

Igf-1r-deficient mice show severe growth retardation and die perinatally. Nestin-cre-mediated conditional knockout of the Igf-1r also results in death shortly after birth but few animals survive up to adulthood [66]. Mice that are heterozygote for the conditional Igf-1r deletion also display severe growth retardation that was studied in detail in the hippocampus. In the postnatal hippocampus all different parts are affected by increased rates of apoptosis rather than by an impaired ability to proliferate through loss of the Igf-1r.

Mutations of the type 2 Igf receptor are lethal but are rescued from this perinatal lethality in Igf-2 and Igf-1r null backgrounds [67]. This observation is attributed to increased Igf-2 signalling due to lack of internalisation of Igf-2, which is thought to be a major function of the Igf-2r. Although general hyperplasia is observed including the brain, Igf-2r-signalling was not further investigated in the brain [67-69].

Deletion of Igf-2 in mice results in severe growth-deficiency, but it was reported that Igf-2-deficient mice do not show striking morphological aberrations [70,71]. However, one source of Igf-2 during development is the choroid plexus, from which it is released into the cerebrospinal fluid (CSF), and CSF-derived Igf-2 is an important signal for cell proliferation of later embryonic precursors that have contact to the ventricular surface [72]. Progenitors of the SVZ, e.g. Tbr-2-expressing cells, do not have contact to the CSF and thus are not influenced by Igf-2-signalling in their proliferation capacity. Increased proliferation of cortical progenitors is dependent on the apical (ventricular) localisation of the Igf-1r that is mediated through the cell polarity protein Pals-1 (Protein Associated with Lin Seven 1) as part of the apical complex. Further support for an Igf-1r-mediated effect of Igf-2-signalling in this context comes from the finding that loss of Pten (Phosphatase and Tensin homolog) opposes the effect of Pals-1-deficiency: Pten-deficient mice have hyperplasic cortices while Pals-1-deficiency results in cortical hypoplasia. The phenotypes are partially reverted through combination of both transgenes [72]. Further downstream signals apart from Igf-1r and PI3K are not analysed in this context.

The function of different Igfbps has been studied through transgenic mouse models. Thereby it turned out, that loss of function mutations do not result in gross morphological changes within the CNS. However, overexpression of Igfbps lead to phenotypes in the CNS, which are exploited to achieve better understanding of IIS within this organ. Overexpression of Igfbp-1 in transgenic mice using either a phosphogylcerate kinase [73] or a methallothionein [74] promoter results in similar phenotypes as observed in adult Igf-1-deficient mice: reduced brain sizes due to loss of mature neurons and decreased progenitor proliferation, impaired myelination as well as decreased activation of GFAP-expressing astrocytes in conditions of injury. However, Igfbp-1 is normally not expressed at detectable levels in the CNS and the observed findings are therefore attributed to the lack of Igf-1 as consequence of increased presence of Igfbp-1. Most of the phenotypes observed in mice overexpressing Igfbps resemble those of loss of Igf-1-signalling, which is mainly characterised by reduced organ size. Whether these phenotypes are exclusively caused by impaired Igf-1-signalling or whether Igfbps have also distinct functions, is so far not resolved [75]. Generally, Igfbp-5 is considered to potentiate Igf-1-signalling, while Igfbp-2 mainly opposes Igf-1 and Igf-2 action [55]. This finding indicates that some Igfbps might exert additional functions that might only be apparent in transgenic mice in which the ligands are mutated as well.

3.3. Insulin/IGF effects in adult neural precursors

Igf-1, though not produced in high amounts in adult rodent brains, is required for normal neuronal functions throughout life. As different source, peripheral Igf-1 is transported to neuronal cells through an uptake from the blood stream (reviewed in [1]). Neural stem cells of the adult hippocampus respond to peripheral administered Igf-1 with increased proliferation as well as neurogenesis but not with astrogenesis [76]. These data were also confirmed *in vitro* using neurospheres generated from the hippocampal dentate gyrus. In this setting, low doses of Igf-1 mediate, and high doses interfere with neuronal differentiation [77]. Igf-1-mediated cell proliferation of adult neuronal progenitor from the hippocampal subgranular zone (SGZ) was also shown in a model of epilepsy [78] as well as in response to physical excercise [79].

Further in vivo evidence for importance of Igf-1-signalling in the adult hippocampus comes from a study of Igf-1-deficient rats. In this context Igf-1 supports survival of newly generated neurons and possibly the maturation of the neuronal phenotype. However, cell proliferation is not affected in this *in vivo* model [80]. Igf-1-instructed differentiation mainly into the oligodendroglial lineage has been shown in rat adult hippocampal NPC [81] (Fig. 3). In this study, withdrawal of proliferation-promoting Fgf-2 is essential to drive NPCs into differen-

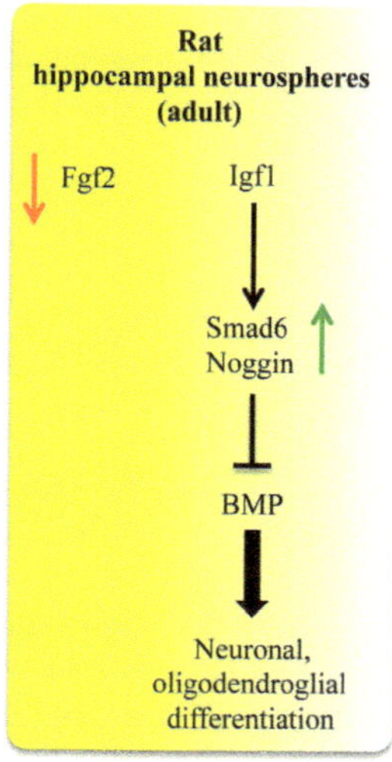

Figure 3. Igf-1 signalling in adult rat hippocampal neurospheres [81].

tiation upon Igf-1. IIS in this setting induces expression of Bmp-antagonists Noggin and Smad6, which are involved in the inhibition of an astrocytic cell fate and in favouring neuronal, but more efficiently oligodendroglial differentiation. Further, this study showed again that Igf-1 has a major impact on cell survival of adult NPCs.

Overexpression of Igf-1 through an Igf-2 promoter element results in increased numbers of neurons in the postnatal mouse hippocampal dentate gyrus. This increase in neurogenesis is transiently accompanied by increased numbers of synapses, which makes it possible that IIS also influences synaptogenesis [82].

Adult rat NPC derived from the subventricular zone proliferate stronger upon an Igf-1 stimulus. This effect is blocked by the presence of Igfbp-3 that also decreases phosphorylation of Akt [83]. Igf-1 signalling under Fgf-2-free conditions in adult subventricular stem cells is also linked to differentiation [84]. Adult mouse NPC are initially cultivated in the presence of Fgf-2. Subsequent withdrawal of Fgf-2 results in neuronal differentiation that is increased by complementation with Igf-1. Blocking of the Igf-1 signal with an antibody reverts the effect [85]. In this setting, the authors also explored the capacity of Igfbp-2 to influence the neurogenic potential of the NPC, since Igfbp-2 complexes with Igf-1 and proteoglycans like heparin in the rat OB [86]. Low doses of exogenous Igfbp-2 increase neuronal differentiation, while application of a blocking Igfbp-2 antibody interferes with this effect. These experiments indicate that Igfbp-2 does not act by sequestering Igf-1 and by limiting its bioavailability, in which scenario Igfbp-2 would have an opposing effect to Igf-1. Instead, both molecules exert the same phenotypic differentiation and this indicates that Igfbp-2 function in this context is more likely a protection of Igf-1 from degradation. It is conceivable that simultaneous interaction of Igfbp-2 with proteoglycans decreases its affinity to Igf-1. The net outcome might be a locally increased amount of free Igf-1 that drives neuronal differentiation of NPC [85]. In another study, differentiation of SVZ NPC was deduced from reduced expression of the stem cell marker Nestin after Igf-1 treatment, but it was not specified whether differentiation of a specific cell lineage was favoured [50].

Further studies in adult mice show that lack of Igf-1 results in disturbed neuroblast exit from the subventricular zone and their subsequent migration to the olfactory bulb through the rostral migratory stream. This Igf-1 function is dependent on PI3-kinase activity and Disabled-1 (Dab-1) phosphorylation via Src-family kinase [87].

Igf-2 is not only provided from the CSF and important for early development of the brain. In addition, adult mouse hippocampal stem cells from the DG also produce Igf-2, and to a much lesser extend Igf-2 is also detected in adult SVZ-derived stem cells [19,88]. Challenging Igf-2 expression through siRNA-mediated approaches as well as treatment of DG-derived NPCs reveals that Igf-2 also influences proliferation. However, SVZ-derived NPCs do not respond with changed proliferation upon Igf-2 knockdown [88]. Igf-2 but not Igf-1 is involved in neuronal survival of newly generated neurons in the adult DG in a model of fear extinction, that is strongly associated with neurogenesis in the hippocampus [31]. Neuronal survival and fear extinction depend on Igf-1r activity and are opposed by increased levels of Igfbp-7. However, Igf-1 does not exert any observable effect in this setting.

FoxO proteins are under the control of IIS and therefore a downstream read-out of this important signalling pathway. GFAP-cre was used to generate a triple allelic knockout of FoxO1, 3, and 4 in adult NPCs. The observed effect on cell proliferation is dependent on the age of the animal or passage of cells in culture. NPCs from young (P8) brains displayed hyperproliferation upon loss of FoxO-proteins and the same was observed for early passages of NPCs in culture. This initial hyperproliferation is followed by decreased doubling times and the depleted progenitor pool results in declining neuronal differentiation. FoxOs balance NPC proliferation and prevent premature loss of NPCs. Microarray studies revealed several cell-cycle regulating genes that are affected in their expression by the loss of FoxO. Furthermore, Aspm (asp (abnormal spindle)-like, microcephaly associated) and anatgonists of the Wnt-signalling cascade, Sfrp-1 (secreted frizzled-related protein) and -2, as well as Sost (sclerostin), are involved in the FoxO-dependent regulation. In this context FoxO might control Wnt-induced cell proliferation by expression of Wnt-antagonists [89].

3.4. Insulin/IGF effects in mature neurons

Igf-1 applied to postnatal cerebellar granule neurons (CGN) prevents cell death, thus establishing IIS as survival factor in mature neurons [90]. Another study described a link of Igf-1-signalling in mature neurons to survival of CGN as well as of cortical neurons. Here, Igf-1 prevents apoptosis through activation of PI3K/Akt, but also through Igf-1r-dependend transactivation of unliganded Pac-1r (PACAP type 1 receptor) via Src-kinase activity [91] (Fig. 4).

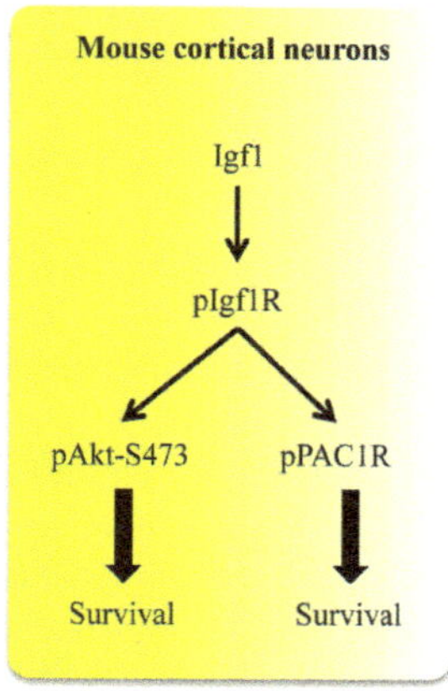

Figure 4. IIS mediated sur-vival of cortical neurons through activation of Akt and PAC-1r [91].

Data from adult Igf-1-deficient mice show however that cerebellar neurons are not affected by the loss of this trophic factor *in vivo* [64]. Contrasting this finding is data showing overexpression of human IGF-1 in mouse through a transgene driven by the mouse Igf-2 promoter [92] that results in cerebellar overgrowth through blockage of the ontogenetic cell death that normally takes place during early postnatal cerebellar development.

Blocking Igf-1 uptake through systemic application of an Igf-1 antibody not only reduces cell proliferation in the adult rat and mouse hippocampus, but is also implicated in synaptic remodelling and interferes with exercise-induced increase of dendritic spines [93]. IIS is also implicated in neuronal maturation and stimulates neurite outgrowth. In postnatal rat slice cultures of the somatosensory cortex, Igf-1-treatment leads to increased apical and basic dendritic branching of pyramidal neurons [94]. As such, Igf-1 is involved in forming mature neuronal networks and ensuring proper information processing. Further data show that Igf-1 mediates axonal growth by inducing plasmalemmal expansions by incorporation of vesicles in the growth cone [95]. This Igf-1-, but not Insulin-dependent effect is mediated by signalling via a growth-cone-specific Igf-1 receptor (βgc), Irs-2, Shp-2, PI3K and Akt. This cascade might also influence dynamics of the cytoskeleton, namely microtubules and actin, both of which are required for axonal growth.

Igf-2 has recently been shown to control the number of synaptic connections and plasticity in mature neurons of the hippocampus [13,14]. Memory enhancement is specifically associated with Igf-2 function. In this context Igf-2 is regulated by CCAAT enhancer binding protein β (C/EBP) in adult rat hippocampus. C/EBP is one of the transcription factors necessary for memory consolidation. In the study of Chen et al. rats are exposed to increased Igf-2 levels in the hippocampus during memory training which results in improved learning [13]. This effect is specific to Igf-2, since injection of Igf-1 did not have any observable effect in this memory consolidation paradigm.

Taken together, IIS has different effects in the developing and mature CNS that vary among the different cell types as summarised in Fig. 5. Differences might be mediated through specific downstream cascades or effector molecules present in only one specific cell or at a specific developmental time point. Another scenario is the cross-talk between IIS and other cytokines that are produced by the organism. Posttranslational modification of the receptors might be another general mechanism that specifies different biological responses to common signal inducers (ligand/receptor) and common intracellular signal transducers. The IGF-1r is sumoylated and modulated in its activity. Sehat et al. showed [96] this sumoylation of the IGF-1 receptor that leads to internalisation of the ligand bound protein complex, which is transduced to the nucleus and binds directly to genomic DNA. Since binding occurs predominantly in intergenic regions, the biological relevance for differential gene transcription has still to be shown. But nevertheless this reflects a possible mechanism through which specificity in activation of different target genes upon the same stimulus might be obtained in different cells or in the same cells at different developmental time points.

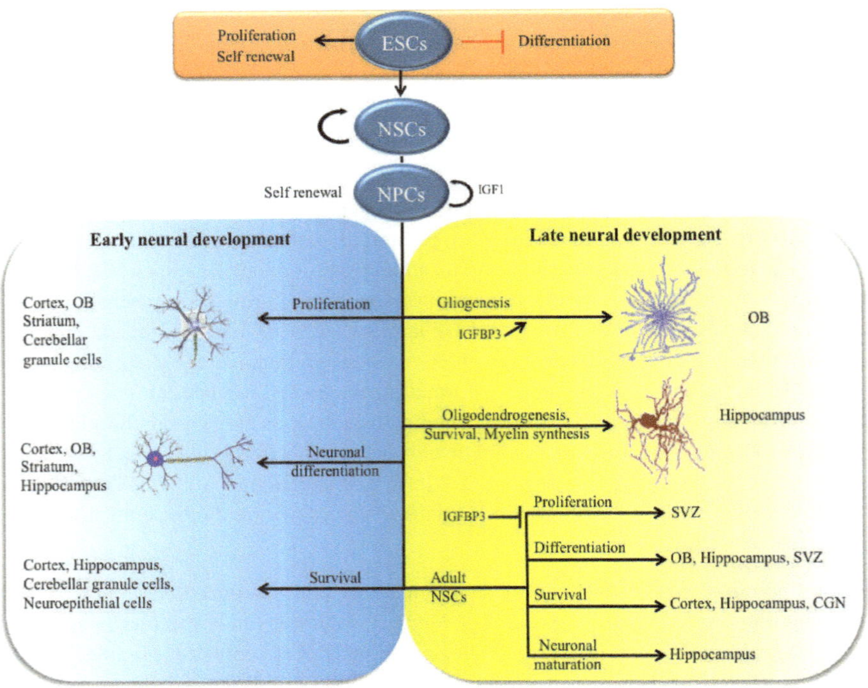

Figure 5. Differences in IIS function in different cell types of the CNS and in developmentThe Insulin-Igf Signalling (IIS) pathway has multiple effects on different cells of the CNS. The effects, beginning from cues for ESC proliferation and self-renewal, transcend to those of proliferation, self-renewal, differentiation and fate determination of NPCs. IIS contributes to either formation of neurons, or glia, oligodendrocytes and myelin.

4. Insulin/IGF-signalling networks

4.1. Signalling networks in neural progenitors and neurons

Igf-1-dependent embryonal NPC proliferation in rat has been shown to be dependent on the PI3K/Akt pathway, but not on the MAPK/Erk branch of signalling. Chemical inhibitors of the latter, U0129 and PD98059, have no effect on NPC proliferation, while PI3K-inhibition through LY294002 interferes with Akt- and downstream Gsk-3β-phosphorylation as well as proliferation. Phosphorylated and thus inactivated Gsk-3β leads to stabilisation of CycD1 (Cyclin D1). Together with increased expression of CycD3, and CycE as cell cycle promoters, decreased expression of inhibitory cell cycle proteins p27 and p57 is observed upon Igf-1-treatment and accounts for the mitogenic effect of Igf-1 [45] (Fig. 6).

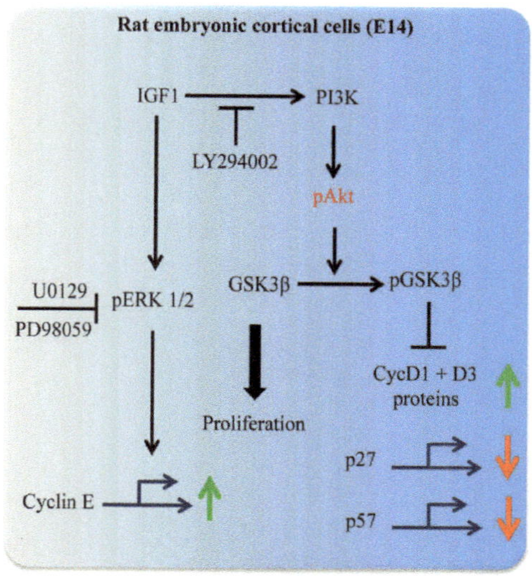

Figure 6. Igf-1-dependent embryonal NPC proliferation in rat [45].

Cortical progenitors isolated from mouse E13.5 brains were investigated with regard to increased Akt-1-signalling. Overexpression of Akt-1 results in increased proliferation as well as survival of progenitors *in vivo* and *in vitro*, consistant with effects of increased IIS. This Akt-1 function does not depend on its action upon p21, but at least in part of mTorc-1, because proliferation is partially hampered through Rapamycin. Survival is not affected through mTorc1 inhibition [97]. Differential downstream signalling of Akt in cortical progenitors is indicated by this study, which also reports that Rapamycin does only block proliferation in a subset of cells at E13.5, and progenitors of later developmental stages are also insensitive to Rapamycin with regard to proliferation (Fig. 7).

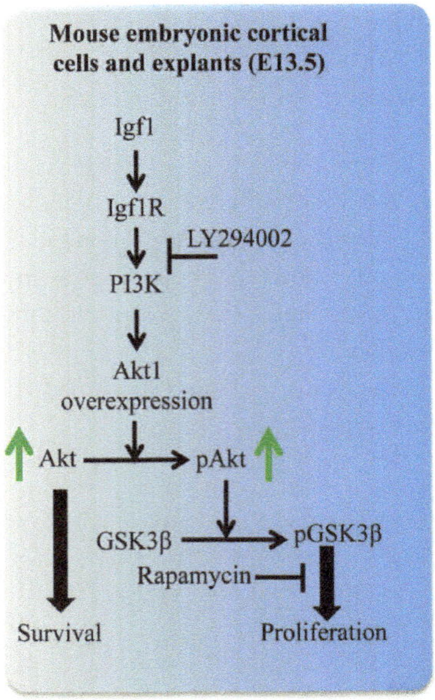

Figure 7. Survival and proliferation upon Igf-1 treat-ment in mouse E13.5 cortical cells [97].

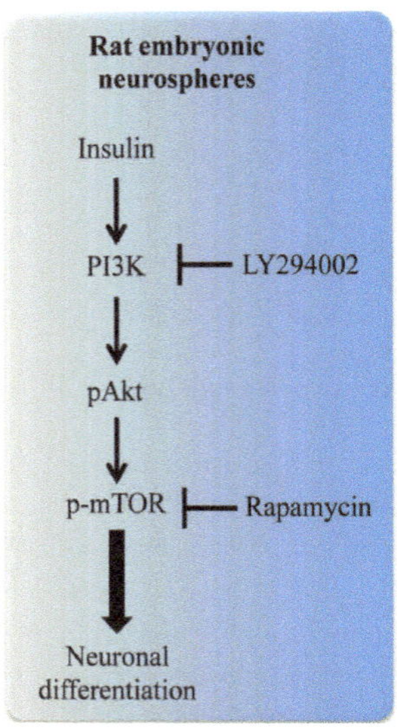

Figure 8. Insulin-dependent neuronal differentiation of embryonic neurosheres [50].

MTorc-1 inhibition through Rapamycin prevents neuronal differentiation of rat embryonic telencephalon-derived neurospheres that is observed in response to Insulin-signalling [53]. In this setting, Insulin-treatment results in phosporylation of mTorSer2448 and of pS670K, and the former is blocked through addition of Rapamycin, indicating that mTorc-1 is implicated in neuronal differentiation. Apoptosis is not observed under these conditions (Fig. 8).

MTor-1-dependent neuronal differentiation is also observed in P19 embryonic carcinoma cells that express Pax-6 as well as Hes-5 upon retinoic acid treatment and initiation of neural differentiation. In this setting, Cdc42 is placed as upstream regulator of mTorc-1, and treatment with Rapamycin abolished Cdc42-mediated neural lineage specification as well as terminal neuronal differentiation [98].

MTorc-1 is also implicated in cell proliferation of rat adult hippocampal progenitors that heavily depend on PI3K-activated Akt-signalling. MTorc-1-dependence is obvious because presence of Rapamycin interfered with increased cell proliferation under Fgf-2-stimulation. Although Igf-1 treatment of these cells did not result in increased proliferation, Igf-1 increases cell division in the presence of Fgf-2 over the rate that is achieved through Fgf-2 alone [99]. Sustained activation of mTor-signalling in mice that are deficient for Tsc-1 results in initially increased proliferation of NPC and premature depletion of the progenitor pool. Self-renewal of Tsc-1-deficient and thus mTor-activated NPC is also dramatically impaired. In addition to increased numbers of cells that differentiate into the neuronal lineage, sustained mTor activity interferes with terminal differentiation of neurons but seems to promote an increase in astrocytes [100]. Increased cell proliferation is also a hallmark of Tsc-2-deficient mouse NPC that are isolated from early (E10.5) developmental time points. This phenotype is also attributed to an activation of mTorc-1-signalling [101].

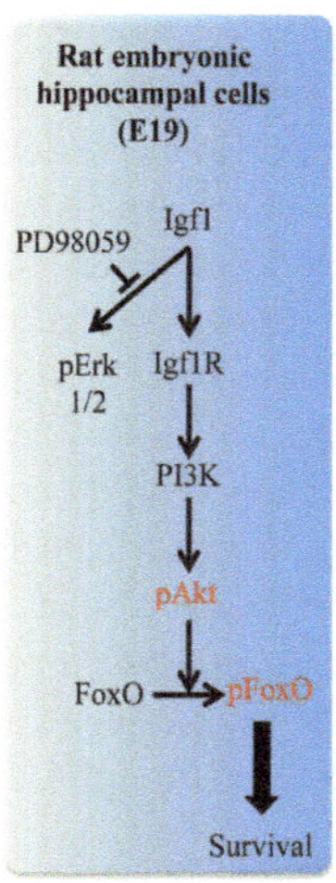

Figure 9. Igf-1-dependent survival of rat hip-pocampal precursors [46].

Igf-1-initiated survival of E19 rat embryonal hippocampal cells is dependent on PI3K-mediated Akt-phosphorylation and subsequent phosphorylation of FoxO3. Phosphorylation of FoxO3 is blocked by LY294002 and partially by Rapamycin, and results in increased survival of hippocampal progenitors. Blocking of MAPK/Erk pathway with PD98059 does not influence survival of these progenitors [46,102] (Fig. 9).

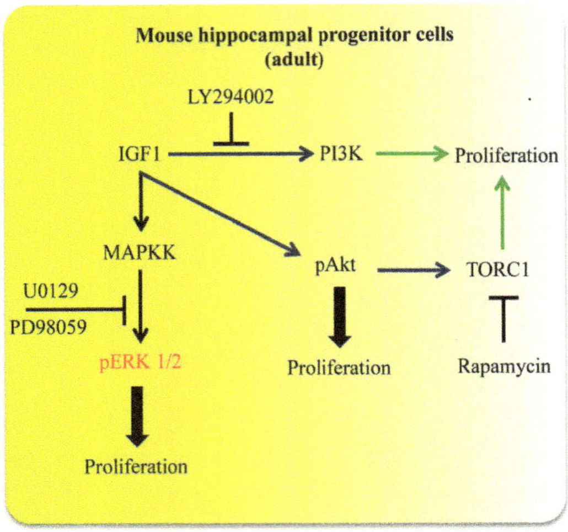

Figure 10. IIS in regulation of proliferation of adult hippocampal progenitors [77, 78].

Igf-1-mediated proliferation of neural progenitors of the adult DG is mainly but not exclusively mediated by MAPK/Erk-signalling, since inhibition of MAPKK/Mek-1/2 through a chemical inhibitor or dominant negative kinases interferes with cell division after Igf-1 treatment. Blocking of PI3 kinase through LY294002 interferes with proliferation even without addition of Igf-1. However, blocking of the Akt-downstream signal through use of a dominant negative kinase also reduces Igf-1-induced mitosis. This finding makes it likely that LY294002-independent activation of Akt might be important for Igf-1-mediated proliferation. Rapamycin does not have significant effects in this setting, making it likely that mTor-complexes are not involved in Igf-1-mediated proliferation of adult hippocampal progenitors [77] (Fig. 10). Further evidence for the implication of Igf-1/MAPK/Erk- signalling in proliferation of adult hippocampal progenitors comes from the study of increased mitosis after a status epilepticus. Here, this lesion activates Igf-1-release from microglia. This increase in Igf-1 results in the activation of the MAPK/Erk-pathway and subsequent cell division. This response is blocked through inhibition of the Igf-1r as well as through U0129-mediated inhibition of the MAPK-pathway [78].

It is interesting to point out that the same biological effect can be achieved through Igf-1 by activating different pathways in different cells: IIS induces proliferation in embryonic rat cortical progenitors in an Erk-independent manner, while Igf-1 signalling induces proliferation of adult hippocampal progenitors via Erk-dependent cytoplasmic downstream signals. On the other hand, IIS mediates different biological effects in similar cells through similar downstream molecules, but at different developmental time points: adult hippocampal neurons respond with proliferation to Igf-1 compared to embryonic hippocampal progenitors that need IIS for their survival. This summary indicates that we still need comprehensive analyses of overlapping or distinct target genes activated through overlapping or distinct signalling pathways during development and in the various cell types of the CNS.

The study of Otaegi et al. of IIS in OBSC also elaborates on downstream signalling by showing that Igf-1 treatment increases phosphorylation of Akt at Ser473 as well as Thr308 which is associated with increased proliferation and neural differentiation [54] (Fig. 11). Pten, that antagonises PI3-kinase induced phosphorylation of phosphatidylinositol (3,4,5)trisphosphate (PtdIns(3,4,5)P3), reduces basal levels of the activating posttranslational modifications of Akt, which are however overridden by presence of Insulin/Igf-1. Nevertheless, overexpression of Pten impaires neural differentiation without affecting progenitor proliferation, and overexpression of a mutant Pten increases OBSC differentiation. Direct inhibition of PI3-kinase through LY294002 interferes with Igf-1-stimulated Akt-phosphorylation and resultes in impaired proliferation as well as neural differentiation. Thus, OBSC differentiation is under control of basic levels of pAkt while increased pAkt-levels through IIS activation affect additionally proliferation.

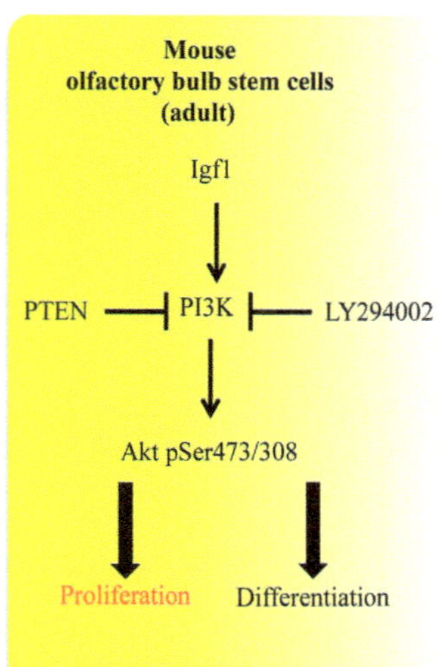

Figure 11. IIS affects proliferation and differentiation in adult OBSC [51].

Early postnatal olfactory bulb neurons do survive upon Igf-1-signalling. In this context, a positive feedback has been proposed between Igf-1 and Bcl-2. Igf-1 increases expression of anti-apoptotic Bcl-2, and overexpression of Bcl-2 *in vivo* results in increased Igf-1 and Igfbp2 [103].

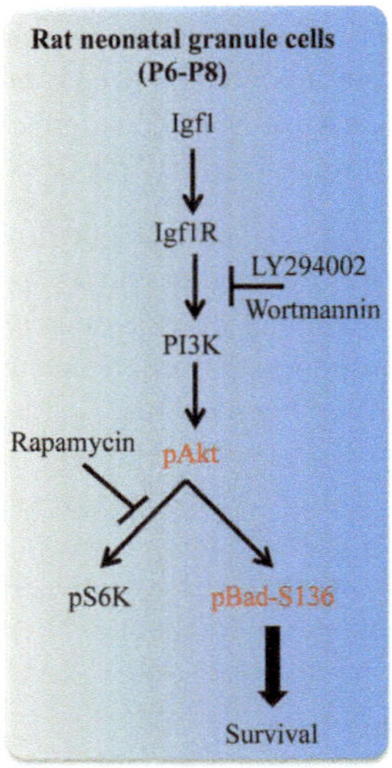

Figure 12. Survival of CGN upon IIS [90, 104, 105].

Igf-1 action as survival factor for postnatal cerebellar granule neurons (CGN) requires different intracellular signalling [90]. In this context, Igf-1 activation of PI3K leads to inhibition of Erk as well as Caspase-3, two pathways exerting different events in cell death, plasma membrane damage and DNA break-down, respectively. Activated PI3K phosphorylates not only Akt but also Protein kinase A (PKA). Whereas pAkt activates Caspase-3 and is leading to DNA break-down, PKA suppresses sustained Erk activation via phosphorylation of cRaf at Ser259 and prevents plasma membrane damage (Fig. 12).

Further studies of Igf-1-dependent survival of rat CGN links PI3K activation of Akt to phosphorylation of Bad at Ser136 that is responsible for releasing anti-apoptotic Bcl-X_L [104,105]. This finding is partially corroborated *in vivo*, where Igf-1 overexpression results in increased levels of Bcl-X_L at early time points (P7) and decreased expression of pro-apoptotic Bax and Bad at P14 and P21. However, the investigation of the phosphorylation status of Bad *in vivo* was not conclusive [92].

Oligodendrogenesis and initiation as well as maintenance of myelination are strongly dependent on IIS. Several mouse models in which normal IIS was manipulated display phenotypes affecting oligodendroglial cells: overexpression of Igf-1 driven by diverse promoters or administration of Igf-1 into the CSF result in increased numbers of oligodendrocytes and myelination [106-108], while loss of Igf-1 leads to impaired and lost myelination [109]. IIS in oligodendrocytes and their precursors is dependent on signalling over the Igf-1r, since Igf-1r-deficient mice show retarded growth and initiation of myelination [110]. This phenotype is not observed in IR-deficient mice and is thus mediated through Igf-1r-signalling [111]. IIS depends on binding of insulin-response substrate (Irs1-4) to the receptors, which results in their respective phosphorylation.

Proliferation of oligodendroglial rat precursors increases in response to Igf-1 and is mediated over a prolonged time period by Pdk-1, Akt Thr308 as well as Ser473 phosphorylation, and pGsk-3β. Igf-1 treatment also activated the Ras/MAPK-pathway as evidenced by increased pErk-1/-2, following a fast kinetic over a short period of time [112]. Inhibition of upstream signalling molecules revealed concerted involvement of PI3K, MAPK as well as Src-kinase in cell cycle progression, and predominance of Akt-mediated signalling. Although so far ill defined, cross-talk among the different signalling pathways activated through Igf-1 is a likely scenario resulting from this study. In continuation of this study it was observed that Igf-1 increases protein synthesis by signalling through PI3K-Akt-mTor-p70S6K-4E-BP1 as well as by activating Ras/MAPK [113]. Transcription was a prerequisite for mTor-1-dependent protein synthesis upon Igf-1 in proliferating oligodendroglial precursors. Early differentiation of the precursors upon Igf-1 also involves transcriptional processes, however subsequent terminal differentiation is independent. This finding indicates different roles for Igf-1 during oligodendroglial cell development.

Further analyses of these potential downstream signalling components reveal that initiation of myelination is coupled to the activity of Irs-2 but not to Irs-1. Irs-2-deficient mice display a defect in timing of myelination and this effect can not be compensated through a simultaneous upregulation of Igf-1r and Irs-1 expression as well as signalling in these mice [111]. Increased Igf-1r signalling is shown through increased levels of pAkt, pGsk-3β and pErk-1/2.

Igf-2 influences proliferation of adult DG progenitors [88]. In this study, knockdown of Igf-2 results in decreased mitosis that is paired with reduced phosphorylation of Irs-1 and Akt. This phenotype is rescued through overexpression of a dominant-active Akt. Blocking of Igf-1r-signalling reduces proliferation that exceeds the drop observed after Igf-2 knockdown. This indicates that NPC proliferation in the adult DG is influenced through Igf-1 and Igf-2 ligands that signal both through the Igf-1r onto Akt.

Signalling of Igf-2 through its cognate Igf-2r has been shown to be important for neuronal maturation with regard to synapse density and spine morphology [14]. Downstream signals included the activation of MAPK/Erk- pathway, since changes at the level of the synapses were inhibited through PD98059.

Igf-2 dependent memory enhancement in adult rat hippocampus requires signalling via the Igf-2r [13]. This Igf-2 effect is associated with *de novo* protein synthesis. Further analyses of the downstream signalling cascade reveales involvement of Gsk-3β, since the Igf-2-specific effect is blocked by the presence of the Gsk-3β-inhibitor SB216763. It was shown that this cascade does not act on a widespread cell level but that it mainly regulates molecular events at specific synapses, e.g. synapses that are "transcriptionally marked" through training. Igf-2 results in increased synaptic activity as revealed by stable long-term potentiation (LTP). The underlying mechanism is therefore deduced to include Igf-2-dependent activation of Gsk-3β that leads to synaptic mobilisation and expression of the AMPA-receptor GluR1.

Igf-2 is further under control of NF-κB transcription factors. Nuclear import of NF-κB is prevented by IκB proteins, which are degraded upon activation of the IκB kinase (IKK) complex. This proteasomal event releases NF-κB into the nucleus. In the adult mouse hippocampus, synaptic IKK/NF-κB signalling is important for function and maturation. Recent data show that Igf-2 is under control of NF-κB-mediated transcriptional regulation [14]. This study shows that Igf-2 increases the number of synapses and of mature spines *in vitro,* while Igf-1 does only have moderate effects in this assay. The Igf-2 effect is predominantly transduced via the Igf-2r and is prevented through MEK inhibitor PD98059, but not through inhibition of Gsk-3β or p38 activity. Corroborating these findings *in vivo,* mice with deficient IKK-2 show reduced Igf-2 expression and pErk1/2 levels [14].

Igf-2-dependent proliferation of mouse CGP is associated with activation of PI3K, but also with mTorc-2 activity that is obvious from increased Akt Ser473 phosphorylation [57]. IIS downstream signalling is followed up to Gsk-3β in this cellular context.

5. Insulin/IGF-signalling cross-talk

5.1. Signalling cross-talk in the central nervous system

In vivo, it is very unlikely that growth factors act alone, but a more likely scenario is the presence of a plethora of signalling molecules and that a phenotypic consequence is a complicated interplay of various signalling pathways. Special emphasise is given to know interactions and cross-talks between such pathways involving IIS, although this is only an emerging field that awaits further studies.

Cultured NPC from the rat adult SVZ respond with neuronal differentiation upon various single stimuli, like Fgf-2, Bdnf, Ngf, and Igf-1. When Fgf-2, Bdnf, and Ngf are applied in combination with Igf-1, significant increases in the number of neurons are observed, indicating synergistic action upon neuronal differentiation [114]. Another study uses immobilised growth factors, alone and in different combinations, on which the authors plated NPC from embryonic rat striatum. Proliferation, neuronal as well as glial differentiation is assessed and reveals that Igf-1 alone mainly drives neuronal differentiation and does not affect proliferation or glial differentiation significantly. In combination with Fgf-2, Igf-1 only slightly increases progenitor states and proliferation, and this effect is even smaller in combination with Egf that also acts mitotic in single treatments. Bdnf increases neuronal differentiation alone, as does Igf-1, however the combination of the two factors results in fewer neurons than single treatments. The differentiation potential of Igf-1 alone is also lowered by presence of the mitotic growth factors Fgf-2 and Egf. Igf-1 alone does not induce glial differentiation. In combination with Cntf that induces astrocytic phenotypes alone, Igf-1 decreases Cntf-mediated differentiation [115].

The cross-talk of IIS with regard to Fgf-2- as well as Egf-signalling mainly influences stem cell proliferation, but whether it is synergistically is not yet totally clear [47,49,50,51,52]. A putative scenario might be that Igf-1 keeps progenitors in a healthy or fit state in which they are ready for further cell divisions, for which Fgf-2 or Egf are the instructive cues. However, withdrawal of Fgf-2 is a prerequisite for neuronal differentiation upon Igf-1 presence [85]. Synergistically, Igf-1-signalling seems to increase the effects of Fgf-2 on NPC proliferation as has been shown in rat adult hippocampal cells. This effect is dependent on PI3K that is activated upon Fgf-2 treatment [99].

Survival of CNS-derived cells is one of the major and comprehensive effects of IIS in the developing and adult organism. IIS is only one of several pathways that influence survival, and thus cross-talk with other pathways might be of principal importance. Bdnf-mediated signalling is one of such pathways that are studied with regard to IIS. No additive function of Bdnf- and Igf-1-mediated survival is reported from different cellular sources [102,116], however other data is contradictory in finding additive affects on prenatal rat hippocampal cell survival [117] that cumulate on increased pGsk-3β. Consistently reported is a stronger survival effect under serum-deprivation for IIS compared to Bdnf. The underlying signalling might again diverge in different cellular systems: hippocampal neurons survive upon Igf-1 and Bdnf through induction of the PI3K-pAkt branch and survival is blocked by LY294002. Activity of the MAPK-pErk1/2 branch does not mediate survival. However, cortical neurons that also depend much stronger on IIS than on Bdnf-signalling for their survival also activate the PI3K-pAkt branch [117], but LY294002 does not completely attribute for survival upon IIS. In addition, Src-kinase is activated in these cortical neurons upon Igf-1, corroborating the finding of an involvement of Pac1-r-signalling in IIS-mediated survival in cortical neurons [91]. Nevertheless, Bdnf and IIS have additive effects in the activation of PI3-K, although this is not detectable on the level of the number of surviving cells. This finding strongly suggests that IIS is overriding the effects of Bdnf in survival of CNS-derived cells. However, one Bdnf effect on hippocampal as well as cortical neurons is to slightly activate Irs-1 and -2 phosphorylation, indicating a potential cross-activation of IIS through Bdnf. Whether this cross-activation is of physiological significance in the presence of Igf-1, remains to be determined.

Studies of neural cell proliferation provide evidence of IIS cross-talk with the Wnt/β-catenin pathway. Nestin-expressing neural progenitors as well as oligodendrocytes express different levels of β-catenin upon Igf-1 deletion or treatment [118,119]. *In vitro*, Igf-1 induces increase of β-catenin as well as CycD1 expression in a PI3K-Akt kinases dependent manner in cultured oligodendrocytes. β-catenin is also known to activate CycD1 and thus defines a point of intersection between IIS and Wnt signalling [118]. Impaired proliferation of NPCs is observed after inactivation of the Igf-1r in Nestin-positive cells. Such NPCs of prenatal mouse brains are dependent on Wnt-signalling when proliferating, and Igf-1r inactivation results in decreased levels of Gsk-3β and β-catenin, but with increased levels of the Wnt-receptor Frizzeled3 and Wnt3a. While the former expression changes are influenced through the Igf-1/PI3K/Akt-pathway, increased levels of Frizzeled3 and Wnt3a are thought to reflect a compensatory regulation stimulated by low levels of β-catenin. Inactivation of Gsk-3β in this setting reverts β-catenin levels and overcomes the block of proliferation as consequence of Igf-1r inactivation.

Overexpression of Igf-1 increases β-catenin-levels and stimulates progenitor proliferation [119]. These experiments clearly establish an important cross-talk to regulate progenitor proliferation in the developing brain.

IIS has also been described to cross-talk with the Tgfβ-pathway in numerous systems [120]. However, a comprehensive analysis of the multiple points of intersections was not published yet for the nervous system. In a general view, Tgfβ-ligands 1, 2, and 3 exert opposing effects compared to IIS. This has been shown for the potential of NPC proliferation and differentiation [121] upon Tgfβ-treatment, since these cells stop proliferating and initiate neuronal differentiation in mouse E16.5 hippocampus and cerebral cortex, *in vitro* and *in vivo*. Proliferation and differentiation of ESCs are also influenced in opposite ways through IIS or Tgfβ-signalling. Smad4-deficient ESC show increased neuronal differentiation, and hereby preferentially in neuronal lineages of the mid- and anterior hindbrain [122]. Further, more serotonergic neurons of the dorsal midbrain are observed in *in vitro* differentiated Smad4-deficient cultures. However, Smad4 is a transcriptional mediator of several members of the Tgfβ-superfamiliy, including Activin-, Gdf-, Nodal-, Tgfβ- as well as Bmp-signalling. Thus, direct correlation to one specific signalling pathway is not achieved in this study. Neural induction of human ESCs is also increased in the presence of the Alk4,5,7 inhibitor SB431542 that interferes with Activin-, Gdf- and Nodal-signalling apart from Tgfβ. Increased differentiation into the neural lineage is assessed by Pax-6 expression which is accompanied by decreased Bmp-4 and increased Noggin expression. These dynamics point to a contribution of several members of the Tgfβ-superfamily of which the Bmp branch has a major contribution [123], but certainly does not act alone. Of further note, neuronal differentiation of ESC cells is not solely dependent on signalling of the above mentioned members of the Tgfβ-superfamily, since deletion of the common effector Smad4 in ESC does not completely abolish the potential for neuronal differentiation [122]. In contrast, IIS keeps ESCs in a proliferative state and is necessary for self-renewal. Whether both pathways cross-talk to suppress the respective other one is not investigated so far, but might be a likely scenario, given the connections described in other cellular lineages.

FoxO and Smad proteins interact and the FoxO/Smad complex is implicated in transcriptional control in early mouse cortical NPCs, thereby defining one point of intersection of IIS and Tgfβ. Smad2 and 3 transcriptions factors are part of the canonical Tgfβ-signalling pathway and are phosphorylated upon binding of Tgfβ-ligands to the Tgfβ-receptor 1 and 2. The phosphorylated proteins bind to Smad4 and together translocate to the nucleus. This Smad complex interacts with FoxO1, 3a, and 4, three TF of the forkhead family that are under influence of IIS. Upon activation of the Igf-1r, FoxO TF are phosphorylated in a PI3K-Akt-dependent manner. This phosphorylation leads to retention of FoxO proteins in the cytoplasm. Thus, IIS opposes transcriptional control through the Tgfβ-pathway by interfering with translocation of cofactors into the nucleus [124].

While survival of cerebellar granule precursors depends on IIS, control of CGP proliferation indicates cross-talk of IIS and Shh-signalling [34,55,125]. Igf/Shh interaction is reported to occur on various levels. The study of Fernandez et al. (2010) suggests that IIS via Igf-1r increases Shh-mediated proliferation, but IIS-mediated proliferation is independent on Shh-signalling. In this setting, Igfbp-5 interfered with Shh-mediated cell proliferation. Igf-2-signalling increases levels of Gli-1, a transcription factor that is mainly activated through Shh-signalling. Gli-1 as well as Gsk-3β are regulators of CycD1, which might be another point of intersection between these two signalling pathways besides regulation of Shh-target Nmyc-1 through Gsk-3β [57,126]. Parathath and colleagues established a role for Irs-1 and mTorc-1 upon Shh-mediated CGP proliferation. This study shows specific upregulation of Irs-1 protein upon Shh that does not result in the activation of Akt. Knockdown of Irs-1 abolishes Shh-mediated CGP proliferation, which is in turn activated upon Irs-1 overexpression. Irs-1 overexpression increases or maintains expression levels of CycD2 and Nmyc-1, which are implicated in cell cycle control. Irs-1 protein stability in CGP is controlled by the negative feed back loop, in which mTorc-1-activation induces p70S6K that phosphorylates Irs-1 and targets Irs-1 for degradation. Shh-dependent increase in Irs-1 is dependent on mTorc-1-inhibition that is followed by suppression of p70S6K-kinase activity [125]. In contrast to this study, Hartmann et al. [57] postulated PI3K/Akt- and synergistically Shh-dependent transcriptional control of Gli-1 and CycD1 as possible lines of interaction.

Although these data corroborate tight connections between Shh and IIS, there is need for further mechanistic investigation to define further knots in the signalling network.

6. Concluding remarks

As pointed out through the many studies of IIS in the CNS, this signalling pathway has an essential role for development and function of this organ. Albeit studied in many laboratories, our understanding of this central signalling pathway is far from being complete. Still we do not understand how the same biological function is achieved by activating different downstream cascades and why it is necessary to have these multiple pathways that respond to one stimulus. We also do not know why different biological functions are the consequence of IIS at different developmental time points in cells from the same part of the brain. In this light it is of major interest that studies are emerging that focus on cross-talks of various stimuli. Exposure to multiple stimuli at a time probably reflects more the natural environment of a developing and mature neural cell than exposure to one single growth factor. It is also of major interest to dissect different functions during development and to define the molecular players involved into functional switches. In this regard it will be important to dissect different subcomplexes of PI3Ks or Akts that might be implicated in IIS. It will be also needed to carefully analyse the balances between the different branches of the signalling cascades and to identify and close further gaps that might be still in the pathways as they are commonly described today. Given the central role of IIS in body development, growth and maintenance, this knowledge will be of utmost interest and will also be exploited for therapeutic medicine in various contexts.

Nomenclature and abbreviations

CA - Cornu ammonis, CGN - Cerebellar granule neurons, CGP - Cerebellar granule precursor, CNS - Central nervous system, CSF - Cerebrospinal fluid, DG - dentate gyrus, ESC - Embryonic Stem Cell, GH - Growth hormone, IIS - Insulin/Igf-signalling, Igf - Insulin like growth factor 1, Igfbp - Insulin like growth factor binding protein, Ir - Insulin receptor, mTOR - mammalian target of rapamycin, NSC - Neural Stem Cell, NPC - Neural Progenitor cell, OB - Olfactory Bulb, OBSC - Olfactory Bulb stem cell, p - phospho-, SGZ - Subgranular zone, SVZ - Subventricular zone, TF - Transcription factor.

Acknowledgements

The author gratefully thanks Dr. K. Thedieck, Dept. of Biology III, Albert-Ludwigs-University Freiburg for conceptualising and discussing this review. I also thank S. Wahane, Dept. of Molecular Embryology, Albert-Ludwigs-University Freiburg for preparing figures for this review.

Author details

Tanja Vogel

Dept. of Molecular Embryology, Institute for Anatomy and Cell Biology, Albert-Ludwigs-University Freiburg, Germany

References

[1] Fernandez AM, Torres-Aleman I. The many faces of insulin-like peptide signalling in the brain. Nat Rev Neurosci. 2012;13(4):225–39.

[2] Pandini G, Frasca F, Mineo R, Sciacca L, Vigneri R, Belfiore A. Insulin/insulin-like growth factor I hybrid receptors have different biological characteristics depending on the insulin receptor isoform involved. J. Biol. Chem. 2002;277(42):39684–95.

[3] Kim JG, Kang MJ, Yoon Y-K, Kim H-P, Park J, Song S-H, et al. Heterodimerization of glycosylated insulin-like growth factor-1 receptors and insulin receptors in cancer cells sensitive to anti-IGF1R antibody. PLoS ONE. 2012;7(3):e33322.

[4] Chiu S-L, Cline HT. Insulin receptor signaling in the development of neuronal structure and function. Neural Dev. 2010;5:7.

[5] Werner H, Weinstein D, Bentov I. Similarities and differences between insulin and IGF-I: structures, receptors, and signalling pathways. Arch. Physiol. Biochem. 2008;114(1):17–22.

[6] Anderson KE, Jackson SP. Class I phosphoinositide 3-kinases. Int. J. Biochem. Cell Biol. 2003;35(7):1028–33.

[7] Pearce LR, Komander D, Alessi DR. The nuts and bolts of AGC protein kinases. Nat. Rev. Mol. Cell Biol. 2010;11(1):9–22.

[8] Dalle Pezze P, Sonntag AG, Thien A, Prentzell MT, Gödel M, Fischer S, et al. A dynamic network model of mTOR signaling reveals TSC-independent mTORC2 regulation. Sci Signal. 2012;5(217):ra25.

[9] Gehart H, Kumpf S, Ittner A, Ricci R. MAPK signalling in cellular metabolism: stress or wellness? EMBO reports. 2010;11(11):834–40.

[10] Taniguchi CM, Aleman JO, Ueki K, Luo J, Asano T, Kaneto H, et al. The p85alpha regulatory subunit of phosphoinositide 3-kinase potentiates c-Jun N-terminal kinase-mediated insulin resistance. Molecular and Cellular Biology. 2007;27(8):2830–40.

[11] Asada S, Daitoku H, Matsuzaki H, Saito T, Sudo T, Mukai H, et al. Mitogen-activated protein kinases, Erk and p38, phosphorylate and regulate Foxo1. Cell. Signal. 2007;19(3):519–27.

[12] Russo VC, Gluckman PD, Feldman EL, Werther GA. The insulin-like growth factor system and its pleiotropic functions in brain. Endocrine Reviews. 2005;26(7):916–43.

[13] Chen DY, Stern SA, Garcia-Osta A, Saunier-Rebori B, Pollonini G, Bambah-Mukku D, et al. A critical role for IGF-II in memory consolidation and enhancement. Nature. 2011;469(7331):491–7.

[14] Schmeisser MJ, Baumann B, Johannsen S, Vindedal GF, Jensen V, Hvalby ØC, et al. IκB kinase/nuclear factor κB-dependent insulin-like growth factor 2 (Igf2) expression regulates synapse formation and spine maturation via Igf2 receptor signaling. Journal of Neuroscience. 2012;32(16):5688–703.

[15] Rajaram S, Baylink DJ, Mohan S. Insulin-like growth factor-binding proteins in serum and other biological fluids: regulation and functions. Endocrine Reviews. 1997;18(6):801–31.

[16] Bondy C, Werner H, Roberts CT, LeRoith D. Cellular pattern of type-I insulin-like growth factor receptor gene expression during maturation of the rat brain: comparison with insulin-like growth factors I and II. NSC. 1992;46(4):909–23.

[17] Bondy CA, Lee WH. Patterns of insulin-like growth factor and IGF receptor gene expression in the brain. Functional implications. Ann. N. Y. Acad. Sci. 1993;692:33–43.

[18] Werther GA, Abate M, Hogg A, Cheesman H, Oldfield B, Hards D, et al. Localization of insulin-like growth factor-I mRNA in rat brain by in situ hybridization--relationship to IGF-I receptors. Mol Endocrinol. 1990;4(5):773–8.

[19] Zhang J, Moats-Staats BM, Ye P, D'Ercole AJ. Expression of insulin-like growth factor system genes during the early postnatal neurogenesis in the mouse hippocampus. J. Neurosci. Res. 2007;85(8):1618–27.

[20] Chernausek SD, Murray MA, Cheung PT. Expression of insulin-like growth factor binding protein-4 (IGFBP-4) by rat neural cells--comparison to other IGFBPs. Regul. Pept. 1993;48(1-2):123–32.

[21] Wood TL, Streck RD, Pintar JE. Expression of the IGFBP-2 gene in post-implantation rat embryos. Development. 1992;114(1):59–66.

[22] Lee WH, Michels KM, Bondy CA. Localization of insulin-like growth factor binding protein-2 messenger RNA during postnatal brain development: correlation with insulin-like growth factors I and II. NSC. 1993;53(1):251–65.

[23] Holmes KM, Annala M, Chua CYX, Dunlap SM, Liu Y, Hugen N, et al. Insulin-like growth factor-binding protein 2-driven glioma progression is prevented by blocking a clinically significant integrin, integrin-linked kinase, and NF-κB network. Proc. Natl. Acad. Sci. U.S.A. National Academy of Sciences; 2012;109(9):3475–80.

[24] Rorive S, Berton A, D'haene N, Takacs CN, Debeir O, Decaestecker C, et al. Matrix metalloproteinase-9 interplays with the IGFBP2-IGFII complex to promote cell growth and motility in astrocytomas. Glia. 2008;56(15):1679–90.

[25] Ikonen M, Liu B, Hashimoto Y, Ma L, Lee K-W, Niikura T, et al. Interaction between the Alzheimer's survival peptide humanin and insulin-like growth factor-binding protein 3 regulates cell survival and apoptosis. Proc. Natl. Acad. Sci. U.S.A. 2003;100(22):13042–7.

[26] Liu B, Lee HY, Weinzimer SA, Powell DR, Clifford JL, Kurie JM, et al. Direct functional interactions between insulin-like growth factor-binding protein-3 and retinoid X receptor-alpha regulate transcriptional signaling and apoptosis. J. Biol. Chem. 2000;275(43):33607–13.

[27] Stenvers KL, Zimmermann EM, Gallagher M, Lund PK. Expression of insulin-like growth factor binding protein-4 and -5 mRNAs in adult rat forebrain. J. Comp. Neurol. 1994;339(1):91–105.

[28] Kang DW, Chung YH, Lee JC, Bang JS, Kim D, Kim SS, et al. Immunohistochemical study on the distribution of insulin-like growth factor-binding protein 4 in the central nervous system of SOD1(G93A) transgenic mice as an in vivo model of amyotrophic lateral sclerosis. Ann. Anat. 2008;190(6):502–9.

[29] Naeve GS, Vana AM, Eggold JR, Verge G, Ling N, Foster AC. Expression of rat insulin-like growth factor binding protein-6 in the brain, spinal cord, and sensory ganglia. Brain Res. Mol. Brain Res. 2000;75(2):185–97.

[30] Bienvenu G, Seurin D, Grellier P, Froment P, Baudrimont M, Monget P, et al. Insulin-like growth factor binding protein-6 transgenic mice: postnatal growth, brain development, and reproduction abnormalities. Endocrinology. 2004;145(5):2412–20.

[31] Agis-Balboa RC, Arcos-Diaz D, Wittnam J, Govindarajan N, Blom K, Burkhardt S, et al. A hippocampal insulin-growth factor 2 pathway regulates the extinction of fear memories. The EMBO Journal. 2011;30(19):4071–83.

[32] Werther GA, Hogg A, Oldfield BJ, McKinley MJ, Figdor R, Allen AM, et al. Localization and characterization of insulin receptors in rat brain and pituitary gland using in vitro autoradiography and computerized densitometry. Endocrinology. 1987;121(4): 1562–70.

[33] Unger J, McNeill TH, Moxley RT, White M, Moss A, Livingston JN. Distribution of insulin receptor-like immunoreactivity in the rat forebrain. NSC. 1989;31(1):143–57.

[34] Fernandez C, Tatard VM, Bertrand N, Dahmane N. Differential modulation of Sonic-hedgehog-induced cerebellar granule cell precursor proliferation by the IGF signaling network. Dev Neurosci. 2010;32(1):59–70.

[35] Wang L, Schulz TC, Sherrer ES, Dauphin DS, Shin S, Nelson AM, et al. Self-renewal of human embryonic stem cells requires insulin-like growth factor-1 receptor and ERBB2 receptor signaling. Blood. 2007;110(12):4111–9.

[36] Watanabe S, Umehara H, Murayama K, Okabe M, Kimura T, Nakano T. Activation of Akt signaling is sufficient to maintain pluripotency in mouse and primate embryonic stem cells. Oncogene. 2006;25(19):2697–707.

[37] Armstrong L, Hughes O, Yung S, Hyslop L, Stewart R, Wappler I, et al. The role of PI3K/AKT, MAPK/ERK and NFkappabeta signalling in the maintenance of human embryonic stem cell pluripotency and viability highlighted by transcriptional profiling and functional analysis. Human Molecular Genetics. 2006;15(11):1894–913.

[38] McLean AB, D'Amour KA, Jones KL, Krishnamoorthy M, Kulik MJ, Reynolds DM, et al. Activin a efficiently specifies definitive endoderm from human embryonic stem cells only when phosphatidylinositol 3-kinase signaling is suppressed. Stem Cells. 2007;25(1):29–38.

[39] Vazin T, Becker KG, Chen J, Spivak CE, Lupica CR, Zhang Y, et al. A novel combination of factors, termed SPIE, which promotes dopaminergic neuron differentiation from human embryonic stem cells. PLoS ONE. 2009;4(8):e6606.

[40] Chen L, Khillan JS. A novel signaling by vitamin A/retinol promotes self renewal of mouse embryonic stem cells by activating PI3K/Akt signaling pathway via insulin-like growth factor-1 receptor. Stem Cells. 2010;28(1):57–63.

[41] Freund C, Oostwaard DW-V, Monshouwer-Kloots J, van den Brink S, van Rooijen M, Xu X, et al. Insulin redirects differentiation from cardiogenic mesoderm and endoderm to neuroectoderm in differentiating human embryonic stem cells. Stem Cells. 2008;26(3):724–33.

[42] Brüning JC, Gautam D, Burks DJ, Gillette J, Schubert M, Orban PC, et al. Role of brain insulin receptor in control of body weight and reproduction. Science. 2000;289(5487):2122–5.

[43] Arsenijevic Y, Weiss S. Insulin-like growth factor-I is a differentiation factor for postmitotic CNS stem cell-derived neuronal precursors: distinct actions from those of brain-derived neurotrophic factor. J. Neurosci. 1998;18(6):2118–28.

[44] Ajo R, Cacicedo L, Navarro C, Sánchez-Franco F. Growth hormone action on proliferation and differentiation of cerebral cortical cells from fetal rat. Endocrinology. 2003;144(3):1086–97.

[45] Mairet-Coello G, Tury A, DiCicco-Bloom E. Insulin-like growth factor-1 promotes G(1)/S cell cycle progression through bidirectional regulation of cyclins and cyclin-dependent kinase inhibitors via the phosphatidylinositol 3-kinase/Akt pathway in developing rat cerebral cortex. Journal of Neuroscience. 2009Jan.21;29(3):775–88.

[46] Zheng W-H, Kar S, Quirion R. Insulin-like growth factor-1-induced phosphorylation of transcription factor FKHRL1 is mediated by phosphatidylinositol 3-kinase/Akt kinase and role of this pathway in insulin-like growth factor-1-induced survival of cultured hippocampal neurons. Mol. Pharmacol. 2002;62(2):225–33.

[47] Drago J, Murphy M, Carroll SM, Harvey RP, Bartlett PF. Fibroblast growth factor-mediated proliferation of central nervous system precursors depends on endogenous production of insulin-like growth factor I. Proc. Natl. Acad. Sci. U.S.A. 1991;88(6): 2199–203.

[48] DiCicco-Bloom E, Black IB. Insulin growth factors regulate the mitotic cycle in cultured rat sympathetic neuroblasts. Proc. Natl. Acad. Sci. U.S.A. 1988;85(11):4066–70.

[49] Arsenijevic Y, Weiss S, Schneider B, Aebischer P. Insulin-like growth factor-I is necessary for neural stem cell proliferation and demonstrates distinct actions of epidermal growth factor and fibroblast growth factor-2. Journal of Neuroscience. 2001;21(18):7194–202.

[50] Kalluri HSG, Vemuganti R, Dempsey RJ. Mechanism of insulin-like growth factor I-mediated proliferation of adult neural progenitor cells: role of Akt. Eur J Neurosci. 2007;25(4):1041–8.

[51] Sato A, Sunayama J, Matsuda K-I, Tachibana K, Sakurada K, Tomiyama A, et al. Regulation of neural stem/progenitor cell maintenance by PI3K and mTOR. Neurosci. Lett. 2010;470(2):115–20.

[52] Vicario-Abejón C, Yusta-Boyo MJ, Fernández-Moreno C, de Pablo F. Locally born olfactory bulb stem cells proliferate in response to insulin-related factors and require

endogenous insulin-like growth factor-I for differentiation into neurons and glia. Journal of Neuroscience. 2003;23(3):895–906.

[53] Han J, Wang B, Xiao Z, Gao Y, Zhao Y, Zhang J, et al. Mammalian target of rapamycin (mTOR) is involved in the neuronal differentiation of neural progenitors induced by insulin. Mol. Cell. Neurosci. 2008;39(1):118–24.

[54] Otaegi G, Yusta-Boyo MJ, Vergaño-Vera E, Méndez-Gómez HR, Carrera AC, Abad JL, et al. Modulation of the PI 3-kinase-Akt signalling pathway by IGF-I and PTEN regulates the differentiation of neural stem/precursor cells. Journal of Cell Science. 2006;119(Pt 13):2739–48.

[55] Ye P, Xing Y, Dai Z, D'Ercole AJ. In vivo actions of insulin-like growth factor-I (IGF-I) on cerebellum development in transgenic mice: evidence that IGF-I increases proliferation of granule cell progenitors. Brain Res. Dev. Brain Res. 1996;95(1):44–54.

[56] Lin X, Bulleit RF. Insulin-like growth factor I (IGF-I) is a critical trophic factor for developing cerebellar granule cells. Brain Res. Dev. Brain Res. 1997;99(2):234–42.

[57] Hartmann W, Koch A, Brune H, Waha A, Schüller U, Dani I, et al. Insulin-like growth factor II is involved in the proliferation control of medulloblastoma and its cerebellar precursor cells. The American Journal of Pathology. 2005;166(4):1153–62.

[58] Nitta A, Zheng W-H, Quirion R. Insulin-like growth factor 1 prevents neuronal cell death induced by corticosterone through activation of the PI3k/Akt pathway. J. Neurosci. Res. 2004;76(1):98–103.

[59] Moosavi M, Maghsoudi N, Zahedi-Asl S, Naghdi N, Yousefpour M, Trounce IA. The role of PI3/Akt pathway in the protective effect of insulin against corticosterone cell death induction in hippocampal cell culture. Neuroendocrinology. 2008;88(4):293–8.

[60] Hodge RD, D'Ercole AJ, O'Kusky JR. Insulin-like growth factor-I accelerates the cell cycle by decreasing G1 phase length and increases cell cycle reentry in the embryonic cerebral cortex. Journal of Neuroscience. 2004;24(45):10201–10.

[61] Popken GJ, Hodge RD, Ye P, Zhang J, Ng W, O'Kusky JR, et al. In vivo effects of insulin-like growth factor-I (IGF-I) on prenatal and early postnatal development of the central nervous system. Eur J Neurosci. 2004;19(8):2056–68.

[62] Hodge RD, D'Ercole AJ, O'Kusky JR. Insulin-like growth factor-I (IGF-I) inhibits neuronal apoptosis in the developing cerebral cortex in vivo. Int. J. Dev. Neurosci. 2007;25(4):233–41.

[63] Hodge RD, D'Ercole AJ, O'Kusky JR. Increased expression of insulin-like growth factor-I (IGF-I) during embryonic development produces neocortical overgrowth with differentially greater effects on specific cytoarchitectonic areas and cortical layers. Brain Res. Dev. Brain Res. 2005;154(2):227–37.

[64] Beck KD, Powell-Braxton L, Widmer HR, Valverde J, Hefti F. Igf1 gene disruption results in reduced brain size, CNS hypomyelination, and loss of hippocampal granule and striatal parvalbumin-containing neurons. Neuron. 1995;14(4):717–30.

[65] Carson MJ, Behringer RR, Brinster RL, McMorris FA. Insulin-like growth factor I increases brain growth and central nervous system myelination in transgenic mice. Neuron. 1993;10(4):729–40.

[66] Liu W, Ye P, O'Kusky JR, D'Ercole AJ. Type 1 insulin-like growth factor receptor signaling is essential for the development of the hippocampal formation and dentate gyrus. J. Neurosci. Res. 2009;87(13):2821–32.

[67] Ludwig T, Eggenschwiler J, Fisher P, D'Ercole AJ, Davenport ML, Efstratiadis A. Mouse mutants lacking the type 2 IGF receptor (IGF2R) are rescued from perinatal lethality in Igf2 and Igf1r null backgrounds. Developmental Biology. 1996;177(2):517–35.

[68] Wang ZQ, Fung MR, Barlow DP, Wagner EF. Regulation of embryonic growth and lysosomal targeting by the imprinted Igf2/Mpr gene. Nature. 1994;372(6505):464–7.

[69] Lau MM, Stewart CE, Liu Z, Bhatt H, Rotwein P, Stewart CL. Loss of the imprinted IGF2/cation-independent mannose 6-phosphate receptor results in fetal overgrowth and perinatal lethality. Genes & Development. 1994;8(24):2953–63.

[70] DeChiara TM, Efstratiadis A, Robertson EJ. A growth-deficiency phenotype in heterozygous mice carrying an insulin-like growth factor II gene disrupted by targeting. Nature. 1990;345(6270):78–80.

[71] Dikkes P, B Jaffe D, Guo W-H, Chao C, Hemond P, Yoon K, et al. IGF2 knockout mice are resistant to kainic acid-induced seizures and neurodegeneration. Brain Research. 2007;1175:85–95.

[72] Lehtinen MK, Zappaterra MW, Chen X, Yang YJ, Hill AD, Lun M, et al. The cerebrospinal fluid provides a proliferative niche for neural progenitor cells. Neuron. 2011;69(5):893–905.

[73] Ni W, Rajkumar K, Nagy JI, Murphy LJ. Impaired brain development and reduced astrocyte response to injury in transgenic mice expressing IGF binding protein-1. Brain Research. 1997;769(1):97–107.

[74] D'Ercole AJ, Dai Z, Xing Y, Boney C, Wilkie MB, Lauder JM, et al. Brain growth retardation due to the expression of human insulin like growth factor binding protein-1 in transgenic mice: an in vivo model for the analysis of igf function in the brain. Brain Res. Dev. Brain Res. 1994;82(1-2):213–22.

[75] Schneider MR, Lahm H, Wu M, Hoeflich A, Wolf E. Transgenic mouse models for studying the functions of insulin-like growth factor-binding proteins. FASEB J. 2000;14(5):629–40.

[76] Aberg MA, Aberg ND, Hedbäcker H, Oscarsson J, Eriksson PS. Peripheral infusion of IGF-I selectively induces neurogenesis in the adult rat hippocampus. Journal of Neuroscience. 2000;20(8):2896–903.

[77] Aberg MAI, Aberg ND, Palmer TD, Alborn A-M, Carlsson-Skwirut C, Bang P, et al. IGF-I has a direct proliferative effect in adult hippocampal progenitor cells. Mol. Cell. Neurosci. 2003;24(1):23–40.

[78] Choi Y-S, Cho H-Y, Hoyt KR, Naegele JR, Obrietan K. IGF-1 receptor-mediated ERK/MAPK signaling couples status epilepticus to progenitor cell proliferation in the subgranular layer of the dentate gyrus. Glia. 2008;56(7):791–800.

[79] Trejo JL, Carro E, Torres-Aleman I. Circulating insulin-like growth factor I mediates exercise-induced increases in the number of new neurons in the adult hippocampus. Journal of Neuroscience. 2001;21(5):1628–34.

[80] Lichtenwalner RJ, Forbes ME, Sonntag WE, Riddle DR. Adult-onset deficiency in growth hormone and insulin-like growth factor-I decreases survival of dentate granule neurons: insights into the regulation of adult hippocampal neurogenesis. J. Neurosci. Res. 2006;83(2):199–210.

[81] Hsieh J, Aimone JB, Kaspar BK, Kuwabara T, Nakashima K, Gage FH. IGF-I instructs multipotent adult neural progenitor cells to become oligodendrocytes. The Journal of Cell Biology. 2004;164(1):111–22.

[82] O'Kusky JR, Ye P, D'Ercole AJ. Insulin-like growth factor-I promotes neurogenesis and synaptogenesis in the hippocampal dentate gyrus during postnatal development. Journal of Neuroscience. 2000;20(22):8435–42.

[83] Kalluri HSG, Dempsey RJ. IGFBP-3 inhibits the proliferation of neural progenitor cells. Neurochem. Res. 2011;36(3):406–11.

[84] Choi K-C, Yoo D-S, Cho K-S, Huh P-W, Kim D-S, Park C-K. Effect of single growth factor and growth factor combinations on differentiation of neural stem cells. J Korean Neurosurg Soc. 2008;44(6):375–81.

[85] Brooker GJ, Kalloniatis M, Russo VC, Murphy M, Werther GA, Bartlett PF. Endogenous IGF-1 regulates the neuronal differentiation of adult stem cells. J. Neurosci. Res. 2000;59(3):332–41.

[86] Russo VC, Bach LA, Fosang AJ, Baker NL, Werther GA. Insulin-like growth factor binding protein-2 binds to cell surface proteoglycans in the rat brain olfactory bulb. Endocrinology. 1997;138(11):4858–67.

[87] Hurtado-Chong A, Yusta-Boyo MJ, Vergaño-Vera E, Bulfone A, de Pablo F, Vicario-Abejón C. IGF-I promotes neuronal migration and positioning in the olfactory bulb and the exit of neuroblasts from the subventricular zone. Eur J Neurosci. 2009;30(5):742–55.

[88] Bracko O, Singer T, Aigner S, Knobloch M, Winner B, Ray J, et al. Gene expression profiling of neural stem cells and their neuronal progeny reveals IGF2 as a regulator of adult hippocampal neurogenesis. Journal of Neuroscience. 2012;32(10):3376–87.

[89] Paik J-H, Ding Z, Narurkar R, Ramkissoon S, Muller F, Kamoun WS, et al. FoxOs cooperatively regulate diverse pathways governing neural stem cell homeostasis. Cell Stem Cell. 2009;5(5):540–53.

[90] Subramaniam S, Shahani N, Strelau J, Laliberte C, Brandt R, Kaplan D, et al. Insulin-like growth factor 1 inhibits extracellular signal-regulated kinase to promote neuronal survival via the phosphatidylinositol 3-kinase/protein kinase A/c-Raf pathway. Journal of Neuroscience. 2005;25(11):2838–52.

[91] Delcourt N, Thouvenot E, Chanrion B, Galéotti N, Jouin P, Bockaert J, et al. PACAP type I receptor transactivation is essential for IGF-1 receptor signalling and antiapoptotic activity in neurons. The EMBO Journal. 2007;26(6):1542–51.

[92] Chrysis D, Calikoglu AS, Ye P, D'Ercole AJ. Insulin-like growth factor-I overexpression attenuates cerebellar apoptosis by altering the expression of Bcl family proteins in a developmentally specific manner. Journal of Neuroscience. 2001;21(5):1481–9.

[93] Glasper ER, Llorens-Martin MV, Leuner B, Gould E, Trejo JL. Blockade of insulin-like growth factor-I has complex effects on structural plasticity in the hippocampus. Hippocampus. 2010;20(6):706–12.

[94] Niblock MM, Brunso-Bechtold JK, Riddle DR. Insulin-like growth factor I stimulates dendritic growth in primary somatosensory cortex. Journal of Neuroscience. 2000;20(11):4165–76.

[95] Laurino L, Wang XX, la Houssaye de BA, Sosa L, Dupraz S, Cáceres A, et al. PI3K activation by IGF-1 is essential for the regulation of membrane expansion at the nerve growth cone. Journal of Cell Science. 2005;118(Pt 16):3653–62.

[96] Sehat B, Tofigh A, Lin Y, Trocmé E, Liljedahl U, Lagergren J, et al. SUMOylation mediates the nuclear translocation and signaling of the IGF-1 receptor. Sci Signal. 2010;3(108):ra10.

[97] Sinor AD, Lillien L. Akt-1 expression level regulates CNS precursors. Journal of Neuroscience. 2004;24(39):8531–41.

[98] Endo M, Antonyak MA, Cerione RA. Cdc42-mTOR signaling pathway controls Hes5 and Pax6 expression in retinoic acid-dependent neural differentiation. J. Biol. Chem. 2009;284(8):5107–18.

[99] Peltier J, O'Neill A, Schaffer DV. PI3K/Akt and CREB regulate adult neural hippocampal progenitor proliferation and differentiation. Dev Neurobiol. 2007;67(10): 1348–61.

[100] Magri L, Cambiaghi M, Cominelli M, Alfaro-Cervello C, Cursi M, Pala M, et al. Sustained activation of mTOR pathway in embryonic neural stem cells leads to develop-

ment of tuberous sclerosis complex-associated lesions. Cell Stem Cell. 2011;9(5):447–62.

[101] Onda H, Crino PB, Zhang H, Murphey RD, Rastelli L, Gould Rothberg BE, et al. Tsc2 null murine neuroepithelial cells are a model for human tuber giant cells, and show activation of an mTOR pathway. Mol. Cell. Neurosci. 2002;21(4):561–74.

[102] Zheng W-H, Quirion R. Comparative signaling pathways of insulin-like growth factor-1 and brain-derived neurotrophic factor in hippocampal neurons and the role of the PI3 kinase pathway in cell survival. J Neurochem. 2004;89(4):844–52.

[103] Baker NL, Carlo Russo V, Bernard O, D'Ercole AJ, Werther GA. Interactions between bcl-2 and the IGF system control apoptosis in the developing mouse brain. Brain Res. Dev. Brain Res. 1999;118(1-2):109–18.

[104] Datta SR, Dudek H, Tao X, Masters S, Fu H, GOTOH Y, et al. Akt phosphorylation of BAD couples survival signals to the cell-intrinsic death machinery. Cell. 1997;91(2): 231–41.

[105] Dudek H, Datta SR, Franke TF, Birnbaum MJ, Yao R, Cooper GM, et al. Regulation of neuronal survival by the serine-threonine protein kinase Akt. Science. 1997;275(5300): 661–5.

[106] Ye P, Carson J, D'Ercole AJ. In vivo actions of insulin-like growth factor-I (IGF-I) on brain myelination: studies of IGF-I and IGF binding protein-1 (IGFBP-1) transgenic mice. J. Neurosci. 1995;15(11):7344–56.

[107] Goddard DR, Berry M, Butt AM. In vivo actions of fibroblast growth factor-2 and insulin-like growth factor-I on oligodendrocyte development and myelination in the central nervous system. J. Neurosci. Res. 1999;57(1):74–85.

[108] Luzi P, Zaka M, Rao HZ, Curtis M, Rafi MA, Wenger DA. Generation of transgenic mice expressing insulin-like growth factor-1 under the control of the myelin basic protein promoter: increased myelination and potential for studies on the effects of increased IGF-1 on experimentally and genetically induced demyelination. Neurochem. Res. 2004;29(5):881–9.

[109] Ye P, Li L, Richards RG, DiAugustine RP, D'Ercole AJ. Myelination is altered in insulin-like growth factor-I null mutant mice. Journal of Neuroscience. 2002;22(14):6041–51.

[110] Zeger M, Popken G, Zhang J, Xuan S, Lu QR, Schwab MH, et al. Insulin-like growth factor type 1 receptor signaling in the cells of oligodendrocyte lineage is required for normal in vivo oligodendrocyte development and myelination. Glia. 2007;55(4):400–11.

[111] Freude S, Leeser U, Müller M, Hettich MM, Udelhoven M, Schilbach K, et al. IRS-2 branch of IGF-1 receptor signaling is essential for appropriate timing of myelination. J Neurochem. 2008;107(4):907–17.

[112] Cui Q-L, Almazan G. IGF-I-induced oligodendrocyte progenitor proliferation requires PI3K/Akt, MEK/ERK, and Src-like tyrosine kinases. J Neurochem. 2007;100(6): 1480–93.

[113] Bibollet-Bahena O, Almazan G. IGF-1-stimulated protein synthesis in oligodendrocyte progenitors requires PI3K/mTOR/Akt and MEK/ERK pathways. J Neurochem. 2009;109(5):1440–51.

[114] Choi K-C, Yoo D-S, Cho K-S, Huh P-W, Kim D-S, Park C-K. Effect of Single Growth Factor and Growth Factor Combinations on Differentiation of Neural Stem Cells. J Korean Neurosurg Soc. 2008;44(6):375.

[115] Konagaya S, Kato K, Nakaji-Hirabayashi T, Arima Y, Iwata H. Array-based functional screening of growth factors toward optimizing neural stem cell microenvironments. Biomaterials. 2011;32(22):5015–22.

[116] Yamada M, Tanabe K, Wada K, Shimoke K, Ishikawa Y, Ikeuchi T, et al. Differences in survival-promoting effects and intracellular signaling properties of BDNF and IGF-1 in cultured cerebral cortical neurons. J Neurochem. 2001;78(5):940–51.

[117] Johnson-Farley NN, Travkina T, Cowen DS. Cumulative activation of akt and consequent inhibition of glycogen synthase kinase-3 by brain-derived neurotrophic factor and insulin-like growth factor-1 in cultured hippocampal neurons. J. Pharmacol. Exp. Ther. 2006;316(3):1062–9.

[118] Ye P, Hu Q, Liu H, Yan Y, D'Ercole AJ. beta-catenin mediates insulin-like growth factor-I actions to promote cyclin D1 mRNA expression, cell proliferation and survival in oligodendroglial cultures. Glia. 2010;58(9):1031–41.

[119] Hu Q, Lee SY, O'Kusky JR, Ye P. Signaling Through the Type 1 Insulin-Like Growth Factor Receptor (IGF1R) Interacts with Canonical Wnt Signaling to Promote Neural Proliferation in Developing Brain. ASN Neuro. 2012.

[120] Danielpour D, Song K. Cross-talk between IGF-I and TGF-β signaling pathways. Cytokine & Growth Factor Reviews. 2006;17(1-2):59–74.

[121] Vogel T, Ahrens S, Buttner N, Krieglstein K. Transforming Growth Factor Promotes Neuronal Cell Fate of Mouse Cortical and Hippocampal Progenitors In Vitro and In Vivo: Identification of Nedd9 as an Essential Signaling Component. Cereb. Cortex. 2010;20(3):661–71.

[122] Sonntag K-C, Simantov R, Björklund L, Cooper O, Pruszak J, Kowalke F, et al. Context-dependent neuronal differentiation and germ layer induction of Smad4-/- and Cripto-/- embryonic stem cells. Mol. Cell. Neurosci. 2005;28(3):417–29.

[123] Li W, Sun W, Zhang Y, Wei W, Ambasudhan R, Xia P, et al. Rapid induction and long-term self-renewal of primitive neural precursors from human embryonic stem cells by small molecule inhibitors. Proc. Natl. Acad. Sci. U.S.A. 2011;108(20):8299–304.

[124] Seoane J, Le H-V, Shen L, Anderson SA, MassaguE J. Integration of Smad and forkhead pathways in the control of neuroepithelial and glioblastoma cell proliferation. Cell. 2004;117(2):211–23.

[125] Parathath SR, Mainwaring LA, Fernandez-L A, Campbell DO, Kenney AM. Insulin receptor substrate 1 is an effector of sonic hedgehog mitogenic signaling in cerebellar neural precursors. Development. 2008;135(19):3291–300.

[126] Kenney AM, Widlund HR, Rowitch DH. Hedgehog and PI-3 kinase signaling converge on Nmyc1 to promote cell cycle progression in cerebellar neuronal precursors. Development. 2004;131(1):217–28.

Chapter 2

Role of TGF-β Signaling in Neurogenic Regions After Brain Injury

Sonia Villapol, Trevor T. Logan and Aviva J. Symes

Additional information is available at the end of the chapter

1. Introduction

In 1928 Santiago Ramón y Cajal penned what became the accepted view about neurons in the central nervous system; *"everything may die, nothing can be regenerated"*. He later exhibited his wisdom by adding; *"It's the job of science to rewrite, if possible, this cruel phrase"* [1]. Up until 20 years ago, the scientific literature had emphasized that neurogenesis only occurs during development with no new neurons generated in the adult mammalian brain. However, since the discovery of adult neurogenesis, an extensive literature has emerged supporting the constant generation of new neurons in two neurogenic regions of the adult brain: the subventricular zone around the lateral ventricles (SVZ) and the subgranular zone (SGZ) of the hippocampal dentate gyrus (DG) [2].

The existence of adult neurogenesis gave hope for recovery and regeneration from the many different insults that can damage the brain. After stroke or traumatic brain injury (TBI), immediate massive necrosis occurs followed by a subsequent prolonged period of inflammation and further neuronal death [3]. Although brain injury induces massive cell loss, it also induces an increase in proliferation of NSCs residing in the neurogenic niches [4]. The environment of the neurogenic niche in adult animals is exquisitely regulated, with a finely-tuned balance of soluble and cell-intrinsic factors that regulate the many different processes that are critical to neurogenesis: cell survival, proliferation, differentiation, and migration [5]. Dramatic changes occur in this environment as a consequence of the injury. The careful regulation of neurogenesis is disrupted by the many different cellular, soluble and vascular signals detected by the different cell types in the SVZ and DG. This major environmental alteration leads to increased proliferation of progenitor cells for long periods after the acute injury, yet the ability of the neural progenitor cells to fully differentiate, migrate and integrate into the lesioned area is limited [6]. Understanding the signals that regulate adult neurogenesis in the naïve and injured animals is key to ultimately being able to harness the potential of neuronal replacement and improve stem cell therapy.

There are many different factors important to regulation of neurogenesis, many of which are discussed in other chapters in this book. Here we will focus on the role of the transforming growth factor-β (TGF-β) superfamily and its associated signaling pathways in regulating neurogenesis after brain injury. Members of this family, including the bone morphogenetic proteins (BMPs), Activin, and TGF-β1, -β2 and -β3 have a profound influence on the neurogenic process in naïve animals [7]. Many of these cytokines are induced by injury and play critical roles in many kinds of brain damage related processes around the lesion [3]. We and others recently started to accumulate data on their induction in the neurogenic niches after different types of injury. Here we will focus on the relevance of their induction in these specific brain regions, and the mechanisms through which they may influence the neurogenic response to injury. As there are significant differences between the behavior of cells contributing to neurogenesis during development and in the adult, we will restrict our analysis to that observed in adult animals after injury. Delineation of the specific role of members of the TGF-β superfamily in injury-induced neurogenesis may provide specific therapeutic targets for enhancing neurogenesis after trauma.

2. The TGF-β superfamily; cytokines, receptors and signaling

The TGF-β cytokine superfamily is a large group of proteins comprising 33 different members that include: bone morphogenetic proteins (BMPs), growth differentiation factors (GDFs), activins, inhibins, nodal, lefty, mülllerian inhibiting substance (MIS) together with the TGF-β proteins [8, 9]. All members of this cytokine family mediate their effects in a broadly analogous manner, binding specific type I and II transmembrane serine threonine kinase receptors and transducing their signal through similar intracellular Smad proteins [10]. These cytokines are divided into two distinct groups: those of the TGF-β/Activin group which mainly signal through the type I receptors ALK4, -5 and -7 activating Smad2 and -3, and those of the BMP/GDF group [11, 12] which employ ALK1, -2, -3 and -6 to activate Smad1, -5 and -8 [13, 14]. The specificity of Smad activation is therefore mainly determined by the identity of the type I receptor used to transduce the cytokine signal [15] (Figure 1).

TGF-β1, -β2 and -β3 together with some GDFs are unique in that they are synthesized as a large precursor molecule that is cleaved but remains non-covalently linked to its latency associated peptides, in either a small or large complex [18]. The bioavailability of TGF-βs is tightly regulated by the release of active TGF-β from these complexes in the extracellular matrix, so synthesis of TGF-β does not necessarily provide a reliable indication of available cytokine to initiate signaling. Similarly, the bioavailability of BMPs is regulated by binding to secreted extracellular antagonists that prevent BMP (and sometimes Activin) from binding to their receptor [19]. Expression levels of endogenous antagonists, including noggin, chordin, follistatin, gremlin and cerberus, thereby regulate the availability, and therefore, active signaling by their associated ligands [20]. TGF-β signaling is the archetype for signaling by

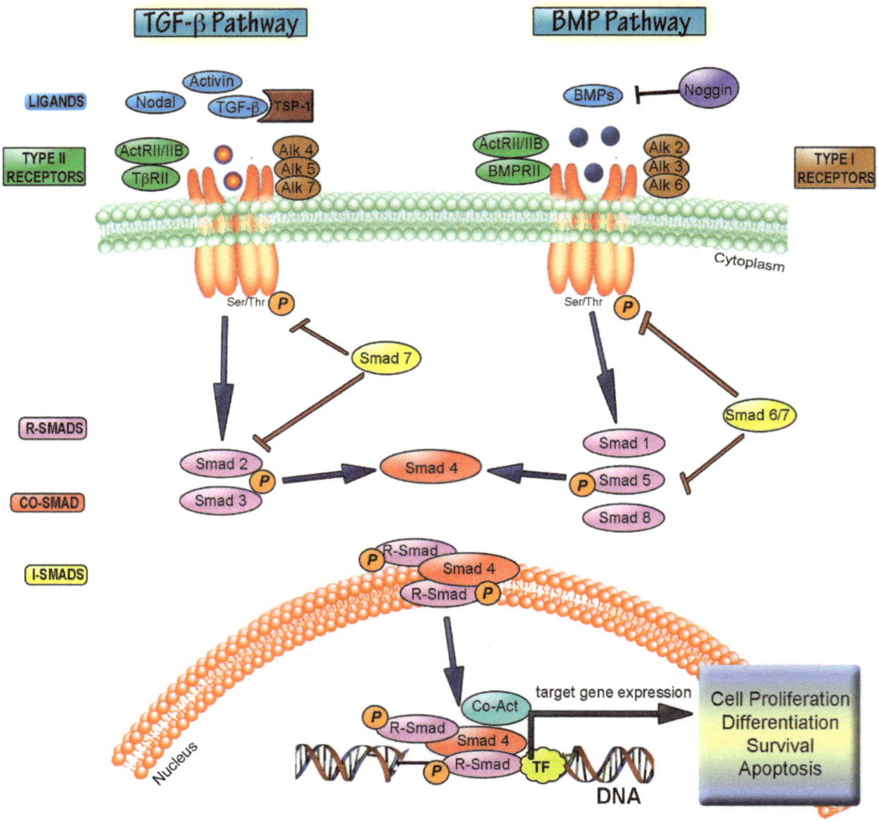

Figure 1. TGF-β superfamily signal transduction. TGF-β, nodal or activin ligands bind to Type II receptors, which then recruit Type I receptors leading to transphosphorylation of type 1 receptors. Activated type I receptors phosphorylate Smad 2/3 (*i.e.* R-Smads) which then complex with the co-Smad, Smad4 and translocate to the nucleus to bind DNA at specific DNA motifs. Smad proteins activate or repress transcription through association with various co-activator (Co-Act) or co-repressor proteins. This pathway is inhibited by Smad7. BMP signaling operates by a similar paradigm. BMP6 and BMP7 bind to their Type II receptor before the complex recruits the Type I receptors, Alk-3 or Alk-6. BMP2 and BMP4, however bind first to their type I receptor before recruiting the type II receptor BMPRII. BMP binding to either receptor can be inhibited by first binding to various extracellular inhibitor proteins, such as noggin. Activation of the receptor complex leads to phosphorylation of the receptors and subsequent phosphorylation of Smad1, Smad5, or Smad8, allowing them to form a complex with Smad4. This heteromeric complex translocates to the nucleus, to target BMP-regulated genes through interaction with co-activators or repressors. Smad 6 and Smad7 may act similarly to inhibit the BMP pathway through interactions with the receptor complex and thus inhibiting R-Smad activation. TGF-β and BMP pathways induce the expression of proteins involved in proliferation, differentiation, survival and apoptosis. The diagram is adapted from [16] and [17].

this cytokine family. TGF-β binds to the constitutively active TGF-β receptor II (TβRII) which can then recruit the type I receptor TGF-β receptor I (TβRI/ALK5). Activation of TβRI by transphosphorylation activates it, initiating downstream signaling [21]. Canonical signaling by these cytokines is through the receptor regulated Smads (R-smads). As previously mentioned, TGF-β and activin signal through activation of Smad2 and Smad3, which are phosphorylated by the Type I receptor, and form a heteromeric complex with the common or co-Smad, Smad4 [22]. This Smad complex translocates to the nucleus where it regulates the transcription of numerous genes in cooperation with other transcription factors, coactivators and corepressors. Inhibitory Smads, or I-smads, are Smad-activated proteins that provide negative feedback to the Smad pathway through a variety of mechanisms [16, 23]. BMP signaling is similar in form to TGF-β signaling, although the specifics of individual receptors and R-Smads (1, 5, 8/9) involved vary according to the specific cytokine. For a full review of signaling and receptor nomenclature by this cytokine family please refer to some excellent reviews [14, 24]. The Smad pathway is by no means the only mechanism through which TGF-β cytokine signals are transduced from the receptor to the nucleus. Smad-independent pathways include activation of MAPKs, Ras/ERK, JNK, p38, PI3K-Akt, NF-kappaB, JAK/STAT, PP2A/S6 phosphatases and small Rho-related GTPases (16, 25). Some of the non-Smad kinases can influence Smad directed signaling by complexing with, or modifying the Smad proteins directly [16, 25]. Another level of control was found when it was shown that TGF-β/BMP signaling is both regulated by, and can regulate transcription of miRNAs [26]. Smads can also influence miRNA biogenesis by binding directly to the pri-miRNA to enhance Drosha processing of these molecules to pre-miRNA [27]. An intricate balance between Smad and non-Smad signaling superimposed on cell intrinsic and environmental conditions determines the specificity and the ultimate response of each cell to TGF-β signaling. Thus, there is a complexity to TGF-β superfamily signaling that befits cytokines that signal to multiple different cell types, in context dependent manners to influence many different physiologic processes [28].

Genetic evidence indicates that TGF-β family members regulate embryonic, perinatal or neonatal development of the mouse embryo. Most mice null for one TGF-β superfamily ligand, receptor, protein or signaling protein fail in either gastrulation or mesoderm differentiation. Table 1 lists known phenotypes of mice that are null for specific proteins in the TGF-β superfamily signaling pathways.

Conventional knockout mouse model of TGF-β proteins	Phenotype	References
TβRI	Failed angiogenesis, Embryonic lethality (E8)	[29]
TβRII	Embryonic lethality (E10.5)	[30]
TβRIII	Failed coronary vessel development accompanied by reduced epicardial cell invasion. Embryonic lethality (E14.5)	[31]
TGFβ-1	Loss of a critical regulator of immune function	[32, 33]
TGFβ-2	Perinatal lethal, craniofacial defects	[34]
TGFβ-3	Perinatal lethal, delayed lung development	[33]

Conventional knockout mouse model of TGF-β proteins	Phenotype	References
Smad1	Embryonic lethality (E10)	[35, 36]
Smad2	Embryonic lethality (E7.5–E12.5)	[37]
Smad3	Viable and fertile. Impaired immune function, including defective neutrophil chemotaxis, and impaired mucosal immunity	[38, 39]
Smad4	Increased number of Olig2-expressing progeny	[40]
Smad5	Embryonic lethality: defective vascular development	[41, 42]
Smad7	Significantly smaller than wild-type mice, died within a few days of birth	[43]
Smad8	Viable and fertile	[41, 44]
BMPRIA	Embryonic lethality (E9.5)	[45]
BMPRIB	Viable and exhibit defects in the appendicular skeleton	[46]
BMPRII	Embryonic lethality (E9.5), arrest at gastrulation	[47]
BMP2	Embryonic lethality (E7.5-10.5), defective cardiac development and have defects in cardiac development	[48]
BMP3	Increased bone density in adult	[49]
BMP4	Embryonic lethality (E6.5-E9.5), no mesoderm differentiation and show little or no mesodermal differentiation	[50]
BMP5	Viable, skeletal and cartilage abnormalities	[51]
BMP6	Viable and fertile; slight delay in ossification.	[52]
BMP7	Perinatal lethal because of poor kidney development, eye defects that appear to originate during lens induction.	[53-56]
BMP8A	Viable: male infertility due to germ cell degeneration	[57]
BMP8B	Viable: male infertility due to germ cell depletion	[58]
BMP15	Viable: female subfertility	[59]
Endoglin	Embryonic lethality (E11.5)	[60, 61]
Activin receptor IA (ALK2)	Embryonic lethality (E9.5)	[62]
Activin receptor IIB (ActR2B)	Perinatal lethal	[63]
Activin-βA	Neonatal lethal, craniofacial defects (cleft palate and loss of whiskers, upper incisors, lower incisors and molars)	[64]

Conventional knockout mouse model of TGF-β proteins	Phenotype	References
Activin-βB	Large litters but delayed parturition; nursing defects; Eye lid closure defects at birth	[65]
Noggin	Perinatal lethal, cartilage hyperplasia	[66]
Follistatin	Neonatal lethal, craniofacial defects, growth retardation and skin defects retardation and skin defects	[67]

Table 1. Phenotype of mice that do not express specific TGF-β ligands, receptors or signaling molecules.

3. TGF-*β* superfamily expression and function in normal adult brain: Role in neurogenesis

Adult neurogenesis involves proliferation of neural stem cells (NSCs), cell cycle exit, differentiation, maturation, and integration into the neural circuits, in a process that is involved in learning and memory in the normal adult brain [68]. The neurogenic niche of the adult forebrain subventricular zone (SVZ) is comprised of three major proliferative cell types; A, B and C. Multipotent, self-renewing type B cells occur earliest in the neurogenic lineage of the SVZ and give rise to the rapidly dividing type C cells, or transit amplifying progenitors. Type A cells or neuroblasts differentiate from Type C cells and are migratory neuronal progenitors with proliferative capacity, which migrate to the olfactory bulb where they differentiate into interneurons (reviewed in [69-71]. In the subgranular zone (SGZ) of the hippocampal dentate gyrus (DG), type 1 and type 2 slowly-dividing progenitors give rise to more rapidly dividing intermediate progenitor cells, and these in turn differentiate into immature neuroblasts, which migrate into the granule cell layer, then differentiate into mature neurons and integrate with the existing hippocampal circuitry [71].

Within the CNS, all three isoforms of TGF-β are produced by both glial and neuronal cells [72]. Immunohistochemical studies show widespread expression of TGF-β2 and -β3 in the developing CNS, and these proteins play a role in regulation of neuronal migration, glial proliferation and differentiation [73-76]. In adult brain, TGF-β receptors are found in all areas of the CNS including the cortex, hippocampus, striatum, brainstem and cerebellum [77, 78]. Immunoreactivity for TβRI and TβRII is detected on neurons, astrocytes and microglia and endothelial cells located in the cortical gray matter, suggesting that almost every cell type in the CNS is a potential target for TGF-β signaling [79].

The TGF-β superfamily and its downstream targets are capable of controlling proliferation, differentiation, maturation and survival of stem cells and precursors in the neurogenic niches of adult brain [18]. TβRI and TβRII are expressed by Nestin-positive type B and C cells in the SVZ [80, 81]. Our data show mRNA expression of TGF-β1, -β2, and -β3 in both the adult SVZ and DG [82]. In the adult human brain, TGF-β1 protein expression has been reported in the hippocampus, and the protein levels significantly increased with the age of the individual [83]. As neurogenesis declines with age [84], it has been suggested that TGF-β is a possible regulator of this age-related decline [83]. Signaling by the Smad2/3 pathway is high in the hippocampus and specifically the dentate gyrus, indicating a role for TGF-β and/or activin in regulation of neurogenesis [85, 86]. When TGF-β protein is overexpressed or infused directly into the lateral ventricles of uninjured animals, hippocampal neurogenesis is dramatically inhibited [81, 87]. This may be due to a direct anti-proliferative effect of TGF-β on type 1 and 2 primary NSCs [17]. A direct effect of TGF-β on NSCs is supported by *in vitro* studies showing that TGF-β1 treatment of cultured adult NSCs induces the cyclin-dependent kinase inhibitor (p21) and leads to cell cycle termination, without altering the differentiation choices of the NSCs [81]. Additionally, overexpression studies lead to increased TGF-β signaling in many different cell types within the neurogenic niche, making the exact contribution of more restricted, endogenous TGF-β difficult to determine. Recent data have suggested that TGF-β signaling at later stages of neurogenesis is critical for newborn neuron survival and maturation in the DG. Conditional deletion of the TβRI (ALK5) gene specifically in immature and mature neurons, leads to decreased neurogenesis and reduced survival of newborn neurons [85]. Thus, TGF-β potentially has opposing roles at different stages of neurogenesis, providing an additional example of the contextual nature of TGF-β action.

Activin receptors are expressed throughout the brain, with strong expression in the neuronal layers of the hippocampus [88-90]. We have found that mRNA for activin-A and for activin's endogenous high affinity inhibitor, follistatin, are expressed in both the SVZ and DG of the adult mouse [82] and several recent reports have demonstrated that activin-A modulates adult neurogenesis [88, 91, 92]. Chronic overexpression of follistatin by neurons of the hippocampus almost entirely ablates adult DG neurogenesis, due to drastically lowered survival of adult-generated neurons [91], although short-term infusion of follistatin does not affect neurogenesis in uninjured animals [88]. Infusion of activin to the lateral ventricle of uninjured mice mildly increases the rate of NSC proliferation and neuron generation in the DG, indicating that activin might stimulate division of NSCs. This effect may be indirect as activin has a potent anti-inflammatory effect in the CNS, and may modulate local microglia to stimulate neurogenesis [88]. Smad3 knockout mice have decreased levels of cell proliferation in the SVZ and along the rostral migratory stream, and decreased levels of olfactory bulb neurogenesis [93]. As these mice have defective signaling by both TGF-β and activin, these data suggest that activin signaling in the SVZ may be the predominant Smad3-utilizing cytokine in defining basal levels of neurogenesis. In the DG pSmad2 is normally absent from Sox2-positive type 1 and 2 primary NSCs in the DG of adult mice [17]. However, Smad3 knockout mice also have reduced proliferation in the DG potentially pointing to a different role for Smad2 and Smad3 in the DG [93].

The BMP family of proteins regulates cell proliferation and fate commitment throughout development and within the adult neurogenic niches [19]. Expression of BMP2, -4 and -7 mRNAs have been reported in neurogenic regions of adult rodent brain [94], and the BMP receptors BMPRIA, -IB and -II are expressed abundantly in neurons, as well as in astrocytes and ependymal cells [95]. All three of these receptors are expressed in type A cells of the SVZ, while type B and C cells express BMPRIA and BMPRII [96]. In the DG, radial stem cells of the SGZ marked with glial fibrillary acidic protein (GFAP) and Nestin or Sox2 primarily express BMPRIA but not BMPRIB, while mature neurons express only BMPRIB [97]. BMP ligands are also expressed in the adult rat brain [98, 99]. BMP2, -4, -6, and -7 are expressed by cells of the SVZ and DG [96, 97]. In the DG, the BMP signal transducer pSmad1 is strongly expressed in non-dividing primary NSCs and neuroblasts, but is absent in dividing primary NSCs [97], while in the SVZ, pSmad1/5/8 has been reported in primary NSCs and transit amplifying progenitors, but not in DCX-positive neuroblasts [40]. The soluble BMP inhibitor noggin is also expressed by ependymal cells of the SVZ [96] and by cells of the DG [100].

Changing the ratio of BMP to noggin alters the rates of NSC proliferation and neurogenesis in adult animals, indicating that these proteins are primary regulators of basal adult neurogenesis [96, 97, 100]. Administration of exogenous BMP4 or BMP7 potently inhibits the division of NSCs and generation of new neurons in vivo and in vitro [96, 97], as does inhibition of noggin expression [101]. Conversely, infusion of noggin or genetic deletion of the BMPRIA receptor causes an increase in NSC proliferation and generation of NeuN-expressing neurons in the DG [96, 97]. However this increase is transient, there is an eventual depletion of the primary NSC pool and a drastically reduced level of neurogenesis [97]. Decreased BMP signaling in the DG is thought to be responsible for increased neurogenesis driven by exercise [102]. It has been proposed that secretion of noggin from ependymal cells inhibits BMP signaling allowing a low level of basal neurogenesis to occur, while BMP signaling maintains the overall quiescence of the primary NSC pool [96, 97, 100]. Exogenous noggin infusion potentially has a different effect on SVZ NSCs, leaving their proliferation rate unaffected, but causing an increase in the generation of oligodendrocyte precursor cells from primary NSCs at the expense of immature neuroblasts [40]. This noggin infusion phenocopies the effect of conditionally deleting Smad4 in NSCs using GLAST-cre [40] and is in contrast to the pro-neurogenic effects of noggin described by Lim et al [96]. Thus, although there is still some controversy in the field it its clear that the balance between BMP and noggin is critical to proper maintenance of the adult NSC population.

4. Expression of TGF-β related cytokines in the adult rodent brain after injury

TGF-β family proteins are present in the brain immediately after injury as they are carried into the wound by the blood [103]. Additionally, extracellular TGF-β proteins are activated and released from their latent protein complexes in the brain parenchyma [104]. Local CNS expression of TGF-β, activin, and BMP proteins is increased after many different injuries [72, 105, 106]. Following acute brain injury, TGF-β1 levels are elevated in astrocytes, microglia, macrophages, neurons, ependymal cells and choroid plexus cells with peak expression around 3 days [107-110]. TGF-β2 and -β3 expression has also been found in astrocytes, microglia, endothelial cells and neurons after both ischemic and TBI [111, 112]. We have recently found TGF-β2 expression in oligodendrocytes in the lesioned cortex and corpus callosum [113]. Ischemic lesions as well as TBI show elevated activin-A mRNA as well as mRNA for the BMPRII receptor [90, 94,

114]. Smad proteins are also upregulated after injury and were mainly located in the cerebral cortex, typically in the nucleus and/or in the cytoplasm of astrocytes, oligodendrocytes or neurons [86, 108, 115, 116]. We have summarized many studies that have examined changes in the TGF-β superfamily of cytokines after central nervous system injury in Table 2.

TGF-β protein	Acute brain Insult (Animal model)	Expression in Brain	Expression in neurogenic niche	Cell types in which protein is expressed	mRNA and/or protein	References
TGF-β1	Ischemia	Cerebral cortex	_____	Microglia, neurons, oligodendrocytes, endothelial cells, astrocytes, macrophages, and ependymal cells	mRNA, protein	[107-110]
	Transient ischemia	Cerebellum, Cerebral cortex	Hippocampus, Subventricular zone	Microglia, T cells, neuroblasts and neurons	mRNA, protein	[117-120]
	Permanent ischemia	Cerebral cortex, Striatum	_____	Neurons, neuroblasts	mRNA, protein	[121-123]
	Bilateral cerebral ischemia	Cerebellum, Cerebral cortex	Dentate gyrus	Neurons, vessels	Protein	[124, 125]
	Hypoxic-ischemic	Cerebral cortex, Corpus callosum	_____	Astrocytes, Microglia and blood vessels	Protein	[126]
	Stab wound	Cerebral cortex	_____	Neurons	Protein	[116]
	Traumatic brain injury	Cerebral cortex	Hippocampus, Subventricular zone	Microglia, astrocytes and neurons	mRNA, protein	[82, 112, 127, 128]
	Excitotoxic lesion (NMDA)	Gray matter surrounding the lesion	_____	Astrocytes, neurons	Protein	[129]
	Triethyltin exposure	Cerebral cortex	Hippocampus	Neurons	mRNA, protein	[130, 131]
	Penetrating brain Injury	Cerebral cortex	_____	Activated glia, meningeal cells, choroid plexus	mRNA, protein	[132]
	Excitotoxic Injury	_____	Hippocampus	Neurons	Protein	[133]
	Irradiation	Cerebral cortex	_____	Macrophages and astrocytes	Protein	[134]

TGF-β protein	Acute brain Insult (Animal model)	Expression in Brain	Expression in neurogenic niche	Cell types in which protein is expressed	mRNA and/or protein	References
	Excitotoxicity with kainic acid	Cerebral cortex	Hippocampus	Microglia/macrophages, neurons and astrocytes	mRNA, protein	[86, 135-137]
	Stab wound	Cerebral cortex	_____	Astrocytes	Protein	[138]
TGF-β2	Ischemia	Cerebral cortex, cerebellum, striatum	Hippocampus	Neurons and endothelial cells, microglia and astrocytes	mRNA, protein	[108, 109, 111]
TGF-β3	Ischemia	Cerebral cortex	Dentate gyrus	Neurons	mRNA, protein	[111]
	Traumatic brain injury	Cerebral cortex	Hippocampus	Astrocytes	Protein	[112]
TβRI	Permanent ischemia	Cerebral cortex	_____	Astrocytes and neurons	mRNA, protein	[122]
TβRII	Ischemia	Cerebral cortex, midbrain, cerebellum, and brainstem	_____	Neurons, astrocytes, microglia, endothelial cells, and other non-neuronal cells found in the choroid plexus	mRNA, protein	[122, 139, 140]
	Traumatic brain injury	Cerebral Cortex	_____	Endothelial cells	Protein	[141]
Smad2	Excitotoxicity	Cerebral Cortex	Hippocampus	Neurons, astrocytes and microglia	Protein	[86]
pSmad2	Stroke	Cerebral Cortex	_____	Astrocytes, activated microglia	Protein	[108]
pSmad 1,5,8	Cuprizone-induced demyelination	_____	Subventricular zone	Oligodendrocytes	mRNA, protein	[115]
BMPRII	Traumatic brain injury	_____	Dentate gyrus	Neurons	mRNA, protein	[90]
BMPs and receptors	Ischemia	Cerebral Cortex, cerebellum	Hippocampus	Neurons	mRNA, protein	[124, 142, 143]
	Bilateral cerebral ischemia	Cerebral cortex, cerebellum	Subventricular zone, dentate gyrus	Neurons	mRNA, protein	[94]
	Traumatic brain injury	Cerebral cortex	Subventricular zone	Astrocytes	mRNA, protein	[144]

TGF-β protein	Acute brain Insult (Animal model)	Expression in Brain	Expression in neurogenic niche	Cell types in which protein is expressed	mRNA and/or protein	References
BMP4	Cuprizone-induced demyelination	-----	Subventricular zone	Astrocytes and oligodendrocytes	mRNA, protein	[115]
BMP7	Traumatic brain injury	Cerebral cortex	-----	Astrocytes	Protein	[144]
	Stroke	Cerebral cortex, corpus callosum	Subventricular zone	Progenitors cells and neurons	Protein	[145]
Noggin	Traumatic brain injury	Cerebral cortex	Subventricular zone	Astrocytes and progenitors cells	Protein	[144]
ActR-1A	Traumatic brain injury	-----	Dentate gyrus	Neurons	mRNA, protein	[90]
Activin	Ischemia	Cerebral Cortex, striatum	Hippocampus	Neurons	mRNA, protein	[89, 146]
	Hypoxia-ischemia	Cerebral Cortex	Dentate gyrus	Microglia and blood vessels	mRNA, protein	[114]
	Excitotoxicity	Amygdala, Piriform cortex, and thalamus	Dentate gyrus	Neurons, blood vessels	mRNA, protein	[105, 146-148]

Table 2. TGF-β superfamily cytokine and signaling intermediate expression after different forms of injury.

Relatively few studies have examined changes in expression of the TGF-β superfamily of cytokines specifically within the neurogenic regions after brain injury. TGF-β1 expression increases in the SVZ [119] and DG [117, 118, 124] after ischemic injury. Its expression is also induced in neurons of the DG after a demyelinating lesion [131] or after local kainic acid injection [133]. Our group recently found that controlled cortical impact injury increased mRNA expression of many TGF-β cytokines, including TGF-β1 and -β2, activin-A, and BMPs -4, -5, -6, and -7 in the DG and SVZ, demonstrating that a distal injury can alter TGF-β signaling pathways in the neurogenic regions [82]. We have observed upregulation of TGF-β1 and -β3 in GFAP and Nestin positive progenitors in the SVZ and DG after TBI (Figure 2 and unpublished data). TβRII is expressed in these Nestin positive progenitors in the lateral SVZ (Figure 2d). Phospho-Smad3 (pSmad3) shows strong nuclear localization in these cells as well (Figure 2i and unpublished data) suggesting a role for TGF-β/activin signaling in the regulation of post-injury neurogenesis. In the DG, TβRII is expressed in GFAP-positive precursors with strong pSmad3 nuclear staining (Figure 2m, 2r) suggesting a similar role for TGF-β cytokines in this neurogenic niche.

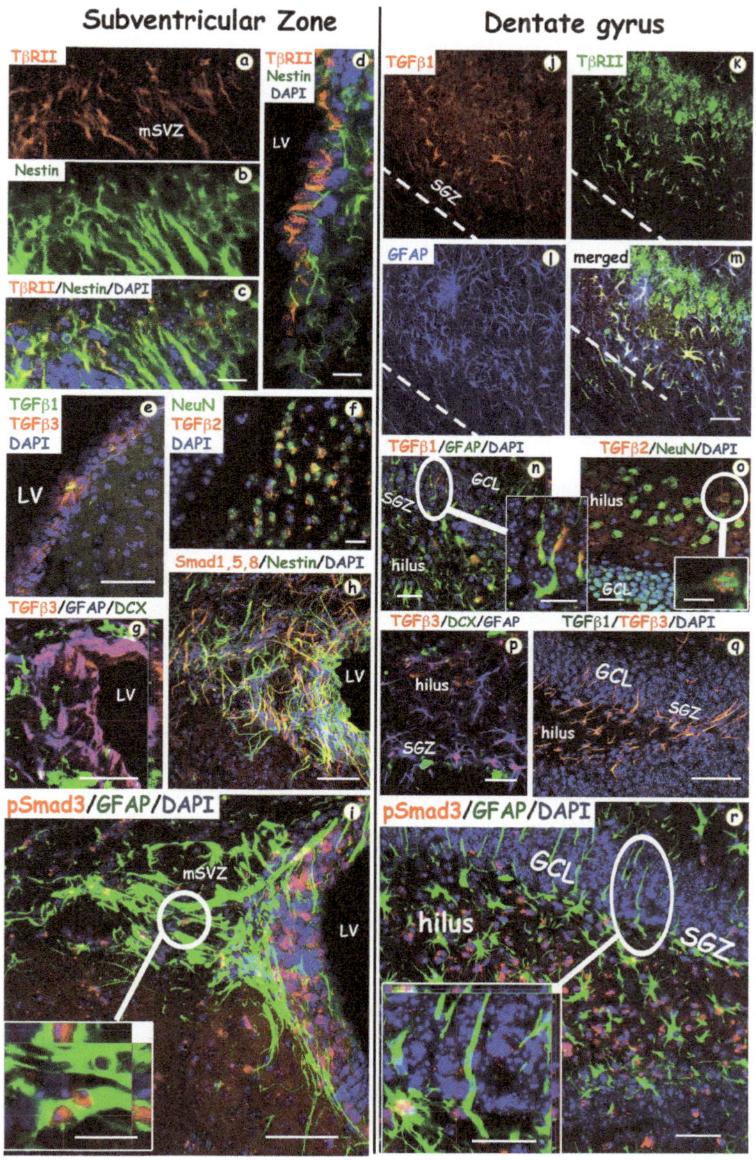

Figure 2. Confocal images of the TGF-β ligands, receptors and signaling proteins in the SVZ and DG in the injured adult mice brain. Double and triple labelled inmmunofluorescence staining for TGF-β proteins and receptors, with the following cell-type specific markers: Nestin (for undifferentiated neuronal precursors), NeuN (for mature neurons), GFAP (for progenitor and astroglial cells), DCX (for neuroblasts). The left column shows coronal sections within

the subventricular zone (SVZ) at 3 (a-g) and 7 (h and i) days after traumatic brain injury (TBI). TβRII (a, red) is expressed in Nestin positive (b, green) neural stem cells (NSCs) in the SVZ, and also in ependymal cells (d), lining the walls of the lateral ventricle (LV). Light TGFβ–1 (green) and predominant TGFβ–3 (red) expression is also found in the walls of the LV where the adult NSCs reside (e). (f) Neurons (NeuN, green) are co-localized with TGFβ–2 (red) in the damaged striatum. (h) The majority of Smad 1,5,8 proteins (red) are co-expressed with Nestin (green). (i) pSmad3 (red) colocalizes with GFAP (green) in the dorsolateral corner of the SVZ. The right column shows coronal sections within the dentate gyrus (DG) of the hippocampus at 3 (j-q) and 7 (r) days after TBI. (j-m) TGFβ–1 (red, j) and TβRII (green) are colocalized in astrocytes (GFAP, blue) in the hilus and GCL (granule cell layer) of the hippocampus (n) TGFβ–1 (red) is co-localized with astrocytes (GFAP positive cells) located in the subgranular zone (SGZ) of the hippocampus. In (o) TGFβ–2 (red) is co-localized with NeuN (green) positive neurons in the hilus of the dentate gyrus. (p) TGFβ–3 (red) is co-localized with GFAP positive (blue) immature progenitors in the SGZ but not with DCX (green) positive neuroblasts. (q) Immunostaining with TGFβ–1 (green) and TGFβ–3 (red) show they are almost entirely colocalized in the SGZ. (r) pSmad3 staining in the nuclei of GFAP positive progenitor cells in the SGZ and hilus of the hippocampus. Scale bars: (c, d, f, (inset in i), m, (inset in n), o, (inset in o), p, (inset in r)) 20 μm; (e, g, h, i, q, r) 50 μm.

Local injury to the hippocampus via saline injection produces a strong induction of activin-βA mRNA in the DG, which can be blocked by inhibiting NMDA receptors [114]. Activin expression in the DG is potently induced by seizures, local excitotoxic lesions, hypoxia/ischemia, TBI or permanent MCAO [89, 114, 146, 148, 149]. Cortical weight drop injury also elevates the expression of the activin receptor ActR-I and the BMP receptor BMPRII in the DG [90]. BMPRII expression is also elevated in the DG after global cerebral ischemia [94], and BMP4 levels increase in the SVZ after a demyelinating lesion [115].

The limited studies available indicate that TGF-β, BMP, and activin signaling may all be active in the neurogenic regions after injury. However, it is currently unclear the manner in which they affect the behavior of neural stem cells. Given that these cytokines clearly regulate adult neurogenesis in the uninjured adult, more research in this area is necessary to fully elucidate the effect of brain injury on these signaling pathways, and the mechanisms through which these changes alter post-injury neurogenesis.

5. Injury-induced neurogenesis and its regulation by TGF-β family proteins

We have described the role of TGF-β proteins in the regulation of neurogenesis under basal conditions. In response to various injuries, the rate of neurogenesis is increased and the fate and migration of the neural progenitors is changed. Cerebral ischemia, excitotoxicity and TBI can all promote neurogenesis in the adult DG and SVZ [88, 150-153]. After injury, the altered environment changes the basic processes of proliferation, differentiation, migration and integration. TGF-β related cytokines have the potential to regulate many of these processes. Alteration in the destination of progenitor cells means that many of the neuroblasts change their usual trajectory and migrate towards and into the lesion [154]. The cell fate of progenitor cells can be altered by the changed environment of the injured brain, in both the neurogenic niche and at the lesion site to which the progenitor cells migrate. The environment around the lesion is now very different than the normal location of these progenitors and thus further differentiation and integration occurs in an entirely unique environment [155]. Additionally, the actions of TGF-β cytokines are highly context dependent, and they can have very different effects in the injured as compared to the uninjured brain.

A major component of the brain post-injury in comparison to the uninjured brain is the inflammatory response, both of local CNS cells and invading macrophages. While the majority of studies have indicated that inflammation is detrimental to neurogenesis, it is now appreciated that the effect of inflammation on neurogenesis is multifaceted [156]. Of particular importance is the response of local microglia and astrocytes in the neurogenic regions. Microglia are potent regulators of neurogenesis, and in certain contexts can powerfully inhibit the process [157]. However microglia have also been shown to promote neurogenesis [158, 159], and studies have described differential action of acute vs. chronically activated microglia on NSC division and neurogenesis, as well as for microglia activated by different mechanisms or by different cytokines [160, 161]. As TGF-β proteins are prominent anti-inflammatory molecules [162], their actions after brain injury can regulate neurogenesis by acting directly on NSCs as well as indirectly through their effects on the glial inflammatory response [163].

Due to their pleiotropic actions, TGF-β superfamily proteins have been investigated as potential treatments for a variety of CNS injuries, and several studies have demonstrated potential uses for these cytokines as therapeutic molecules (see Table 3). They have also provided insights into the action of these molecules as regulators of neural stem/progenitor cell (NSPC) proliferation and differentiation, with respect to both endogenous and transplanted stem cell populations.

TGF-β related protein	Animal Model	Mode of administration	Effect on cell proliferation and neurogenesis	Behavioral Outcome	Reference
TGFβ-1	Transient ischemia	Intranasal aerosol spray	Decreased NSC proliferation and induce the number of DCX expressing neuronal precursors	Reduced Neurological Severity Score deficits	[164]
	Adrenalectomy	Intraventricular infusion	Decreased the percentage of dividing cells which co-express PSA-NCAM in the DG	None measured	[163]
	Adrenalectomy	Adenoviral overexpression	Increased NSC proliferation and neurogenesis in the SVZ	None measured	[165]
	Prenatal LPS inflammation	Adult adenoviral overexpression	Inhibited chronic microglial activation and restored neurogenesis	None measured	[166]
	Naïve animals	Injected into the cerebrospinal fluid	Number of proliferating cells in the hippocampus and in the lateral ventricle wall is substantially reduced, fewer neuronal precursor cells	None measured	[81]

TGF-β related protein	Animal Model	Mode of administration	Effect on cell proliferation and neurogenesis	Behavioral Outcome	Reference
Noggin	Naïve animals	Transgenic astrocytic overexpression	Decreased DG cell proliferation and generation of neuroblasts and neurons	None measured	[87]
	Permanent MCAO	Transgenic neuronal overexpression	Increased immature oligodendrocyte generation	Reduced motor deficits	[167]
	Naïve animals	Intraventricular infusion	Promoted neuronal differentiation of SVZ precursor cells transplanted to the striatum	None measured	[96]
	Cuprizone-induced corpus callosum demyelination	Intraventricular infusion	Decreased astrocyte and increased oligodendrocyte generation from the SVZ	None measured	[115]
	Spinal cord injury	Overexpression by transplanted NPCs.	Increased neuronal and oligodendroglial differentiation of transplanted NPCs	Improved motor recovery	[168]
BMP7	Transient ischemia	Intraventricular infusion	Increased SVZ proliferation and neurogenesis	Reduced motor deficits	[145]
	Naïve animals	Intraventricular infusion	Inhibited SVZ proliferation	None measured	[96]
Chordin	Lysolectithin-induced corpus callosum demyelination	Intraventricular infusion	Increased NPCs migrating to lesion, and increased oligodendrocyte differentiation	None measured	[169]
Activin-A	Excitotoxic hippocampal lesion	Continuous intraventricular infusion	Decreased astrocyte and microglial inflammation, and increases neurogenesis	None measured	[88]
	Naïve mice	Transgenic overexpression	Increases new neuron survival	Reduced anxiety-like behavior	[91]
Activin-A or Activin-B	Naïve mice	ICV injection	Not examined	Reduced depression-like behavior	[170]
Follistatin	Excitotoxic hippocampal lesion	Continuous intraventricular infusion	Increased NSC proliferation and neurogenesis.	None measured	[88]
	Naïve mice	Transgenic overexpression	Potently inhibited neurogenesis	Increased anxiety-like behavior	[91]

Table 3. Therapeutic application of TGF-β proteins in the normal and injured brain that affect neurogenesis.

5.1. TGF-β1

TGF-β1 treatment improves the outcome in several models of injury as it is strongly neuroprotective [76, 133, 171, 172] and in certain circumstances can promote neurogenesis after injury. After middle cerebral artery occlusion (MCAO) in mice, intranasal treatment with TGF-β1 increases the number of proliferative DCX-positive neural progenitors and the number of new neurons in the SVZ and striatum, while decreasing the fraction of proliferative cells that express GFAP [119]. After adrenalectomy, TGF-β also stimulates neurogenesis. TGF-β1 expression is upregulated and is necessary for the increased rates of neurogenesis in the SVZ and DG caused by adrenalectomy [163]. In this model TGF-β mediated downregulation of microglial activation and proliferation may be partially responsible for the increased neurogenesis [163, 165]. TGF-β1 can also inhibit chronic microglial activation induced by prenatal LPS exposure, and ameliorate the LPS-mediated decrease in neurogenesis [166] suggesting that the anti-inflammatory action of TGF-β participates in its pro-neurogenic effects. Conversely, in naïve animals intracerebroventricular infusion of TGF-β1 lowered the number of DCX-positive neuronal precursors in the neurogenic niches. This reduced level of proliferation in the TGF-β1 infused brains was strongly correlated with an increased accumulation of pSmad2 in Sox2/GFAP expressing cells of the SGZ [81]. Transgenic overexpression of TGF-β1 in naïve mice also leads to reduce neurogenesis [87]. The opposite effects of TGF-β1 in injured as compared to naïve animals illustrate the difficulty in assigning one specific role to TGF-β1 due to its context-dependent effects. Chronic inflammation, either after lesion or in neurodegenerative disease, provides a different environment for the consequences of TGF-β signaling. The anti-inflammatory actions of TGF-β can have an important role in influencing neurogenic processes, independent of direct effects on neural progenitor cells. Dysregulation of TGF-β signaling is being acknowledged as a potential source for chronic inflammation. Indeed, aberrant TGF-β signaling and consequent accumulation of activated microglia in the neurogenic regions may play an important role in the progression of Alzheimer's disease [171, 173].

5.2. Activin

Recent studies have demonstrated a critical role for activin signaling as a modulator of adult neurogenesis [91] in addition to its well-established role as a neuroprotective molecule [174, 175]. After local excitotoxic injury to the hippocampus, ablating activin signaling by infusion of the activin inhibitor follistatin potently inhibits post-injury neurogenesis and exacerbates the inflammatory response of astrocytes and microglia. Conversely, infusion of activin-A facilitates neurogenesis and represses gliosis [88]. Perhaps related to its effects on neurogenesis, activin can also regulate anxiety and depression-like behavior in rodents, and the activin pathway may be a useful therapeutic target for treating depression. Hippocampal infusion of activin-A or activin-B reduces measures of depression in a forced swim test, with a similar efficacy to that of the antidepressant fluoxetine [170]. Further, transgenic mice which overexpress activin-A, have decreased anxiety measures in spontaneous place preference tests, while mice which overexpress follistatin, display the reverse [91].

5.3. BMPs

In the naïve rodent, BMPs usually act to suppress neurogenesis in the SVZ and DG whereas the BMP inhibitor noggin promotes it [96]. In contrast, inhibition of BMP signaling by upregulation of the BMP inhibitor chordin after lysolecithin-induced demyelination of the corpus callosum, led to redirection of SVZ precursors away from a neuronal lineage towards that of oligodendrocytes [169]. This change in differentiation potential was accompanied by a change in the migration pattern of the SVZ precursors, away from the rostral migratory stream, and towards the corpus callosum. Injury-induced changes in expression of regulatory factors often alter the normal pattern of cell differentiation and migration [176, 177]. In a different model of demyelination, cuprizone-induced upregulation of BMP-4 resulted in more SVZ precursors becoming astrocytes, with a concomitant reduction in the number of mature oligodendrocytes [115]. Intraventricular infusion of noggin in this model increased the generation of oligodendrocytes from the SVZ [115] illustrating that inhibition of BMP signaling has the potential to promote remyelination in models of multiple sclerosis. The astrogliogenic potential of BMP has been demonstrated in multiple studies, where various precursors are pushed towards the astrocytic lineage [168, 178]. This is also true with transplanted neural stem cells or mesenchymal stem cells, where BMPs around the implantation site push the transplanted cells towards astrocytes [179]. If these cells are being used to enhance repair after spinal cord or TBI, inhibition of BMP becomes an attractive option to promote neuronal or oligodendrocyte differentiation rather than that of astrocytes. In contrast to all these studies, one group has shown that BMP-7 has neuroprotective properties which may enhance the survival of immature neurons [142, 180]. In one study, infusion of BMP-7 into the lateral ventricles of rats 24 hours after transient MCAO led to increased numbers of proliferating NSCs and more mature neurons generated in the SVZ while also facilitating behavioral recovery [145]. However, a different group has shown that transgenic expression of the BMP-inhibitor noggin in neurons after permanent MCAO in the mouse enhances functional recovery [167]. These conflicting data illustrate the sometimes confusing nature of the literature whereby BMP effects, similar to those of TGF-β are extremely contextual and are dependent on the exact model used. Overall, although some BMPs may have neuroprotective properties, the vast majority of the literature supports the view that BMP induction after injury is not beneficial for recovery, and that inhibition of BMP signaling may have therapeutic potential.

6. Future therapeutic strategies

In spite of extensive research in the field of brain injury or stroke, there is little effective treatment for these injuries [182]. Many of the neuroprotective treatments that have been successful in rodents have failed in clinical trials [183]. Harnessing the regenerative capacity of the adult brain is one strategy for repairing and replacing injured tissue, together with enhancing neurotrophic support of existing neurons to promote survival [184, 185]. A complementary strategy also under development is transplantation of neural stem cells or committed progenitors into the lesion. However, when multipotent NSCs were implanted

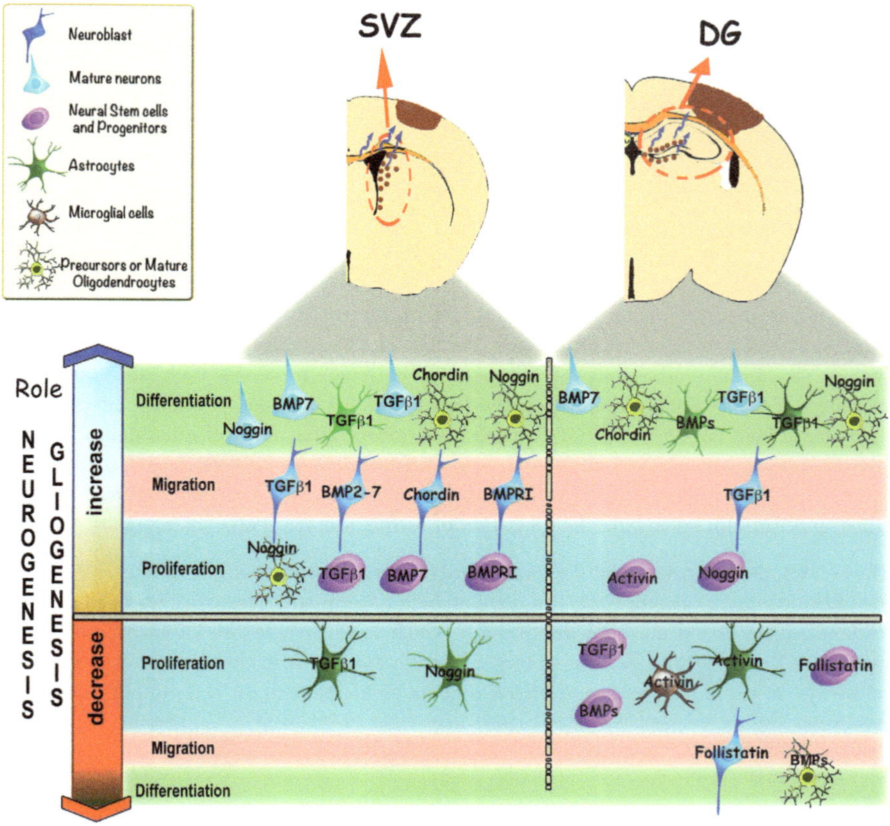

Figure 3. Modulation of neurogenesis and gliogenesis after adult brain injury by members of the TGF-β cytokine superfamily. In the top panel, the dentate gyrus (DG) in the hippocampus and subventricular zone (SVZ) of the lateral ventricles are shown after damage to the cerebral cortex. Note the proliferation and migration of cells from the SVZ and DG towards the infarcted area (blue arrows). Red dots represent proliferating and migrating neural stem cells and progenitors cells (NSPCs) located in these neurogenic regions. In the bottom panel, the role of TGF-β proteins at different stages of neurogenesis or gliogenesis after adult brain injury is illustrated. Proliferation, migration or differentiation are induced or inhibited by growth factors, such as: TGF-β, BMPs proteins, Activin, Follistatin or Noggin. After injury to the brain, TGF-β1 can increase proliferation of NSPCs and induce the differentiation of neuroblasts into neurons within the SVZ, [119]. BMP7 can induce neural stem cell proliferation, neuronal migration and differentiation [145]; other BMPs proteins (BMP2-7) also can stimulate neuronal migration [94]. The BMP inhibitor proteins noggin and chordin promote NSPC migration and oligodendrocyte proliferation and differentiation, while decreasing astrocyte proliferation [115, 169]. After injury to the brain, within the DG TGF-β1 can reduce the proliferation of immature neurons while increasing neuronal migration and differentiation [165, 166]. BMP7 can enhance NSPC proliferation and neuronal differentiation [96, 145]. Noggin can also increase NSPC proliferation [169]. Generally, BMPs can increase astroglial differentiation and inhibit oligodendrocyte generation, and the BMP inhibitors Chordin and Noggin can facilitate oligodendrocyte differentiation and proliferation [181]. Activin can induce NSPCs proliferation, and decrease microglial and astroglial proliferation. The activin antagonist, follistatin, reduces proliferating NSPCs and migrating neuroblasts [88]. In summary, the proliferation, migration and differentiation of cells in the SVZ and the DG may be influenced by the spatial and temporal expression profile of these TGF-β proteins after brain injury.

directly into non-neurogenic regions in the injured brain, such as in the cortex or striatum, they failed to generate neurons but instead generated glial cells [186, 187]. Endogenous neural progenitors also are limited in their differentiation potential, presumably because the post-lesion environment is one that supports glial differentiation in preference to that of neurons [188]. As TGF-β family members can promote astrogliogenesis [189, 190], it would seem that in some circumstances, inhibition of specific cytokine signals would increase neuronal differentiation. A further consideration for repair and neuronal survival is promotion of oligodendrocyte survival and differentiation, since remyelination is critical to continued survival and function of many neurons. Inhibition of BMP action through infusion of noggin can promote oligodendrocyte differentiation after demyelination [115]. Inflammation after injury is yet one more factor that alters the environment for regeneration. Although often thought of as a short-lived phenomenon, there can be longer lasting inflammatory changes that persist months after injury [191]. One of the major problems with development of members of the TGF-β superfamily or their inhibitors for therapeutic use are the pleiotropic nature of their effects. Thus TGF-β1 itself is neuroprotective and anti-inflammatory, which should promote recovery, but it inhibits proliferation of precursors, and also promotes development of the glial scar through upregulation of many extracellular matrix molecules, and through enhancing the migration of astrocytes [128, 192].

These cytokines act in a context dependent and concentration dependent manner, which adds an additional layer of complexity. To develop better therapeutic strategies we need a deeper understanding of the mechanisms through which the many actions of each cytokine are mediated. We may then be able to target specific molecules in the downstream signaling pathways, to avoid the pleiotropic effects that are emblematic of the activity of this cytokine family.

Acknowledgements

This study was supported by grant from the Center for Neuroscience and Regenerative Medicine (CNRM). SV is supported by a CNRM postdoctoral fellowship. The opinions and assertions contained herein are the private opinions of the authors and are not to be construed as reflecting the views of the Uniformed Services University of the Health Sciences or the US Department of Defense.

Author details

Sonia Villapol, Trevor T. Logan and Aviva J. Symes

Department of Pharmacology and Center for Neuroscience and Regenerative Medicine, Uniformed Services University of the Health Sciences, Bethesda, MD, USA

References

[1] Berciano J, Lafarga M, Berciano M: Santiago Ramon y Cajal. *Neurologia* 2001, 16(3): 118-121.

[2] Alvarez-Buylla A: Mechanism of neurogenesis in adult avian brain. *Experientia* 1990, 46(9):948-955.

[3] Parent JM: Injury-induced neurogenesis in the adult mammalian brain. *Neuroscientist* 2003, 9(4):261-272.

[4] Whitney NP, Eidem TM, Peng H, Huang Y, Zheng JC: Inflammation mediates varying effects in neurogenesis: relevance to the pathogenesis of brain injury and neurodegenerative disorders. *J Neurochem* 2009, 108(6):1343-1359.

[5] Hagg T: Molecular regulation of adult CNS neurogenesis: an integrated view. *Trends Neurosci* 2005, 28(11):589-595.

[6] Kronenberg G, Reuter K, Steiner B, Brandt MD, Jessberger S, Yamaguchi M, Kempermann G: Subpopulations of proliferating cells of the adult hippocampus respond differently to physiologic neurogenic stimuli. *J Comp Neurol* 2003, 467(4):455-463.

[7] Mackowiak M, Chocyk A, Markowicz-Kula K, Wedzony K: Neurogenesis in the adult brain. *Pol J Pharmacol* 2004, 56(6):673-687.

[8] Massague J, Cheifetz S, Ignotz RA, Boyd FT: Multiple type-beta transforming growth factors and their receptors. *J Cell Physiol Suppl* 1987, Suppl 5:43-47.

[9] Massague J: Receptors for the TGF-beta family. *Cell* 1992, 69(7):1067-1070.

[10] Wrighton KH, Feng XH: To (TGF)beta or not to (TGF)beta: fine-tuning of Smad signaling via post-translational modifications. *Cell Signal* 2008, 20(9):1579-1591.

[11] Umulis D, O'Connor MB, Blair SS: The extracellular regulation of bone morphogenetic protein signaling. *Development* 2009, 136(22):3715-3728.

[12] Miyazono K, Maeda S, Imamura T: BMP receptor signaling: transcriptional targets, regulation of signals, and signaling cross-talk. *Cytokine Growth Factor Rev* 2005, 16(3): 251-263.

[13] Ross S, Hill CS: How the Smads regulate transcription. *Int J Biochem Cell Biol* 2008, 40(3):383-408.

[14] Heldin CH, Moustakas A: Role of Smads in TGFbeta signaling. *Cell Tissue Res* 2012, 347(1):21-36.

[15] Derynck R, Feng XH: TGF-beta receptor signaling. *Biochim Biophys Acta* 1997, 1333(2):F105-150.

[16] Derynck R, Zhang YE: Smad-dependent and Smad-independent pathways in TGF-beta family signalling. *Nature* 2003, 425(6958):577-584.

[17] Kandasamy M, Reilmann R, Winkler J, Bogdahn U, Aigner L: Transforming Growth Factor-Beta Signaling in the Neural Stem Cell Niche: A Therapeutic Target for Huntington's Disease. *Neurol Res Int* 2011, 2011:124256.

[18] Moustakas A, Heldin CH: The regulation of TGFbeta signal transduction. *Development* 2009, 136(22):3699-3714.

[19] Mehler MF, Mabie PC, Zhang D, Kessler JA: Bone morphogenetic proteins in the nervous system. *Trends Neurosci* 1997, 20(7):309-317.

[20] Walsh DW, Godson C, Brazil DP, Martin F: Extracellular BMP-antagonist regulation in development and disease: tied up in knots. *Trends Cell Biol* 2010, 20(5):244-256.

[21] Kang JS, Liu C, Derynck R: New regulatory mechanisms of TGF-beta receptor function. *Trends Cell Biol* 2009, 19(8):385-394.

[22] Kretzschmar M, Massague J: SMADs: mediators and regulators of TGF-beta signaling. *Curr Opin Genet Dev* 1998, 8(1):103-111.

[23] Vogt J, Traynor R, Sapkota GP: The specificities of small molecule inhibitors of the TGFss and BMP pathways. *Cell Signal* 2011, 23(11):1831-1842.

[24] de Caestecker M: The transforming growth factor-beta superfamily of receptors. *Cytokine Growth Factor Rev* 2004, 15(1):1-11.

[25] Zhang YE: Non-Smad pathways in TGF-beta signaling. *Cell Res* 2009, 19(1):128-139.

[26] Saj A, Lai EC: Control of microRNA biogenesis and transcription by cell signaling pathways. *Curr Opin Genet Dev* 2011, 21(4):504-510.

[27] Davis BN, Hilyard AC, Nguyen PH, Lagna G, Hata A: Smad proteins bind a conserved RNA sequence to promote microRNA maturation by Drosha. *Mol Cell* 2010, 39(3):373-384.

[28] Wharton K, Derynck R: TGFbeta family signaling: novel insights in development and disease. *Development* 2009, 136(22):3691-3697.

[29] Larsson J, Goumans MJ, Sjostrand LJ, van Rooijen MA, Ward D, Leveen P, Xu X, ten Dijke P, Mummery CL, Karlsson S: Abnormal angiogenesis but intact hematopoietic potential in TGF-beta type I receptor-deficient mice. *Embo J* 2001, 20(7):1663-1673.

[30] Oshima M, Oshima H, Taketo MM: TGF-beta receptor type II deficiency results in defects of yolk sac hematopoiesis and vasculogenesis. *Dev Biol* 1996, 179(1):297-302.

[31] Hill CR, Sanchez NS, Love JD, Arrieta JA, Hong CC, Brown CB, Austin AF, Barnett JV: BMP2 signals loss of epithelial character in epicardial cells but requires the Type III TGFbeta receptor to promote invasion. *Cell Signal* 2012, 24(5):1012-1022.

[32] Shull MM, Ormsby I, Kier AB, Pawlowski S, Diebold RJ, Yin M, Allen R, Sidman C, Proetzel G, Calvin D *et al*: Targeted disruption of the mouse transforming growth factor-beta 1 gene results in multifocal inflammatory disease. *Nature* 1992, 359(6397): 693-699.

[33] Kulkarni AB, Huh CG, Becker D, Geiser A, Lyght M, Flanders KC, Roberts AB, Sporn MB, Ward JM, Karlsson S: Transforming growth factor beta 1 null mutation in mice causes excessive inflammatory response and early death. *Proc Natl Acad Sci U S A* 1993, 90(2):770-774.

[34] Sanford LP, Ormsby I, Gittenberger-de Groot AC, Sariola H, Friedman R, Boivin GP, Cardell EL, Doetschman T: TGFbeta2 knockout mice have multiple developmental defects that are non-overlapping with other TGFbeta knockout phenotypes. *Development* 1997, 124(13):2659-2670.

[35] Huang S, Tang B, Usoskin D, Lechleider RJ, Jamin SP, Li C, Anzano MA, Ebendal T, Deng C, Roberts AB: Conditional knockout of the Smad1 gene. *Genesis* 2002, 32(2): 76-79.

[36] Tremblay KD, Dunn NR, Robertson EJ: Mouse embryos lacking Smad1 signals display defects in extra-embryonic tissues and germ cell formation. *Development* 2001, 128(18):3609-3621.

[37] Heyer J, Escalante-Alcalde D, Lia M, Boettinger E, Edelmann W, Stewart CL, Kucherlapati R: Postgastrulation Smad2-deficient embryos show defects in embryo turning and anterior morphogenesis. *Proc Natl Acad Sci U S A* 1999, 96(22):12595-12600.

[38] Datto MB, Frederick JP, Pan L, Borton AJ, Zhuang Y, Wang XF: Targeted disruption of Smad3 reveals an essential role in transforming growth factor beta-mediated signal transduction. *Mol Cell Biol* 1999, 19(4):2495-2504.

[39] Yang X, Letterio JJ, Lechleider RJ, Chen L, Hayman R, Gu H, Roberts AB, Deng C: Targeted disruption of SMAD3 results in impaired mucosal immunity and diminished T cell responsiveness to TGF-beta. *Embo J* 1999, 18(5):1280-1291.

[40] Colak D, Mori T, Brill MS, Pfeifer A, Falk S, Deng C, Monteiro R, Mummery C, Sommer L, Gotz M: Adult neurogenesis requires Smad4-mediated bone morphogenic protein signaling in stem cells. *J Neurosci* 2008, 28(2):434-446.

[41] Arnold SJ, Maretto S, Islam A, Bikoff EK, Robertson EJ: Dose-dependent Smad1, Smad5 and Smad8 signaling in the early mouse embryo. *Dev Biol* 2006, 296(1): 104-118.

[42] Chang H, Brown CW, Matzuk MM: Genetic analysis of the mammalian transforming growth factor-beta superfamily. *Endocr Rev* 2002, 23(6):787-823.

[43] Tojo M, Takebe A, Takahashi S, Tanaka K, Imamura T, Miyazono K, Chiba T: Smad7-deficient mice show growth retardation with reduced viability. *J Biochem* 2012, 151(6): 621-631.

[44] Huang Z, Wang D, Ihida-Stansbury K, Jones PL, Martin JF: Defective pulmonary vascular remodeling in Smad8 mutant mice. *Hum Mol Genet* 2009, 18(15):2791-2801.

[45] Mishina Y, Suzuki A, Ueno N, Behringer RR: Bmpr encodes a type I bone morphogenetic protein receptor that is essential for gastrulation during mouse embryogenesis. *Genes Dev* 1995, 9(24):3027-3037.

[46] Yi SE, Daluiski A, Pederson R, Rosen V, Lyons KM: The type I BMP receptor BMPRIB is required for chondrogenesis in the mouse limb. *Development* 2000, 127(3): 621-630.

[47] Beppu H, Kawabata M, Hamamoto T, Chytil A, Minowa O, Noda T, Miyazono K: BMP type II receptor is required for gastrulation and early development of mouse embryos. *Dev Biol* 2000, 221(1):249-258.

[48] Zhang H, Bradley A: Mice deficient for BMP2 are nonviable and have defects in amnion/chorion and cardiac development. *Development* 1996, 122(10):2977-2986.

[49] Daluiski A, Engstrand T, Bahamonde ME, Gamer LW, Agius E, Stevenson SL, Cox K, Rosen V, Lyons KM: Bone morphogenetic protein-3 is a negative regulator of bone density. *Nat Genet* 2001, 27(1):84-88.

[50] Winnier G, Blessing M, Labosky PA, Hogan BL: Bone morphogenetic protein-4 is required for mesoderm formation and patterning in the mouse. *Genes Dev* 1995, 9(17): 2105-2116.

[51] King JA, Marker PC, Seung KJ, Kingsley DM: BMP5 and the molecular, skeletal, and soft-tissue alterations in short ear mice. *Dev Biol* 1994, 166(1):112-122.

[52] Solloway MJ, Dudley AT, Bikoff EK, Lyons KM, Hogan BL, Robertson EJ: Mice lacking Bmp6 function. *Dev Genet* 1998, 22(4):321-339.

[53] Dupe V, Ghyselinck NB, Thomazy V, Nagy L, Davies PJ, Chambon P, Mark M: Essential roles of retinoic acid signaling in interdigital apoptosis and control of BMP-7 expression in mouse autopods. *Dev Biol* 1999, 208(1):30-43.

[54] Wawersik S, Purcell P, Rauchman M, Dudley AT, Robertson EJ, Maas R: BMP7 acts in murine lens placode development. *Dev Biol* 1999, 207(1):176-188.

[55] Dudley AT, Lyons KM, Robertson EJ: A requirement for bone morphogenetic protein-7 during development of the mammalian kidney and eye. *Genes Dev* 1995, 9(22): 2795-2807.

[56] Luo G, Hofmann C, Bronckers AL, Sohocki M, Bradley A, Karsenty G: BMP-7 is an inducer of nephrogenesis, and is also required for eye development and skeletal patterning. *Genes Dev* 1995, 9(22):2808-2820.

[57] Galloway SD, Maughan RJ: The effects of substrate and fluid provision on thermoregulatory and metabolic responses to prolonged exercise in a hot environment. *J Sports Sci* 2000, 18(5):339-351.

[58] Ying Y, Liu XM, Marble A, Lawson KA, Zhao GQ: Requirement of Bmp8b for the generation of primordial germ cells in the mouse. *Mol Endocrinol* 2000, 14(7): 1053-1063.

[59] Yan C, Wang P, DeMayo J, DeMayo FJ, Elvin JA, Carino C, Prasad SV, Skinner SS, Dunbar BS, Dube JL *et al*: Synergistic roles of bone morphogenetic protein 15 and growth differentiation factor 9 in ovarian function. *Mol Endocrinol* 2001, 15(6):854-866.

[60] Ray BN, Lee NY, How T, Blobe GC: ALK5 phosphorylation of the endoglin cytoplasmic domain regulates Smad1/5/8 signaling and endothelial cell migration. *Carcinogenesis* 2010, 31(3):435-441.

[61] Li DY, Sorensen LK, Brooke BS, Urness LD, Davis EC, Taylor DG, Boak BB, Wendel DP: Defective angiogenesis in mice lacking endoglin. *Science* 1999, 284(5419): 1534-1537.

[62] Mishina Y, Crombie R, Bradley A, Behringer RR: Multiple roles for activin-like kinase-2 signaling during mouse embryogenesis. *Dev Biol* 1999, 213(2):314-326.

[63] Matzuk MM, Kumar TR, Shou W, Coerver KA, Lau AL, Behringer RR, Finegold MJ: Transgenic models to study the roles of inhibins and activins in reproduction, oncogenesis, and development. *Recent Prog Horm Res* 1996, 51:123-154; discussion 155-127.

[64] Ferguson CA, Tucker AS, Christensen L, Lau AL, Matzuk MM, Sharpe PT: Activin is an essential early mesenchymal signal in tooth development that is required for patterning of the murine dentition. *Genes Dev* 1998, 12(16):2636-2649.

[65] Vassalli A, Matzuk MM, Gardner HA, Lee KF, Jaenisch R: Activin/inhibin beta B subunit gene disruption leads to defects in eyelid development and female reproduction. *Genes Dev* 1994, 8(4):414-427.

[66] Brunet LJ, McMahon JA, McMahon AP, Harland RM: Noggin, cartilage morphogenesis, and joint formation in the mammalian skeleton. *Science* 1998, 280(5368):1455-1457.

[67] Matzuk MM, Lu N, Vogel H, Sellheyer K, Roop DR, Bradley A: Multiple defects and perinatal death in mice deficient in follistatin. *Nature* 1995, 374(6520):360-363.

[68] Emsley JG, Mitchell BD, Kempermann G, Macklis JD: Adult neurogenesis and repair of the adult CNS with neural progenitors, precursors, and stem cells. *Prog Neurobiol* 2005, 75(5):321-341.

[69] Kazanis I, Lathia J, Moss L, ffrench-Constant C: The neural stem cell microenvironment. In: *StemBook.* Cambridge (MA); 2008.

[70] Ihrie RA, Alvarez-Buylla A: Lake-front property: a unique germinal niche by the lateral ventricles of the adult brain. *Neuron* 2011, 70(4):674-686.

[71] Ming GL, Song H: Adult neurogenesis in the mammalian brain: significant answers and significant questions. *Neuron* 2011, 70(4):687-702.

[72] Vivien D, Ali C: Transforming growth factor-beta signalling in brain disorders. *Cytokine Growth Factor Rev* 2006, 17(1-2):121-128.

[73] ten Dijke P, Arthur HM: Extracellular control of TGFbeta signalling in vascular development and disease. *Nat Rev Mol Cell Biol* 2007, 8(11):857-869.

[74] Flanders KC, Ludecke G, Engels S, Cissel DS, Roberts AB, Kondaiah P, Lafyatis R, Sporn MB, Unsicker K: Localization and actions of transforming growth factor-beta s in the embryonic nervous system. *Development* 1991, 113(1):183-191.

[75] Unsicker K, Meier C, Krieglstein K, Sartor BM, Flanders KC: Expression, localization, and function of transforming growth factor-beta s in embryonic chick spinal cord, hindbrain, and dorsal root ganglia. *J Neurobiol* 1996, 29(2):262-276.

[76] Dobolyi A, Vincze C, Pal G, Lovas G: The neuroprotective functions of transforming growth factor Beta proteins. *Int J Mol Sci* 2012, 13(7):8219-8258.

[77] Flanders KC, Ren RF, Lippa CF: Transforming growth factor-betas in neurodegenerative disease. *Prog Neurobiol* 1998, 54(1):71-85.

[78] Blottner D, Wolf N, Lachmund A, Flanders KC, Unsicker K: TGF-beta rescues target-deprived preganglionic sympathetic neurons in the spinal cord. *Eur J Neurosci* 1996, 8(1):202-210.

[79] De Groot CJ, Montagne L, Barten AD, Sminia P, Van Der Valk P: Expression of transforming growth factor (TGF)-beta1, -beta2, and -beta3 isoforms and TGF-beta type I and type II receptors in multiple sclerosis lesions and human adult astrocyte cultures. *J Neuropathol Exp Neurol* 1999, 58(2):174-187.

[80] Miller MW: Expression of transforming growth factor-beta in developing rat cerebral cortex: effects of prenatal exposure to ethanol. *J Comp Neurol* 2003, 460(3):410-424.

[81] Wachs FP, Winner B, Couillard-Despres S, Schiller T, Aigner R, Winkler J, Bogdahn U, Aigner L: Transforming growth factor-beta1 is a negative modulator of adult neurogenesis. *J Neuropathol Exp Neurol* 2006, 65(4):358-370.

[82] Logan V, Symes: TGF-β superfamily gene expression and induction of the Runx1 transcription factor in adult neurogenic regions after brain injury. *Submitted* 2012.

[83] Werry EL, Enjeti S, Halliday GM, Sachdev PS, Double KL: Effect of age on proliferation-regulating factors in human adult neurogenic regions. *J Neurochem* 2010, 115(4): 956-964.

[84] Artegiani B, Calegari F: Age-related cognitive decline: can neural stem cells help us? *Aging (Albany NY)* 2012, 4(3):176-186.

[85] He Y, Yung A, Wyss-Coray T: TGF-β signaling in newborn neurons is required for their survival and maturation in the adult dentate gyrus. In: *Society for Neuroscience: 2012*. 823.808.

[86] Luo J, Lin AH, Masliah E, Wyss-Coray T: Bioluminescence imaging of Smad signaling in living mice shows correlation with excitotoxic neurodegeneration. *Proc Natl Acad Sci U S A* 2006, 103(48):18326-18331.

[87] Buckwalter MS, Yamane M, Coleman BS, Ormerod BK, Chin JT, Palmer T, Wyss-Coray T: Chronically increased transforming growth factor-beta1 strongly inhibits hippocampal neurogenesis in aged mice. *Am J Pathol* 2006, 169(1):154-164.

[88] Abdipranoto-Cowley A, Park JS, Croucher D, Daniel J, Henshall S, Galbraith S, Mervin K, Vissel B: Activin A is essential for neurogenesis following neurodegeneration. *Stem Cells* 2009, 27(6):1330-1346.

[89] Bottner M, Dubal DB, Rau SW, Suzuki S, Wise PM: Stroke injury in rats causes an increase in activin A gene expression which is unaffected by oestradiol treatment. *J Neuroendocrinol* 2006, 18(2):97-103.

[90] Lewen A, Soderstrom S, Hillered L, Ebendal T: Expression of serine/threonine kinase receptors in traumatic brain injury. *Neuroreport* 1997, 8(2):475-479.

[91] Ageta H, Murayama A, Migishima R, Kida S, Tsuchida K, Yokoyama M, Inokuchi K: Activin in the brain modulates anxiety-related behavior and adult neurogenesis. *PLoS One* 2008, 3(4):e1869.

[92] Gokoffski KK, Wu HH, Beites CL, Kim J, Kim EJ, Matzuk MM, Johnson JE, Lander AD, Calof AL: Activin and GDF11 collaborate in feedback control of neuroepithelial stem cell proliferation and fate. *Development* 2011, 138(19):4131-4142.

[93] Wang Y, Symes AJ: Smad3 deficiency reduces neurogenesis in adult mice. *J Mol Neurosci* 2010, 41(3):383-396.

[94] Charytoniuk DA, Traiffort E, Pinard E, Issertial O, Seylaz J, Ruat M: Distribution of bone morphogenetic protein and bone morphogenetic protein receptor transcripts in the rodent nervous system and up-regulation of bone morphogenetic protein receptor type II in hippocampal dentate gyrus in a rat model of global cerebral ischemia. *Neuroscience* 2000, 100(1):33-43.

[95] Miyagi M, Mikawa S, Hasegawa T, Kobayashi S, Matsuyama Y, Sato K: Bone morphogenetic protein receptor expressions in the adult rat brain. *Neuroscience* 2011, 176:93-109.

[96] Lim DA, Tramontin AD, Trevejo JM, Herrera DG, Garcia-Verdugo JM, Alvarez-Buylla A: Noggin antagonizes BMP signaling to create a niche for adult neurogenesis. *Neuron* 2000, 28(3):713-726.

[97] Mira H, Andreu Z, Suh H, Lie DC, Jessberger S, Consiglio A, San Emeterio J, Hortiguela R, Marques-Torrejon MA, Nakashima K *et al*: Signaling through BMPR-IA regulates quiescence and long-term activity of neural stem cells in the adult hippocampus. *Cell Stem Cell* 2010, 7(1):78-89.

[98] Sato T, Mikawa S, Sato K: BMP2 expression in the adult rat brain. *J Comp Neurol* 2010, 518(22):4513-4530.

[99] Mikawa S, Wang C, Sato K: Bone morphogenetic protein-4 expression in the adult rat brain. *J Comp Neurol* 2006, 499(4):613-625.

[100] Bonaguidi MA, Peng CY, McGuire T, Falciglia G, Gobeske KT, Czeisler C, Kessler JA: Noggin expands neural stem cells in the adult hippocampus. *J Neurosci* 2008, 28(37): 9194-9204.

[101] Fan X, Xu H, Huang Y, Cai W: A combined in situ hybridization and RT-PCR method to detect spatial and temporal patterns of Noggin gene expression in embryonic and postnatal rat hippocampus. *Brain Res Brain Res Protoc* 2004, 13(2):99-105.

[102] Gobeske KT, Das S, Bonaguidi MA, Weiss C, Radulovic J, Disterhoft JF, Kessler JA: BMP signaling mediates effects of exercise on hippocampal neurogenesis and cognition in mice. *PLoS One* 2009, 4(10):e7506.

[103] Lenzlinger PM, Morganti-Kossmann MC, Laurer HL, McIntosh TK: The duality of the inflammatory response to traumatic brain injury. *Mol Neurobiol* 2001, 24(1-3): 169-181.

[104] Annes JP, Munger JS, Rifkin DB: Making sense of latent TGFbeta activation. *J Cell Sci* 2003, 116(Pt 2):217-224.

[105] Jankowsky JL, Patterson PH: The role of cytokines and growth factors in seizures and their sequelae. *Prog Neurobiol* 2001, 63(2):125-149.

[106] McCoy MK, Tansey MG: TNF signaling inhibition in the CNS: implications for normal brain function and neurodegenerative disease. *J Neuroinflammation* 2008, 5:45.

[107] Logan A, Frautschy SA, Gonzalez AM, Sporn MB, Baird A: Enhanced expression of transforming growth factor beta 1 in the rat brain after a localized cerebral injury. *Brain Res* 1992, 587(2):216-225.

[108] Doyle KP, Cekanaviciute E, Mamer LE, Buckwalter MS: TGFbeta signaling in the brain increases with aging and signals to astrocytes and innate immune cells in the weeks after stroke. *J Neuroinflammation* 2010, 7:62.

[109] Stoll G, Schroeter M, Jander S, Siebert H, Wollrath A, Kleinschnitz C, Bruck W: Lesion-associated expression of transforming growth factor-beta-2 in the rat nervous system: evidence for down-regulating the phagocytic activity of microglia and macrophages. *Brain Pathol* 2004, 14(1):51-58.

[110] Dobbertin A, Schmid P, Gelman M, Glowinski J, Mallat M: Neurons promote macrophage proliferation by producing transforming growth factor-beta2. *J Neurosci* 1997, 17(14):5305-5315.

[111] Vincze C, Pal G, Wappler EA, Szabo ER, Nagy ZG, Lovas G, Dobolyi A: Distribution of mRNAs encoding transforming growth factors-beta1, -2, and -3 in the intact rat

brain and after experimentally induced focal ischemia. *J Comp Neurol* 2010, 518(18): 3752-3770.

[112] Villapol S, Yaszemski AK, Logan TT, Sanchez-Lemus E, Saavedra JM, Symes AJ: Candesartan, an Angiotensin II AT(1)-Receptor Blocker and PPAR-gamma Agonist, Reduces Lesion Volume and Improves Motor and Memory Function After Traumatic Brain Injury in Mice. *Neuropsychopharmacology* 2012.

[113] Villapol S, Flanders K, Symes AJ: TGF-β family proteins expression after traumatic brain injury in mice. unpublished.

[114] Lai M, Sirimanne E, Williams CE, Gluckman PD: Sequential patterns of inhibin subunit gene expression following hypoxic-ischemic injury in the rat brain. *Neuroscience* 1996, 70(4):1013-1024.

[115] Cate HS, Sabo JK, Merlo D, Kemper D, Aumann TD, Robinson J, Merson TD, Emery B, Perreau VM, Kilpatrick TJ: Modulation of bone morphogenic protein signalling alters numbers of astrocytes and oligodendroglia in the subventricular zone during cuprizone-induced demyelination. *J Neurochem* 2010, 115(1):11-22.

[116] Wang Y, Moges H, Bharucha Y, Symes A: Smad3 null mice display more rapid wound closure and reduced scar formation after a stab wound to the cerebral cortex. *Exp Neurol* 2007, 203(1):168-184.

[117] Wiessner C, Gehrmann J, Lindholm D, Topper R, Kreutzberg GW, Hossmann KA: Expression of transforming growth factor-beta 1 and interleukin-1 beta mRNA in rat brain following transient forebrain ischemia. *Acta Neuropathol* 1993, 86(5):439-446.

[118] Lehrmann E, Kiefer R, Finsen B, Diemer NH, Zimmer J, Hartung HP: Cytokines in cerebral ischemia: expression of transforming growth factor beta-1 (TGF-beta 1) mRNA in the postischemic adult rat hippocampus. *Exp Neurol* 1995, 131(1):114-123.

[119] Ma M, Ma Y, Yi X, Guo R, Zhu W, Fan X, Xu G, Frey WH, 2nd, Liu X: Intranasal delivery of transforming growth factor-beta1 in mice after stroke reduces infarct volume and increases neurogenesis in the subventricular zone. *BMC Neurosci* 2008, 9:117.

[120] Becker KJ, McCarron RM, Ruetzler C, Laban O, Sternberg E, Flanders KC, Hallenbeck JM: Immunologic tolerance to myelin basic protein decreases stroke size after transient focal cerebral ischemia. *Proc Natl Acad Sci U S A* 1997, 94(20):10873-10878.

[121] Wang X, Yue TL, White RF, Barone FC, Feuerstein GZ: Transforming growth factor-beta 1 exhibits delayed gene expression following focal cerebral ischemia. *Brain Res Bull* 1995, 36(6):607-609.

[122] Vivien D, Bernaudin M, Buisson A, Divoux D, MacKenzie ET, Nouvelot A: Evidence of type I and type II transforming growth factor-beta receptors in central nervous tissues: changes induced by focal cerebral ischemia. *J Neurochem* 1998, 70(6):2296-2304.

[123] Ishibashi S: [Immunomodulation by inducing tolerance to E-selectin and adult neurogenesis after stroke]. *Rinsho Shinkeigaku* 2010, 50(11):882-885.

[124] Martinez G, Carnazza ML, Di Giacomo C, Sorrenti V, Vanella A: Expression of bone morphogenetic protein-6 and transforming growth factor-beta1 in the rat brain after a mild and reversible ischemic damage. *Brain Res* 2001, 894(1):1-11.

[125] Haqqani AS, Nesic M, Preston E, Baumann E, Kelly J, Stanimirovic D: Characterization of vascular protein expression patterns in cerebral ischemia/reperfusion using laser capture microdissection and ICAT-nanoLC-MS/MS. *FASEB J* 2005, 19(13): 1809-1821.

[126] Li JJ, Lu J, Kaur C, Sivakumar V, Wu CY, Ling EA: Effects of hypoxia on expression of transforming growth factor-beta1 and its receptors I and II in the amoeboid microglial cells and murine BV-2 cells. *Neuroscience* 2008, 156(3):662-672.

[127] Huang RQ, Cheng HL, Zhao XD, Dai W, Zhuang Z, Wu Y, Liu Y, Shi JX: Preliminary study on the effect of trauma-induced secondary cellular hypoxia in brain injury. *Neurosci Lett* 2010, 473(1):22-27.

[128] Yin J, Sakamoto K, Zhang H, Ito Z, Imagama S, Kishida S, Natori T, Sawada M, Matsuyama Y, Kadomatsu K: Transforming growth factor-beta1 upregulates keratan sulfate and chondroitin sulfate biosynthesis in microglias after brain injury. *Brain Res* 2009, 1263:10-22.

[129] Acarin L, Gonzalez B, Castellano B: Neuronal, astroglial and microglial cytokine expression after an excitotoxic lesion in the immature rat brain. *Eur J Neurosci* 2000, 12(10):3505-3520.

[130] Mehta PS, Bruccoleri A, Brown HW, Harry GJ: Increase in brain stem cytokine mRNA levels as an early response to chemical-induced myelin edema. *J Neuroimmunol* 1998, 88(1-2):154-164.

[131] Bruccoleri A, Brown H, Harry GJ: Cellular localization and temporal elevation of tumor necrosis factor-alpha, interleukin-1 alpha, and transforming growth factor-beta 1 mRNA in hippocampal injury response induced by trimethyltin. *J Neurochem* 1998, 71(4):1577-1587.

[132] Krieglstein K, Strelau J, Schober A, Sullivan A, Unsicker K: TGF-beta and the regulation of neuron survival and death. *J Physiol Paris* 2002, 96(1-2):25-30.

[133] Boche D, Cunningham C, Gauldie J, Perry VH: Transforming growth factor-beta 1-mediated neuroprotection against excitotoxic injury in vivo. *J Cereb Blood Flow Metab* 2003, 23(10):1174-1182.

[134] Kim SH, Lim DJ, Chung YG, Cho TH, Lim SJ, Kim WJ, Suh JK: Expression of TNF-alpha and TGF-beta 1 in the rat brain after a single high-dose irradiation. *J Korean Med Sci* 2002, 17(2):242-248.

[135] Morgan TE, Nichols NR, Pasinetti GM, Finch CE: TGF-beta 1 mRNA increases in macrophage/microglial cells of the hippocampus in response to deafferentation and kainic acid-induced neurodegeneration. *Exp Neurol* 1993, 120(2):291-301.

[136] Aronica E, van Vliet EA, Mayboroda OA, Troost D, da Silva FH, Gorter JA: Upregulation of metabotropic glutamate receptor subtype mGluR3 and mGluR5 in reactive astrocytes in a rat model of mesial temporal lobe epilepsy. *Eur J Neurosci* 2000, 12(7): 2333-2344.

[137] Jarvela JT, Lopez-Picon FR, Plysjuk A, Ruohonen S, Holopainen IE: Temporal profiles of age-dependent changes in cytokine mRNA expression and glial cell activation after status epilepticus in postnatal rat hippocampus. *J Neuroinflammation* 2011, 8:29.

[138] Schachtrup C, Ryu JK, Helmrick MJ, Vagena E, Galanakis DK, Degen JL, Margolis RU, Akassoglou K: Fibrinogen triggers astrocyte scar formation by promoting the availability of active TGF-beta after vascular damage. *J Neurosci* 2010, 30(17): 5843-5854.

[139] Wyss-Coray T, Mucke L: Inflammation in neurodegenerative disease--a double-edged sword. *Neuron* 2002, 35(3):419-432.

[140] Wyss-Coray T, Feng L, Masliah E, Ruppe MD, Lee HS, Toggas SM, Rockenstein EM, Mucke L: Increased central nervous system production of extracellular matrix components and development of hydrocephalus in transgenic mice overexpressing transforming growth factor-beta 1. *Am J Pathol* 1995, 147(1):53-67.

[141] Fee DB, Sewell DL, Andresen K, Jacques TJ, Piaskowski S, Barger BA, Hart MN, Fabry Z: Traumatic brain injury increases TGF beta RII expression on endothelial cells. *Brain Res* 2004, 1012(1-2):52-59.

[142] Chang CF, Lin SZ, Chiang YH, Morales M, Chou J, Lein P, Chen HL, Hoffer BJ, Wang Y: Intravenous administration of bone morphogenetic protein-7 after ischemia improves motor function in stroke rats. *Stroke* 2003, 34(2):558-564.

[143] Harvey BK, Hoffer BJ, Wang Y: Stroke and TGF-beta proteins: glial cell line-derived neurotrophic factor and bone morphogenetic protein. *Pharmacol Ther* 2005, 105(2): 113-125.

[144] Hampton DW, Asher RA, Kondo T, Steeves JD, Ramer MS, Fawcett JW: A potential role for bone morphogenetic protein signalling in glial cell fate determination following adult central nervous system injury in vivo. *Eur J Neurosci* 2007, 26(11):3024-3035.

[145] Chou J, Harvey BK, Chang CF, Shen H, Morales M, Wang Y: Neuroregenerative effects of BMP7 after stroke in rats. *J Neurol Sci* 2006, 240(1-2):21-29.

[146] Mukerji SS, Katsman EA, Wilber C, Haner NA, Selman WR, Hall AK: Activin is a neuronal survival factor that is rapidly increased after transient cerebral ischemia and hypoxia in mice. *J Cereb Blood Flow Metab* 2007, 27(6):1161-1172.

[147] Zheng F, Adelsberger H, Muller MR, Fritschy JM, Werner S, Alzheimer C: Activin tunes GABAergic neurotransmission and modulates anxiety-like behavior. *Mol Psychiatry* 2009, 14(3):332-346.

[148] Tretter YP, Hertel M, Munz B, ten Bruggencate G, Werner S, Alzheimer C: Induction of activin A is essential for the neuroprotective action of basic fibroblast growth factor in vivo. *Nat Med* 2000, 6(7):812-815.

[149] Christensen KV, Leffers H, Watson WP, Sanchez C, Kallunki P, Egebjerg J: Levetiracetam attenuates hippocampal expression of synaptic plasticity-related immediate early and late response genes in amygdala-kindled rats. *BMC Neurosci* 2010, 11:9.

[150] Parent JM, Lowenstein DH: Seizure-induced neurogenesis: are more new neurons good for an adult brain? *Prog Brain Res* 2002, 135:121-131.

[151] Thored P, Heldmann U, Gomes-Leal W, Gisler R, Darsalia V, Taneera J, Nygren JM, Jacobsen SE, Ekdahl CT, Kokaia Z *et al*: Long-term accumulation of microglia with proneurogenic phenotype concomitant with persistent neurogenesis in adult subventricular zone after stroke. *Glia* 2009, 57(8):835-849.

[152] Arvidsson A, Collin T, Kirik D, Kokaia Z, Lindvall O: Neuronal replacement from endogenous precursors in the adult brain after stroke. *Nat Med* 2002, 8(9):963-970.

[153] Urrea C, Castellanos DA, Sagen J, Tsoulfas P, Bramlett HM, Dietrich WD: Widespread cellular proliferation and focal neurogenesis after traumatic brain injury in the rat. *Restor Neurol Neurosci* 2007, 25(1):65-76.

[154] Zhang RL, Zhang ZG, Chopp M: Neurogenesis in the adult ischemic brain: generation, migration, survival, and restorative therapy. *Neuroscientist* 2005, 11(5):408-416.

[155] Massouh M, Saghatelyan A: De-routing neuronal precursors in the adult brain to sites of injury: role of the vasculature. *Neuropharmacology* 2010, 58(6):877-883.

[156] Ekdahl CT: Microglial activation - tuning and pruning adult neurogenesis. *Front Pharmacol* 2012, 3:41.

[157] Monje ML, Toda H, Palmer TD: Inflammatory blockade restores adult hippocampal neurogenesis. *Science* 2003, 302(5651):1760-1765.

[158] Aarum J, Sandberg K, Haeberlein SL, Persson MA: Migration and differentiation of neural precursor cells can be directed by microglia. *Proc Natl Acad Sci U S A* 2003, 100(26):15983-15988.

[159] Ziv Y, Ron N, Butovsky O, Landa G, Sudai E, Greenberg N, Cohen H, Kipnis J, Schwartz M: Immune cells contribute to the maintenance of neurogenesis and spatial learning abilities in adulthood. *Nat Neurosci* 2006, 9(2):268-275.

[160] Cacci E, Ajmone-Cat MA, Anelli T, Biagioni S, Minghetti L: In vitro neuronal and glial differentiation from embryonic or adult neural precursor cells are differently affected by chronic or acute activation of microglia. *Glia* 2008, 56(4):412-425.

[161] Nakanishi M, Niidome T, Matsuda S, Akaike A, Kihara T, Sugimoto H: Microglia-derived interleukin-6 and leukaemia inhibitory factor promote astrocytic differentiation of neural stem/progenitor cells. *Eur J Neurosci* 2007, 25(3):649-658.

[162] Makwana M, Jones LL, Cuthill D, Heuer H, Bohatschek M, Hristova M, Friedrichsen S, Ormsby I, Bueringer D, Koppius A *et al*: Endogenous transforming growth factor beta 1 suppresses inflammation and promotes survival in adult CNS. *J Neurosci* 2007, 27(42):11201-11213.

[163] Battista D, Ferrari CC, Gage FH, Pitossi FJ: Neurogenic niche modulation by activated microglia: transforming growth factor beta increases neurogenesis in the adult dentate gyrus. *Eur J Neurosci* 2006, 23(1):83-93.

[164] Ma YP, Ma MM, Ge S, Guo RB, Zhang HJ, Frey WH, 2nd, Xu GL, Liu XF: Intranasally delivered TGF-beta1 enters brain and regulates gene expressions of its receptors in rats. *Brain Res Bull* 2007, 74(4):271-277.

[165] Mathieu P, Piantanida AP, Pitossi F: Chronic expression of transforming growth factor-beta enhances adult neurogenesis. *Neuroimmunomodulation* 2010, 17(3):200-201.

[166] Graciarena M, Depino AM, Pitossi FJ: Prenatal inflammation impairs adult neurogenesis and memory related behavior through persistent hippocampal TGFbeta1 downregulation. *Brain Behav Immun* 2010, 24(8):1301-1309.

[167] Samanta J, Alden T, Gobeske K, Kan L, Kessler JA: Noggin protects against ischemic brain injury in rodents. *Stroke* 2010, 41(2):357-362.

[168] Setoguchi T, Nakashima K, Takizawa T, Yanagisawa M, Ochiai W, Okabe M, Yone K, Komiya S, Taga T: Treatment of spinal cord injury by transplantation of fetal neural precursor cells engineered to express BMP inhibitor. *Exp Neurol* 2004, 189(1):33-44.

[169] Jablonska B, Aguirre A, Raymond M, Szabo G, Kitabatake Y, Sailor KA, Ming GL, Song H, Gallo V: Chordin-induced lineage plasticity of adult SVZ neuroblasts after demyelination. *Nat Neurosci* 2010, 13(5):541-550.

[170] Dow AL, Russell DS, Duman RS: Regulation of activin mRNA and Smad2 phosphorylation by antidepressant treatment in the rat brain: effects in behavioral models. *J Neurosci* 2005, 25(20):4908-4916.

[171] Caraci F, Battaglia G, Bruno V, Bosco P, Carbonaro V, Giuffrida ML, Drago F, Sortino MA, Nicoletti F, Copani A: TGF-beta1 pathway as a new target for neuroprotection in Alzheimer's disease. *CNS Neurosci Ther* 2011, 17(4):237-249.

[172] Li LY, Li JL, Zhang HM, Yang WM, Wang K, Fang Y, Wang Y: TGFbeta1 Treatment Reduces Hippocampal Damage, Spontaneous Recurrent Seizures, and Learning Memory Deficits in Pilocarpine-Treated Rats. *J Mol Neurosci* 2012.

[173] El Khoury J, Luster AD: Mechanisms of microglia accumulation in Alzheimer's disease: therapeutic implications. *Trends Pharmacol Sci* 2008, 29(12):626-632.

[174] Florio P, Gazzolo D, Luisi S, Petraglia F: Activin A in brain injury. *Adv Clin Chem* 2007, 43:117-130.

[175] Luisi S, Florio P, Reis FM, Petraglia F: Expression and secretion of activin A: possible physiological and clinical implications. *Eur J Endocrinol* 2001, 145(3):225-236.

[176] Goings GE, Sahni V, Szele FG: Migration patterns of subventricular zone cells in adult mice change after cerebral cortex injury. *Brain Res* 2004, 996(2):213-226.

[177] Sun J, Zhou W, Sha B, Yang Y: Ischemia induced neural stem cell proliferation and differentiation in neonatal rat involved vascular endothelial growth factor and transforming growth factor-beta pathways. *Brain Dev* 2010, 32(3):191-200.

[178] Cao QL, Zhang YP, Howard RM, Walters WM, Tsoulfas P, Whittemore SR: Pluripotent stem cells engrafted into the normal or lesioned adult rat spinal cord are restricted to a glial lineage. *Exp Neurol* 2001, 167(1):48-58.

[179] Wang Y, Cheng X, He Q, Zheng Y, Kim DH, Whittemore SR, Cao QL: Astrocytes from the contused spinal cord inhibit oligodendrocyte differentiation of adult oligodendrocyte precursor cells by increasing the expression of bone morphogenetic proteins. *J Neurosci* 2011, 31(16):6053-6058.

[180] Chang CF, Morales M, Chou J, Chen HL, Hoffer B, Wang Y: Bone morphogenetic proteins are involved in fetal kidney tissue transplantation-induced neuroprotection in stroke rats. *Neuropharmacology* 2002, 43(3):418-426.

[181] Voumvourakis KI, Antonelou R, Kitsos DK, Stamboulis E, Tsiodras S: TGF-beta/BMPs: crucial crossroad in neural autoimmune disorders. *Neurochem Int* 2011, 59(5): 542-550.

[182] Loane DJ, Faden AI: Neuroprotection for traumatic brain injury: translational challenges and emerging therapeutic strategies. *Trends Pharmacol Sci* 2010, 31(12):596-604.

[183] Marklund N, Hillered L: Animal modelling of traumatic brain injury in preclinical drug development: where do we go from here? *Br J Pharmacol* 2011, 164(4):1207-1229.

[184] Wang Y, Lin SZ, Chiou AL, Williams LR, Hoffer BJ: Glial cell line-derived neurotrophic factor protects against ischemia-induced injury in the cerebral cortex. *J Neurosci* 1997, 17(11):4341-4348.

[185] Yagi T, Jikihara I, Fukumura M, Watabe K, Ohashi T, Eto Y, Hara M, Maeda M: Rescue of ischemic brain injury by adenoviral gene transfer of glial cell line-derived neurotrophic factor after transient global ischemia in gerbils. *Brain Res* 2000, 885(2): 273-282.

[186] Seidenfaden R, Desoeuvre A, Bosio A, Virard I, Cremer H: Glial conversion of SVZ-derived committed neuronal precursors after ectopic grafting into the adult brain. *Mol Cell Neurosci* 2006, 32(1-2):187-198.

[187] Joannides AJ, Webber DJ, Raineteau O, Kelly C, Irvine KA, Watts C, Rosser AE, Kemp PJ, Blakemore WF, Compston A *et al*: Environmental signals regulate lineage

choice and temporal maturation of neural stem cells from human embryonic stem cells. *Brain* 2007, 130(Pt 5):1263-1275.

[188] Teng FY, Hor CH, Tang BL: Emerging cues mediating astroglia lineage restriction of progenitor cells in the injured/diseased adult CNS. *Differentiation* 2009, 77(2):121-127.

[189] Gomes WA, Mehler MF, Kessler JA: Transgenic overexpression of BMP4 increases astroglial and decreases oligodendroglial lineage commitment. *Dev Biol* 2003, 255(1): 164-177.

[190] Bain JM, Ziegler A, Yang Z, Levison SW, Sen E: TGFbeta1 stimulates the over-production of white matter astrocytes from precursors of the "brain marrow" in a rodent model of neonatal encephalopathy. *PLoS One* 2010, 5(3):e9567.

[191] Loane DJ, Byrnes KR: Role of microglia in neurotrauma. *Neurotherapeutics* 2010, 7(4): 366-377.

[192] Nishiyama A: Glial progenitor cells in normal and pathological states. *Keio J Med* 1998, 47(4):205-208.

Chapter 3

The Role of Smad Proteins for Development, Differentiation and Dedifferentiation of Neurons

Uwe Ueberham and Thomas Arendt

Additional information is available at the end of the chapter

1. Introduction

The development of the nervous system, neuralization of ectodermal cells, specification of cell types as well as generation of neurological diseases are closely linked to Smad proteins, which play a central role by integrating TGFβ and BMP signalling with other essential pathways. Due to new findings on Smad activity in neurons and the nervous system, which comprises new roles for brain plasticity and functions, independent of the canonical signalling pathways, we reconsider their relevance for neuronal differentiation and dedifferentiation processes and as therapeutic targets for treatment of neurological diseases. In this chapter we develop a view at Smad molecules, which attributes them a basic significance and allow proving their specific contextual molecular, cellular and tissue relationships. In order to facilitate the understanding of the complex Smad network in the nervous system an overview of the canonical Smad signalling pathway is briefly summarized in the following paragraph.

Smads are phylogenetic old proteins, which are mediating intracellular signalling of the large group of solube TGFβ ligands (Figure 1), containing transforming growth factor βs (TGFβs), bone morphogentic proteins (BMPs), growth and differentiation factors (GDFs), Müllerian inhibitory factors (MISs), activins and inhibins [4]. Ligand binding to activated heteromeric receptor complexes, recruited from seven type I and five type II serine/threonine receptors, results in the specific phosphorylation of receptor-associated Smads (R-Smads) at two C-terminal serine residues.

Activin, nodal and TGFβ activate R-Smad2 and 3, while BMP acts by R-Smad1,5 and 8 phosphorylation. In the cytoplasm non-phosphorylated R-Smads are sequestrated by interacting with specific retention proteins e.g. SARA (Smad anchor for receptor activation) [5], endofin [8], tubulin [3], actin, myosin [11] or filamin [12]. Inhibitory Smad(I-Smad)6 and 7 negatively regulate R-Smad signalling by competing for binding to activated type I receptor and inhibiting R-Smad phosphorylation. I-Smads can also prevent R-Smad complexing to the co-operating Smad(Co-Smad)4, which is required for the nuclear translocation of activated R-Smads to subsequently control Smad sensitive promoter activity. Moreover, I-Smads support recruitment of HECT-type E3-ubiquitin ligases Smurf1/2, which allow type I receptor ubiquitination and its degradation. Members of HECT-type and RING-type E3 ubiquitin ligases have also been implicated in Smad degradation [13]. Regulating Smad activity allows the control of highly complex developmental networks, e.g. the patterning of ventro-lateral mesoderm, the decisive development of epidermal/neural cell lineages including the induction and establishment of neural plate border, the dorso-ventral patterning of the neural tube, or the migration of neural crest cells [18-21].

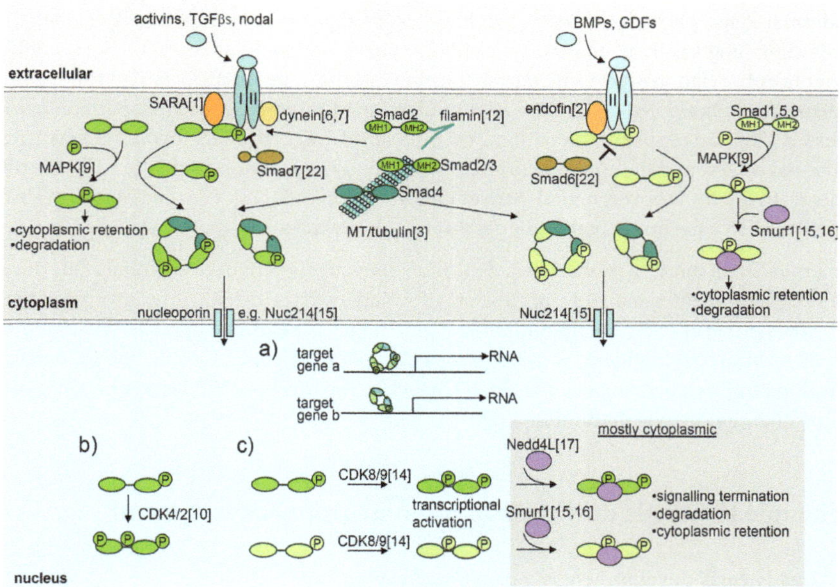

Figure 1. Synopsis of canonical Smad signalling. The upper panel shows the binding of ligands belonging to the TGFβ superfamily to their serine/threonine kinase receptors types I and II, leading to intracellular activation of R-Smads by receptor type I induced phosphorylation of the C-terminal Smad motif SSXS. The left and right receptor complexes represent the TGFβ/activin/nodal linked Smad2/3 signalling and the BMP/GDF linked Smad1/5/8 signalling, respectiviely. The middle panel also displays a set of relevant binding partners of Smad proteins and shows the generation of heterotrimer or heterodimer Smad complexes consisting of C-terminally phosphorylated R-Smads and Co-Smad4, which are transported into the nucleus to excert their transcriptional activity by binding to susceptible promoter sequences (a). In (b) and (c) examples of the agonist-induced Smad linker phosphorylation mediated by cyclin-dependent kinases are shown, which increases Smad transcriptional activity prior to signal termination and Smad degradation [14, 17]. In contrast, the MAPK triggered linker phosphorylation of Smads in cytoplasm diminishes the receptor type I responsible Smad phosphorylation and favours the cytoplasmic retention and degradation of Smad. More information is provided in the main text.*Note*: Numbers in square brackets indicate relevant references included in the reference list provided at the chapters end.*Abbreviations*: CDK, cyclin-dependent kinase; dynein, dynein light chain km23-1 or km23-2; MAPK, mitogen activated protein kinase; MT, microtubuli; Nedd4L, neuronal precursor cell expressed developmentally down-regulated 4-like ubiquitin ligase; Nuc214, nucleoporin 214; SARA, Smad achor for receptor activation; Smurf1, HECT-domain ubiquitin ligase Smurf1.

In R-Smads a linker region, located between the highly conserved N-terminal MH1- and the C-terminal MH2 region (MH represents Mad homology), is rich in potential serine/threonine phosphorylation sites. Several kinases (e.g. MAPK, GSK, CDKs, CamKII, SGK1) can phosphorylate the linker region and determine cellular distribution or protein stability of Smads [14,23-26]. Linker phosphorylation by mitogen-activated protein kinases (MAPKs) restricts Smad1 activity by enabling Smurf1 binding, causing polyubiquitination and inhibiting interaction of Smad1 with nuclear transclocation factor Nup214, thus leading to Smad1 degradation or cytoplasmic retention [15].

A similar mechanism acts on Smad2 and 3, where ubiquitination is controlled by ubiquitin ligase Nedd4L [17]. A sustained MAPK activation, as reported from dissociated embryonic ectodermal cells, phosphorylates Smad linker and interrupt a continuing BMP mediated Smad1 signalling finally resulting in neuralisation of dissociated Xenopus [27]. Remarably, if linker phosphorylation is performed by extracellular signal regulated kinase (Erk) at nuclearly localized phosphorylated Smad, the duration of Smad targeted gene transcription can be increased [28]. Linker phosphorylation by CDK8 and CDK9 promotes both, the Smad transcriptional action, and the cooperation with YAP, an effector of the Hippo organ size control pathway, to finally suppress neural differentiation of stem cells [14]. The data demonstrate the particular role of the linker region for distinct Smad functions.

Numerous Smad binding proteins (e.g. Ski, SnoN) effectively influence essential steps during neural development mostly by repression of Smad activity [29-33]. The group of Smad interacting proteins (SIP), containing several zinc finger proteins, complex to Smad and can directly or indirectly regulate its transcription efficiency [34]. For example, the induction of neuroectoderm is dependent on SIP1 [35-37], which is also involved in the myelination process and the oligodendrocyte maturation [38].

2. The role of Smads during neural/non-neuronal development

2.1. Already early development requires Smad expression

During early ontogenesis, development and aging as well as prior to individual cell death Smad proteins differentially affect cellular function, depending on time and local partners. Already at very early stages of postnatal rat development Smads1-7 were detectable in the ovary [39]. At all stages of follicular development (e.g. in primordial, primary and secondary follicles) Smad proteins are present in oocytes as well as in granulosa cells and theca cells, though with different concentrations [39-41]. While Smad3,6 and 8 content did not change, the expression of Smad1,2,4,5,6 and 7 seems to be regulated in ovary [39]. In mice oocytes a clear and persistent nuclear localization of phosphorylated Smad1,5,9 and Smad2,3 demonstrates activated activin/GDF9/nodal/TGFβ and BMP/MIS pathways, respectively, and confirms oocytes as a major target for Smad signalling pathways [42]. Smad proteins play also important roles already during maturation of human oocytes [43]. In unfertilized oocytes, Smad2 and 3 and TGFβ receptors I and II are present [44]. After fertilization at the 4-cell and 8-cell stages Smad2 and 3 are also present, while neither of the TGFβ receptors is detectable. Later on in the blastocyte stage Smad2 and 3 kept present and TGFβ receptor I again appears [44]. Human granulosa cells express Smad1-7 and 9, but Smad2,3, and 4 with the highest expression levels [45]. A mutual interaction between oocytes and granulosa cells is necessary for normal folliculogenesis. However, if Smad4 is deleted in granulosa cells infertility results, while deletion of Smad4 in oocytes only marginally effects the primordial follicle stage [46]. However, Smad2 reduction in zebrafish oocytes completely blocks activin A-induced oocyte maturation and a Smad2 knockdown decreases basal and hCG-induced oocyte maturation demonstrating a key role of Smads during oocyte maturation [47].

2.2. Gastrulation and neurulation

2.2.1. Suppression of Smad signalling specifies neuroectoderm generation

Initially, the ectoderm cells in Xenopus are pluripotent until gastrulation [48]. Early gastrulation steps are characterized by the formation of mesenchymal cells and the induction of mesoderm in the marginal-zone by an epithelial-to-mesenchymal transition (EMT) process, which involves activation of Smad2,3,4 signalling by TGFβ/nodal ligands after binding to corresponding receptors [49-53].

Mesoderm induction requires a subtle coordination of the canonical TGFβ/nodal signalling, with Smad4 as a key player. However, initially it was shown, that a simple ectopic Smad4 expression in the Xenopus animal cap was inefficient to induce mesoderm [54], due to its binding to ectodermin, a RING-type ubiquitin ligase, which is highly expressed in the animal cap [53]. Ectodermin limits Smad4 function via antagonizing nuclear accumulation of Smad4 and supporting Smad4 degradation by ubiquitin-proteosome pathway [53]. By this, ectodermin ensures that ectoderm cells do only develop to a mesodermal lineage, but also supports neural differentiation of ectoderm towards neuroectodermal fates by interfering with BMP signalling via limiting Smad4 function [53]. However, the stable presence of soluble BMP which prevents the execution of an intrinsic program of ectodermal cells to form neural tissue can also be undermined by the release of BMP antagonists as noggin, chordin, follistatin or cerberus, which however, allows creation and development of neural cells. This interrelation is basically reflected in the 'default model' of neural induction [55,56]. Confirming this model it was shown, that the simultaneous depletion of BMP2, BMP4 and BMP7 induces massive brain formation [57]. Accordingly, during early gastrulation-stage of chick embryo Smad1,5,8 signalling is undetectable [21] but is activated at neurula stage. So, phosphorylated Smad1 becomes detectable only at late gastrulation stages in the posterior territory of the embryo [21].

The default model has been further modified due to experiments showing that inhibition of BMP/Smad1 signalling, e.g. by Smad6, was insufficient to induce neural markers efficiently [58], while the additional suppression of Smad2 was sufficient [59]. Moreover, stimulation of Smad2 signalling blocks neural induction even at gastrula stages and indicate prospective neural cells to further undergo mesodermal and non-neural fates [59]. These data are supported by experiments in sea urchin embryos showing that Smad2 and 3 suppress neural differentiation in the oral ectoderm [60].

Remarkably, conversely, it has also been suggested from very early studies on Smad2$^{+/-}$; Smad3$^{-/-}$ mutants in zebrafish showing anterior truncations [49], that Smad2 and Smad3, which are mainly effectors of TGFβ/nodal pathways, are also positively involved in neural development [61]. Dominant negative Smad3 mutants inhibit the expression of early neural markers sox2 and sox3 at the onset of gastrulation and lead to reduction of anterior and posterior neuroectodermal markers otx2 and hoxb1b, respectively, during late gastrulation. Accordingly, elevated Smad2 and Smad3 activities increased sox2 and sox3 expression, probably at least partly due to its positive impact on chordin expression, which is a BMP antagonist [61]. In mouse embryo BMP signalling also inhibits premature neural differentiation, but in contrast to Xenopus [62] and chick [63,64] FGF signalling seems additionally required to induce neural differentiation [65].

In summary, the data indicate that simultaneous suppression of both Smad1,5,8 and Smad2,3 pathways, e.g. suppression of mesoderm- and ectoderm-inducing Smad signals, respectively, are required for neural induction. In principle, the `dual Smad inhibition` method is adopted for induction of efficient neuralization of human (-induced) pluripotent stem cells (hiPSCs, hPSCs) [66,67].

2.2.2. *Neural tube closure*

To establish a precise borderline between neuroectoderm (containing low BMP2/4 levels) and non-neuroectoderm (containing high BMP2/4 levels) regions during early neurulation, specific strategies are required and examined in urchin embryos, where Fez, a zinc finger protein, drops down the BMP controlled pSmad1,5,8 levels [68]. It is probable that Fez acts as a transcriptional repressor of Smad or interferes with genes attenuating intracellular BMP signalling e.g. SIP1, Smurf1, Ski or SnoN.

Once the neuroectoderm forming is initiated a flat neural plate rolls up, the process of neural plate folding proceeds and is finished by neural tube closure [69]. The closure of neural tube is a complex process involving hinge points (HP), representing specialized neural plate cells. The cells of ventral midline/median hinge point (MHP) as well as both dorso-lateral hinge points (DLHPs) are affected by dynamic BMP signalling [70-73]. Folding of neural plate is connected with a two-dimentionally spatiotemporal gradient of phosphorylated Smad1,5,8 (pSmad1,5,8) [71,73]. While initially a mosaic labelling of pSmad1,5,8 was observed at the apical surface of the presumptive neuroectoderm later two intersecting Smad gradients were exerted: a lateromedial gradient with the lowest pSmad1,5,8 expression at the MHP and a second gradient along the apicobasal axis of the presumptive midbrain plate with mosaic expression in apical nuclei [71]. Some of the apical pSmad1,5,8 positive cells proliferate and thus support the neural fold elevation [71]. Disturbances of the phosphorylation state of Smad1,5,8 alter midbrain shape by multiple hinge-like invaginations but do not affect the ventral cell-fate specification [71]. However, the extent of Smad1,5,8 phosphorylation seems to control MHP formation during neurulation in vertebrates. The correct MHF formation is obviously directly linked to the pSmad1,5,8 controlled regulation of apicobasal polarity of neural plates cells. After phosphorylation, Smad1,5,8 interact with the PAR3-PAR6-aPKC complex and stabilizes linked tight junctions, while inversely low pSmad1,5,8 phosphorylation supports re-arrangement of neural plate cells, a prerequisite for MHP formation and neural fold elevation [72].

2.2.3. *Patterning and developing of the spinal cord*

After closure, the neural tube starts to develop the spinal cord pattern along its dorso-ventral axis which is essentially established by the expression of Wnt and BMPs, the main roof plate morphogens, and sonic hedgehog (SHH) and TGFβs, the morphogens released from the floor plate [74-76]. On the basis of provided intricated morphogenic gradients functionally distinct neurons are generated.

Both roof plate derived BMP6 and BMP7 are evoking Smad1,5,8 phosphorylation and subsequent induction of distinct dorsal interneurons (dI) via BMP receptor I activation [77-79]. While the BMP7/pSmad1,5 activated induction of dI1, dI3 and dI5 is independent of the patterned expression of progenitor proteins, e.g. Pax7, Gsh1/2 or Olig3, a Smad regulated expression of specific proneural proteins, e.g. cAth, and cAscl1, is required [79]. The patterning of dorsal progenitor proteins could be associated with other BMPs, e.g. BMP4 [80]. Smad1 and Smad5 activity seems to be important for the maintenance of neural cells as committed progenitors, because the loss of Smad1,5 reduced the total number of newly generated neurons and forces cell cycle exit and premature neurogenesis of neural progenitors [79]. The inhibitory Smad6 also promotes the neuronal differentiation in the spinal cord by interfering with Wnt-signalling [81]. Hazen and colleagues demonstrated, that the inhibitory Smad6 and Smad7 function to restrict the action of roof plate released BMPs to distinct dorsal interneurons and participate in the determination of dI4-dI6 spinal neuron number [82].

However, the subsequent orientation of spinal neurons is also controlled by BMP7 but not via activation of Smad signalling instead using phosphoinosite-3-kinase (PI3K) activation by the BMP receptor type II [77]. Nevertheless, Smad6 most potently allows blocking dI1 axon outgrowth [82].

While Smad3 was also expressed in the developing spinal cord, Smad2 was not detected [83]. Contrasting to Smad1,5,8, the expression of Smad3 in the developing spinal cord depends on progenitor proteins, e.g. Nkx6.1, Olig2, Nkx2.2, which directs the Smad3 expression mainly to discrete ventral progenitor domains [83]. Smad3 activity in turn reduces expression of progenitor proteins and promotes activation of neuronal differentiation, e.g. by supporting cell cycle exit via activating of $p27^{Kip1}$ expression [83]. The Smad3 expression is sufficient to promote differentiation of ventral and various dorsal interneurons, while differentiation of motor neurons is impaired. Therefore Smad3 expression is excluded in the prospective motor neuron progenitor cells [83].

2.2.4. *Induction of neural crest (NC)*

Multipotent embryonic cells of the dorsal region of the neural tube, an area existing immediately before forming the neural plate border (NPB), are the origin of neural crest cells (NC) that migrate to initiate a panel of diverse derivatives including various non-neural but also neural cells e.g. sensory neurons of the peripheral nervous system. The combination of several signalling pathways is required [84] for a timely and locally well tuned progression. Besides Wnt signalling a major role in NC induction plays canonical BMP signalling [85-90] combined with FGF signalling [21,91]. The inductive step of NPB development during gastrulation requires a concerted action of activated Wnt signals and inhibition of BMP signalling represented by low Smad1,5,8 activity. Later, when neurulation proceeds and NC develops from NPB, activated Wnt signals cooperate with a robust Smad1,5,8 activation in NPB. While during the inductive step of NC gastrulation FGF downregulates Smad1,5,8 activity by triggering MAPK, the catalysed phosphorylation of Smad1,5,8 linker region is nearly completely absent in NPB during neurulation. In consequence, a strongly elevated Smad1,5,8 signalling is observed suggesting a ´two step model of NC development´ with respect to activated Smad1,5,8 signalling [21].

2.3. Peripheral nervous system (PNS)

The further outcome of NC cells including the generation of the PNS also strongly depends on Smad signalling. Interestingly, Smad expression regulates both the formation of neurons of PNS as well as early stages of peripheral glial development.

Precursors that emigrate from the neural crest to the bowel generates the enteric nervous system (ENS) belonging to PNS. If fetal enteral neural crest-derived cells (ENCDC) of gut are exposed to BMP2 or BMP4 phosphorylated Smad1 translocates to the nucleus and the cells develop processes, indicating an essential role of Smad phosphorylation for neuron induction in the gut [92]. However, Smad phosphorylation alone is not sufficient to direct development of ENCDC towards ENS neurons or glial cells but requires further factors e.g. glial growth factor 2 (GGF2) [93]. Moreover, besides generation, also maturation of enteric neurons (as well as regulation of gliogenesis) during postnatal development is Smad-dependent. This function was identified because mice lacking in the homeodomain interacting protein kinase 2 (HIPK2), which can interact with Smad1, Smad2 and Smad3 [94] and therefore control transcription of subsequent Smad-dependent promoters, are characterized by a progressive loss of enteric neurons and an arrest in synaptic maturation postnatally. Additionally, in the HIPK2$^{-/-}$ mice the remaining enteric neurons exhibit an increased number of cells with nuclear Smad1,5,8 phosphorylation [95]. Interestingly, both in the enteric nervous system and in the midbrain [96], HIPK2 reduction severely reduces survival of dopaminergic neurons through interference with Smad signalling pathways, regulated by BMP2/4 or TGFβ, respectively. Whether altered Smad signalling, affected by HIPK2, is also responsible for Parkinson´s disease and would allow to develop a therapeutic intervention has to be investigated in the future.

Recent data demonstrate, that Smad1 signalling by BMP2 induction is implicated in differentiation of primary enteric neurons to catecholaminergic (TH expression) but not to cholinergic (ChAT expression) neuronal subtypes [97].

Peripheral glia precursors derived from neural-crest and exhibiting characteristic expression of immature glia markers e.g. nestin, are critically influenced by BMP2/Smad signalling. Using Smad1 activation, neural-crest precursor cells, that begin to develop along glial pathway are kept in an undifferentiated immature multipotent state, thus allowing migration to their postmigratory locations [98] where they later acquire myelinating properties. Smad-linked activation of GFAP promoter is part of this process [99]. Generally, oligodendroglial differentiation of precursor cells is actively suppressed by BMPs concomitant with the stimulation of astrocytic differentiation [100]. Accordingly, BMP4-activation directs progenitor cells in vivo to commit to the astrocytic rather than the oligodendroglial lineage [101].

3. Specific cell types and the role of Smad expression for their induction and maintenance

3.1. Cell type decision, maturation and differentiation

Both generation and differentiation of neurons in the brain (CNS) comprises several different and complex principles. The initial proliferation of neural precursor cells is followed by the decision to specify neuronal or glial outcome. Afterwards, the primary neurogenesis of neuronal progenitors involves migration, settlement and stopping proliferation by cell cycle exit to enter a terminal differentiation pathway. Many of these basic biological routes as well as further differentiation steps, e.g. dendritic and axonal growth and orientating, synapse formation and myelination depend on Smad proteins. The parallel occurrence of long term and acute Smad-dependent processes require a distinct contextual organisation. For example, in the developing brain an important neural stem cell is provided by radial glia cells which can generate both glial cells and neurons. While TGFβ promoted differentiation of radial glia into astrocytes is mainly regulated by activation of MAPK signalling, neurogenesis is controlled by the interplay of Smad2,3 activity and PI3K activity [102].

3.1.1. Glial cells

Radial glial cells can function as neuronal precursors and also control migration of neurons during cerebral cortex development [103]. Developing neurons are also actively implicated in the radial glial cell fate commitment [104]. Using TGFβ release, neurons can activate Smad signalling in radial glia cells and support their transformation to astrocytes [105] and also induces astrocytic differentiation and GFAP expression [106-109].

Moreover, endothelial cells also promote astrocytic differentiation by BMP-induced Smad signalling, but inhibit oligodendrocyte differentiation of postnatal cortical progenitors [110], and therefore participate in the sequential order of the two macroglial cell gliogenesis. The function of BMP/Smad signalling to drive precursors to astrocytic fate seems a common feature [111,112] which is also involved in CNS injury processes where oligodendrocyte precursors are driven towards type II astrocytes [113]. Accordingly, inhibition of BMP induced nuclear translocation of phospho-Smad1 by FGF2 activated MAPK activity is linked to Smad4 dissociation from Olig2 promoter and results in upregulation of oligodendrogenesis [114]. The very importance of a spatially and temporally regulated BMP induced Smad activation for the fate of neurogenic precursor cells was shown in chick spinal cord. At embryonic day 5, in neuroepithelial progenitors, astrocyte marker expression was inhibited and at embryonic day 6 it was promoted initiating a gliogenic period [115].

3.1.2. Neurons

The commitment of cell fates in the nervous system is strongly dependent on Smad2,3 signalling cascade. However, there have been contradictory results on the role of Smad3 for neuronal precursor proliferation and their differentiation, indicating a complex Smad signalling network dependent on local, temporal and contextual characteristics.

Some reports show, that TGFβ, which activates Smad3 signalling, diminishes neurogenesis in hippocampus after its chronical increase [116], and in SVZ and DG after intracerebroventricular TGFβ1 infusion [117] and promotes neuronal differentiation from hippocampal and cortical progenitors [118]. An clear inhibitory function of Smad3 on neural precursor proliferation was shown in the developing spinal cord [119], where Smad3 also promotes differentiation and influences the fate of selected neurons. The antiproliferative role of Smad3 and Smad4 plays a role during early-postnatal differentiation of cerebellar neurons into postmitotic neurons, where TGFβ stimulation induces nuclear translocation of phosphorylated Smads and induction of cyclin-dependent kinase inhibitors p21, p27 and markers of neuronal maturity [120].

However, other reports show that TGFβ increased neurogenesis in DG after adrenalectomy [121] or in SVZ after stroke [122].

To clarify the relevance of Smad3 for adult neurogenesis Smad3 null mice were studied [123,124]. These mice show decreased neurogenesis in the DG and the SVZ and exhibit a thinner and more disorganized rostral migratory stream (RMS) of neuronal precursor cells (NPC). Using RMS NPCs migrate from SVZ to reach the olfactory bulb, where they differentiate into granular and periglomerular neurons. Though a decreased number of proliferating cells demonstrates the requirement of Smad3 for maintaining a proper cell division rate in SVZ, the neuronal fate is not altered by Smad3 deficiency [123].

For differentiation of mesencephalic progenitors into dopaminergic (DA) neurons a concerted interaction of Smad2,3 signalling and p38 MAPK-pathways by TGFβ receptor stimulation is necessary. Accordingly, treatment of ventral mesencephalic neural progenitors with TGFβ increased the number of tyrosine-hydroxylase (TH)-positive cells [125]. Though not required for the neurogenesis, the survival of midbrain dopaminergic neurons depends on function of the homeodomain interacting protein kinase 2 (HIPK2), which interacts with R-Smads to activate TGFβ responsive genes [96]. Loss of HIPK2 increases apoptosis in DA neurons during development. Nevertheless, apoptosis of specific neural progenitors during neural differentiation also involves Smad phosphorylation as shown for Smad1,5,8 [126,127].

In vitro, treatment of ventral mesencephalic cells with BMP5,6 and 7 also significantly increased the number of TH-positive neurons via Smad phosphorylation and nuclear translocation [128], while the neurotrophin growth/differentiation factor 5 (GDF5) induced Smad pathway promotes neuronal but not dopaminergic differentiation [129]. Remarkably, the in vitro generation of functional dopaminergic substantia nigra neurons for transplantation requires a protocol which uses the temporarily and contextually distinct roles of Smad proteins: Firstly, the dual inhibition of Smad signalling in embryonic stem cells is required to allow induction of floor plate cell state which then passes over to midbrain floor plate cell state.

Secondly, an activation of Smad signalling using TGFβ pathway is necessary to finally obtain dopaminergic neurons suitable to threat Parkinson´s like symptoms [130].

In the developing cerebellum, Smad1 is expressed in the external germinal layer and Smad5 is synthesized in newly differentiated granule neurons. In the granule precursor cells, Smad5 overexpression is sufficient to initiate differentiation [131]. In mice lacking Smad4, a decreased number of cerebellar Purkinje cells and parvalbumin-positive interneurons [132] is found while no alterations of proliferation of neuronal precursor cells were detectable. Loss of Smad4 also reduces differentiation of noradrenergic neurons [133].

Basal forebrain cholinergic neurons are essentially involved in the organisation of cortical brain structures, learning and memory. Smad1-5 are expressed in basal forebrain from embryonic day 14 to the adult age [134]. An intact canonical TGFβ/Smad2,3 cascade is important for the function of cholinergic neurons. Smad signalling mediates rapid inhibition of calcium influx in cholinergic basal forebrain neurons [135]. The sleep/wake circadian rhythm controlled by cholinergic neurons of the pedunculopontine nucleus (PPT) is also dependent on phosphorylation levels of Smad2 and Smad3. Overactivation of Smad2,3 signalling resulting in increased nuclear translocation is linked to sleep/wake circadian rhythm amplitude deficits [136]. BMP9 driven Smad1,5 phosphorylation and their formation of complexes with Smad4 are involved in the induction of the cholinergic phenotype in the basal forebrain [134,137]. Moreover, only in postmitotic cholinergic neurons, this pathway induces NGF expression, an autocrine/paracrine cholinergic trophic factor, which stimulates ACh production [138]. Accordingly, it is of therapeutic relevance for treatment of Alzheimer´s disease, that BMP9/Smad1,5 signalling can prevent lesion-evoked impairment of the cholinergic septo-hippocampal neurons in adult mice [139]. The basal forebrain cholinergic neuron specific gene expression pattern is also basically linked to an interaction of Smad and Sizn1 (Smad-interacting zinc finger protein), a factor which causes mental retardation if mutated [140,141].

3.2. Axon and synapse formation

Induction of axons and orienting of axon responses are controlled by several Smad molecules of both the BMP and the TGFβ/activin pathways in a timely and spatially organized manner. Several different neuronal/neural cell types use individual aspects of the Smad machinery.

3.2.1. Basic role of Smads for neuritic outgrowth

In PC12 cells, which are initially derived from neural crest cells and are used as model system for neuronal differentiation, BMP2 induces neurite outgrowth [142] by activation of TAK1/p38 kinase signalling pathway [143,144], which is in turn tightly controlled by the simultaneous, also BMP2-induced expression of the inhibitory Smad6 and Smad7 [142] performed via activation of Smad1,5,8 pathway. The inhibitory Smads are considered to inversely inhibit BMP signalling in a concerted action by repressing Smad1,5,8, mediating BMP receptor degradation by Smurf1 [16,145], and by physical interaction with TAK1-binding protein, which finally reduces the p38-mediated neuritic outgrowth [143,144]. Neurotrophin 3 induced neuritic outgrowth is potentiated by BMP4/6 induced phosphorylation of Smad1,5,8 and their subsequent inhibition of MEK in chicken neurons [146].

Otherwise, BMP2 inhibits neuritic outgrowth and differentiation of motor neuron-like NSC-34 cells by activation of Smad1,5,8-dependent signalling and subsequent Id genes activation, which are main targets of Smad signalling and which negatively regulate differentiation of various cells including neurogenic precursors and motor-neuron precursors [147].

3.2.2. Subtle control of axonal morphogenesis

The axonal morphogenesis is strongly influenced by the TGFβ-regulated signalling protein Smad2. Endogenous Smad2 is constitutively activated and its phosphorylated form is nuclearly localized in human and mouse hippocampal and cortical neurons [148,149] and in primary granule neurons of rat cerebellum [150]. In granule neurons Smad2 can form a physical complex with the endogenous transcriptional modulator SnoN, which is also nuclearly localized and strongly enhances axonal growth [151] and neuronal branching [152] by regulating a large number of neuronal genes [153]. SnoN ubiquitination and degradation is controlled by the nuclear ubiquitin ligase Cdh1-anaphase-promoting complex (Cdh1-APC), which physically interact with nuclear SnoN thus suppressing axonal growth. [151,154]. Obviously Smad2 binding to SnoN facilitates the ability of Cdh1-APC to control SnoN degradation. Consequently, if phosphorylation levels of Smad2 are reduced, SnoN levels increased and axonal growth is stimulated which allow therapeutic potential after brain injury [150]. The constitutive neuronal expression of axonal growth inhibitors e.g. Smad2, Smad3 [148] and Cdh1 [155] and the reduced expression of axon growth promoters (SnoN) in terminally differentiated neurons [150] generate an intrinsic axon growth inhibition control, allowing a balance between steady state and neuronal plasticity.

3.2.3. Axonal regeneration

Axonal regeneration requires the reversal of an age-dependent loss of intrinsic axonal growth capability [156,157]. In dorsal root ganglion cells (DRG), which possess two branches of a initially unipolar axon, (a) a central branch containing in the spinal cord and (b) a peripheral branch innervating sensory targets, the axotomy of the peripheral branch requires function of transcription factor Smad1 for successful regeneration [158]. While in embryonic DRG neurons during the phase of active axon growth Smad1 RNA and protein were strongly expressed and found abundantly C-terminally phosphorylated in the nuclei (while Smad8 expression was low and Smad5 expression was concentrated to the periventricular zone), in adult DRG neurons Smad1 phosphorylation was diminished [159]. However, after axotomy, the induction and nuclear translocation of Smad1 precedes the onset of axonal extension and are maintained over longer time, demonstrating the importance of Smad1 for the perpetuation of the activated axonal growth program [158]. Interestingly, Smad1-dependent axonal growth program is an intrinsic feature of DRG neurons which functions independently of extracellular BMP. Until now, the detailed underlying mechanism for BMP-independent Smad1 phosphorylation is not completely elucidated. It is possible, that endogenous cytoplasmic kinases or intracellularly available BMP/BMP-receptor complexes might be involved. The ligand-independent C-terminal phosphorylation of the SSXS domain of Smad2 and Smad3 was already reported [160] suggesting a possible extracellular ligand-independent universal strategy. Probably, Smad1 signalling is also involved in the axonogenesis of many other classes of neurons, e.g. Purkinje cells, retinal ganglionic, olfactory and motor neurons which were already found positively labelled for pSmad1 immunoreactivity [159]. Due to the possible linker phosphorylation of Smad1 by several kinases (e.g. MAPK, GSK, CDK), the molecule might serve as an integrator of various pathways relevant for axon growth and regeneration [14,23-26]. However, for clinical and therapeutic relevance, the transduction of adeno-associated vector encoded BMP4 allows stimulation of Smad1 phosphorylation and activation of axonal growth independent of axotomy and also promotes sensory axon regeneration after axotomy [159]. At least partly BMP effects are dependent on its binding to repulsive guidance molecules [161].

While Smad1 positively supports axonal growth, the inhibitory Smad6 can block axon outgrowth, as shown for post-mitotic dI1 axons of the spinal cord [82] and therefore exert roles in spatially limiting the influence of BMP signalling on neurons.

In Drosophila, Smad2 is involved in motor neuron axon guidance, as null mutants of Smad2 exhibit axon guidance defects [162]. It is suggested, that a chemoattractant signal of TGFβ superfamily members provided by muscle cells might guide motor axons to their appropriate innervation sites.

3.2.4. R-Smads and Co-Smads exert neuronal plasticity

The development of peripheral tissues is connected to axonal growth of peripheral nerves, linking sensory information to the spinal cord via neuronal cell bodies localized in ganglia. After initial axon extension for trigeminal sensory neurons in mice, a Smad4-dependent retrograde signalling from developing face to the neuronal nuclei was found, which control the expression of genes in neurons of the trigeminal ganglion in dependence on their position. Extrinsic signals released from developing craniofacial tissue, e.g. BMP4, activate phosphorylation of Smad1,5,8 at the axon terminals and selectively retrogradely signals this information to selected trigeminal neuronal cell bodies thus inducing spacially patterned expression of further transcription factors along the dorso-ventral axis of the trigeminal ganglion [163]. A comparable retrograde mechanism based on dSmad2 was found in R7 axons in the Drosophila visual system, where activin, secreted from the R7 cells growth cone in an autocrine manner, activates its receptor and initiates intracellular Smad2 phosphorylation. The pSmad2 complexes to the nuclear import adaptor Importin-α3, shuttles to the nucleus and reduces growth cone motility and synaptogenesis via transcriptional regulation of several target genes [164]. Already in Drosophila, a retrograde Smad-based signalling of the BMP homolog Gbb regulates synaptic growth in presynaptic motor neurons [165]. The underlying mechanism for the retrograde Smad-based signalling was recently examined for the BMP4 signalling system. Ji and colleagues (2012) discovered that endosomes carrying the BMP-signalling complex containing phosphorylated Smad1,5,8, are essentially linked to a BDNF-induced axonal or growth cone translation of Smad proteins to retrogradely control transcription in trigeminal neurons [166,167]. This `two-target-derived signalling' integrates neurotrophin and BMP signals on the level of Smad proteins, which are axonally translated on demand. This process is involved in the acquisition of positional identity markers during trigeminal ganglia development and selectively works in ophthalmic and maxillary but not in mandibular axons obviously due to the failure of BDNF in the mandibular target field [166]. The underlying mechanism suggests to re-evaluate the role and extent of Smad based transcriptional regulation. (1) Nearly all cellular surfaces/membranes, including dendrites, axons, growth cones and spines might receive information which could be integrated by Smad signalling. (2) The retrograde transport of other ligands of the TGFβ group was already reported, e.g. TGFβ2 in normal and injured motor neurons [168], implicating the question whether axonal Smad signalling is involved in injury-response. (3) The mechanism might work with all those extracellular and also intracellular factors that affect Smad translation, and might at least partly explain neurodegenerative disorders, which are characterized by disturbed axonal transport and/or neurotrophin deficiency at neuronal terminals

The specific structure of axons and the axonal transport of Smad signals [166] as well as simple translocation of receptor phosphorylated Smads from cytoplasmic receptor site into the nucleus require intact microtubule network. Phosphorylated Smad2 is transported using microtubules by support of kinesin-1 and kinesinATPase activity [169] and also requires dynein light chain km23-1 [6], whereas pSmad3 transport was dependent on km23-2 function [170]. Additionally retrograde axonal transport of phosphorylated Smads, which is necessary for transition of axonal synaptic BMP-like ligand mediated phosphorylation of Smads in Drosophila, also depends on an intact function of p150Glued protein. P150Glued is a component of the dynactin complex, which is necessarily involved in synapse assembly and stability [171]. However, a p150Glued knockdown induced disruption of synaptic homeostasis can be rescued by activation of Smad signalling at the soma [172,173], confirming the important role of nuclear phosphorylated Smad to synaptic homeostasis.

3.2.5. Astrocytic and oligodenrocytic Smad signalling influences neuronal axonal growth

Astrocytes surrounding synapses are also target of neuronal activity. Glial metabotropic glutamate 2/3 receptor activation by neuronally released glutamate induces astrocytic TGFβ1 secretion, leading to GFAP gene activation and astrocyte differentiation involving astrocytic Smad signalling pathways [174].

Chondroitin sulphate proteoglycans (CSPG), mainly synthesized by astrocytes, can inhibit axonal growth and regeneration. After traumatic brain injury or disruptions of the blood brain barrier, mature or fibrinogen-coupled latent TGFβ is released into the CNS and increases the CSPG expression by a Smad signalling manner in astrocytes [175,176]. Both astrocytic Smad2 and Smad3 expression and phosphorylation leads to inhibition of neuronal outgrowth and is required for astrocytic neurocan synthesis, whereas phosphacan only requires Smad2 [175,176]. Reduced Smad3 levels selectively reduced induction of chondroitin-4- sulphotransferase 1 and the amount of 4-sulfated CSPGs secreted by astrocytes and also promoted axonal growth of neurons which were fed on these astrocytes [175]. Taxol treatment of astrocytes can reduce CSPG expression by interfering with kinesin-1-dependent pSmad transport into the nucleus [177] and improve axon regeneration after spinal cord injury.

The Smad-interacting-protein 1 (Sip1) is an essential modulator for CNS myelination. In oligodendrocytes, it functions in a dual-mode manner by repressing the differentiation inhibitory signals of the BMP-receptor activated Smad1,5,8 activity [178] and activating oligodendrocytes-promoting factors, thus controlling proper myelination in the CNS [38].

3.3. Smads contribute to synapse formation and synaptic transmission processes

Synapse formation and remodelling are results of intrinsic programs and environmental insults. Synapses are characterized by close cell-to-cell communications, which also include synaptic transmission and signalling processes mediated by growth factors e.g. members of the TGFβ superfamily. In spinster a mutation of the inhibitory Smad Dad (Daughters against dpp) causes synaptic overgrowth [179]. A well investigated synaptic system is the neuromuscular junction (NMJ) of Drosophila, showing the involvement of Smad proteins in synapse function both in pre- and in postsynaptic cells. The release of muscular BMP4-type ligand Gbb, which is required for intact function of a large part of postsynaptic muscles [165], allows its binding to a presynaptic receptor consisting of one type I and one type II receptor, Sax or Tkv and Wit, respectively [180,181], and the subsequent phosphorylation of the R-Smad, Mothers against dpp (Mad) [165]. Activated Mad is responsible for presynaptic nuclear propagation of the postsynaptic muscular BMP signals and finally for regulating synapse growth, morphology and function of motor-neurons at least partly by altering transcription [165,180,182]. The retrograde transport of Mad utilizes microtubule motor proteins, e.g. dynein complexes, and is sensitive to disruption of dynein motor function [165]. The Drosophila Co-Smad/Smad4 homolog Medea (Med) is also necessary for presynaptic BMP signalling cascade and essential for synaptic growth [183]. Both, Med and Mad mutants, exhibit defects in neurotransmitter release and synaptic ultrastructure [165,183]. It is suggested that an equilibrium exist between the binding of presynaptic phosphorylated Mad to Med and the binding of Med to the RING finger E3 ubiquitin ligase Hiw [184], which regulate the synaptic growth in NMJ [183].

Additionally to the retrograde neuronal Mad/Med-mediated Gbb signalling, anterogradely released TGFβ type ligands activate Mad phosphorylation at the postsynaptic density (PSD) zone of postsynaptic muscles and NMJ depolarization supports Mad nuclear transition in the muscles [185]. In summary, a mutual information flow of neuron and muscle on each physiological state and the synaptic cleft situation is essentially controlled by specific R- and Co-Smad signalling in both cellular systems.

Importantly, the activation of Mad phosphorylation and nuclear translocation by the BMP ligand Gbb directs the expression of synaptic homeostasis independently of synaptic growth control in Drosophila [173]. However, retrograde transport of Mad, which was phosphorylated at the periphery of the axon terminal due to synaptic Gbb binding, mediates synaptic homeostasis. Remarkably, Gbb induced phosphorylation of Mad at the soma site of the neuron compensate for a disturbed retrograde axonal pMad transport completely [173]. The release of muscular Gbb into the synaptic cleft at the periphery to activate neuronal retrograde pMad transport, can be regulated by activin, which controls the muscular Gbb synthesis by recruiting the Drosophila dSmad2 [186]. Cdc42-interacting protein 4 (dCIP4) which is also localized postsynaptically at the NMJs co-regulates the phosphorylation of neuronal Mad levels by inhibiting postsynaptic Gbb secretion [187].

These data indicate, that both activin and BMP directed R-Smad signalling controls synaptic function at NMJ and affects the development of synaptic homeostasis.

4. Role of Smads for neurological disorders

Several neurological diseases are characterized by disturbed cellular or subcellular Smad localization and show artificial Smad sequestration or deposition. Especially in neurodegenerative and motor neuron diseases a disruption of Smad controlled transcriptional machinery was reported.

Neurodegenerative diseases are characterised by selective and progressive loss of specific populations of neurones. Four disease-classes are proposed based on four major affected proteins, tau, βA4-amyloid (βA4), α-synuclein and TDP-43, and therefore, neurodegenerative diseases can roughly be classified into four main groups: amyloidosis, tauopathies, synucleinopathies and TDP-43 proteinopathies (for review see [188]). Recent data indicate, that in all four disease groups Smad proteins are essentially involved in the disease progression, finally indicating a remarkable commonness of these diseases.

4.1. Alzheimer´s disease

Alzheimer´s disease (AD), representing a mixture of both amyloidosis and tauopathy, is a severe neurodegenerative disorder and the most common cause of dementia in the elderly. Typical clinical symptoms are memory loss, disturbed activities of daily life and deficiency of social competence. Common morphological correlates to the clinical features are extracellular βA4-plaque depositions, intraneuronal tau pathology, neuronal cell death, and cell cycle activation [189].

In AD, we identified a strong disturbance of the normal constitutive nuclear localization of phosphorylated Smad2 and Smad3 in hippocampal and cortical neurons [148], which subsequently was confirmed by others [190,191]. In AD brain, a strong colocalization of pSmad2,3 with intracellular neurofibrillary tangles (NFTs) in neurons and with βA4-amyloid plaques in addition to a sequestration of pSmad2,3 in cytoplasmic granular vesicles is detectable [148]. Additionally a significant reduction of Smad2,3,4, which are involved in activation of cell cycle proteins was described. Smad4 directly controls cyclin-dependent kinase 4 (CDK4) expression in neuronal cells and is involved in cell cycle activation of neurons in AD brain [192]. It is quite possible, that the recently identified TGFβ1-induced antiapoptotic factor (TIAF1), which can bind and block Smad4-dependent promoter activation [193], participates in the cytoplasmic Smad sequestration in AD neurons and suppresses Smad-regulated promoter activation. Environmental stress or TGFβ1, can induce TIAF aggregation, which in turn removes soluble Smad4, induces apoptosis and activates βA4 generation and its aggregation [193].

A reason for the intraneuronal dislocation of Smads could be due to the disturbed nucleocytoplasmic transport in hippocampal AD neurons [194,195]. The inner nuclear membrane comprises integral proteins, e.g. MAN1, which regulate Smad phosphorylation and nuclear translocation [196], while the outer nuclear membrane is directly continuous with the rough endoplasmic reticulum. Both membranes are separated by nuclear core complexes, which also control nucleocytoplasmic shuttling of Smad2 [197]. Altered nuclear membrane integrity [195] might provoke misrouting of phosphorylated Smads into the associated ER compartment, indicated by the co-localization of phosphorylated Smad2 granules with a luminal marker protein of the ER, protein disulphide isomerase [148,198]. ER containing Smad2 could be secreted and thus explain the extracellular association of pSmad2,3 with amyloid plaques [148,190]. Alternatively, pSmad2 could interact in early endosomes with βA4-peptides which are accumulating in the early stages of AD [199], and there also meet BACE, the β-secretase, generating β-amyloid peptides [200], activated TGFβ receptors type I and II as well as SARA, a Smad anchor for receptor activation [201-203]. It is also possible, that early endosomes can fuse to the ER thus allowing a direct route of Smad proteins to the lumen of the ER [204,205].

However, activation of cell cycle is a hallmark of AD and (1) probably supports hyperphosphorylation of tau protein which leads to generation of neurofibrillary tangles and (2) increases neuronal apoptosis by phosphorylation of retinoblastoma protein and activation of E2F based apoptotic impacts (for review see [206]. Hyperphosphorylation of tau affects the neuronal Smad2,3 localization, diminishes its nuclear concentration and thus impedes with transcriptional Smad functions as shown after βA4 treatment of primary neurons [207]. NFT formation in AD brain disturbs common intra-neuronal transport mechanisms [208]. This disturbance could also interfere with retrograde Smad signalling which could be suggested for hippocampal neurons but so far has only demonstrated for Drosophila motor neurons [173]. Moreover, we also suggest, that the principle of the two-target-derived signalling integrating neurotrophin (BDNF) and Smad pathway found in rat trigeminal neurons [166,167] might also play a role for AD progression, because BDNF is deficient in entorhinal cortex and hippocampus in AD [209,210]. Finally, a disturbed nuclear Smad localization might influence competence of neurons to express synaptic homeostasis and plasticity, both processes are well investigated for Drosophila motor neurons.

Pathogenic reduction of neuronal Smads can also support activation of neuronal cell cycle, resulting in neuronal apoptosis [211] e.g. by repression of cyclin-dependent kinase inhibitors (CDIs) $p15^{Ink4B}$, $p16^{Ink4A}$, or $p21^{Cip}$, which expression is controlled by TGFβ/Smad signalling [212-214]. Though the increased levels of TGFβ1 in AD [215,216] does not seem to be able to compensate for the compromised canonical neuronal Smad pathway [148,190], astrocytes were shown responsive to this growth factor, which induces amyloid precursor protein (APP) expression in cooperation with Sp1 [217] and CTCF [218]. Altered APP cleavage by the concerted action of α-, β- and γ-secretases is a main aspect of AD pathology and results in the generation of the pathogenetic βA4 peptide 1-42, which is neurotoxic and leads to βA4-amyloid plaques. Whether βA4 peptide 1-42 can further suppress neuronal TGFβ1/Smad2,3 signalling by activation of the inhibitory Smad7 in neurons as already shown for human monocytes cannot be excluded [219].

Clearance of βA4 peptide was reported by microglia cells [220]. TGFβ released by neurons or astrocytes stimulates βA4 peptide uptake through Smad3-dependent increased scavenger receptor SR-A expression and increased phagocytosis [221]. Though the microglial capacity to remove βA4-plaques is limited [222], peripheral phagocytes, migrating into the brain if their Smad2,3 signalling is blocked at the expense of Smad1,5,8 phosphorylation, might perform this task successfully [223].

In other tauopathies, e.g. Pick disease, progressive supranuclear palsy, and corticobasal degeneration, cytoplasmic phospho-tau bound pSmad2,3 was also identified, though reduced nuclear pSmad levels were not found [224] suggesting a different impact on Smad signalling in these diseases compared to AD.

4.2. Parkinson´s disease

Parkinson´s disease (PD) is a progressive neurodegenerative disorder which is characterized by dopaminergic neurodegeneration in the substantia nigra (SN) pars compacta. The closely associated loss of dopaminergic inputs into the striatum results in failure of motor programmes (e.g. voluntary movements) and initiates a striatal plastic change [225,226]. The gradual loss of dopaminergic neurons is linked to an increase of dopamine turnover [227,228]. α-synuclein (α-syn) is the major protein component of Lewy bodies, a hallmark of PD. It can aggregate to form toxic oligomers and fibrillar structures [226,229].

It was shown, that the TGFβ3-Smad-HIPK2 pathway is important for the survival of dopaminergic neurons during development [96,230]. However, recently, a very specific and important role of Smad3 for the nigrostriatal system was explored in a Smad3 null mouse model representing an exciting model of PD [231]. These animals show a reduced number of dopaminergic neurons in the rostral SN, resulting from a postnatal neurodegenerative process. The selective pro-survival effect of Smad3 for SN dopaminergic neurons was emphasized by stereological quantifications showing no alterations of the striatal neuronal number. In Smad3 null mice a diminished trophic support provided by Erk1/2 signalling and a reduced astrocytic support to nigral dopaminergic neurons was detected [231]. Though striatal dopamine levels were not changed in Smad3 null mice, a strong increase of DA metabolism, including elevated monoamine-oxidase (MAO) levels were identified, resembling PD findings [232]. Finally, increased expression and aggregation of α-syn in neurites and cell bodies of several telencephalic, mesencephalic and rombencephalic brain regions and in fibres of the primary and secondary motor cortex were found [231]. Two possible functional Smad3-based circuits are suggested. Either Smad3 might directly regulate the α-syn transcription, which further allows modulating DA metabolism, or the Smad3 deficiency caused elevated DA catabolism generates oxidative stress which allow toxic aggregation of α-syn. The data qualify Smad3 as a possible target for PD therapy. Interestingly, the currently pursued target to re-implant dopaminergic neurons is also based on modification of Smad signalling during their in vitro establishment [130,233].

4.3. Motor neuron diseases

As mentioned above, Smads are essentially controlling the plasticity of NMJ, the intra-axonal transport and affect axonal repair processes. Accordingly, selective motor neuron diseases exhibit disturbances of Smad signalling, e.g. spinal muscular atrophy, [234], spinal bulbar muscular atrophy [235] or amyotrophic lateral sclerosis (ALS).

ALS is a progressive neurodegenerative disease, which targets upper and lower motor neurons. In the primary motor cortex and the anterior horn of the spinal cord, motor neurons disappear and the pyramidal tract degenerates [236-238]. The remaining motor neurons exhibit inclusion bodies e.g. Bunina bodies, hyaline and skein-like inclusions. The pathological transactive response DNA-binding protein with a molecular weight of 43 kDa (TDP-43) was shown to be the major disease protein in ALS. Recently, increased nuclear immunoreactivity for pSmad2,3 in motor neurons was reported from sporadic ALS patients in spinal cord [239]. Motor neurons, where a colocalization of TDP-43 and pSmad2,3 in skeine-like and round hyaline inclusions was detected [239], show reduced nuclear pSmad2,3 immunoreactivity [240]. Obviously a disruption of Smad signalling by Smad segregation, comparable to AD or several tauopathies, enhances the loss of motor neuron function. Smad4 seems actively involved in the control of motor function as targeted disruption of Smad4 demonstrates [132]. Probably, increased nuclear pSmad2,3 content in the remaining ALS motor neurons indicates an endogenously initiated approach to a functional improvement. Experiments with an ALS mouse model support this hypothesis, because TGFβ2 administration ameliorated the motor performance of the mice [241]. A reduction of TDP-43 containing aggregates by Smad2 overexpression confirms in vitro a protective role of activated Smad signalling in ALS [242].

In summary, initiation and/or progression of many neurological disorders are directly linked to altered Smad signalling, comprising cytoplasmic Smad aggregation/sequestration, and nuclear reduction, disruption of transcriptional machinery and stimulating proapoptotic signalling, therefore disturbing biological processes, which are essential for all phases of nervous system development and homeostasis.

Acknowledgements

This manuscript was supported by the Project BBZ09: 14494 (University Leipzig) and the AFI-Project 984 000-150.

Author details

Uwe Ueberham* and Thomas Arendt

*Address all correspondence to: Uwe.Ueberham@medizin.uni-leipzig.de

Department for Molecular and Cellular Mechanisms of Neurodegeneration, Paul Flechsig Institute for Brain Research, University Leipzig, Leipzig, Germany

References

[1] Tsukazaki T, Chiang TA, Davison AF, Attisano L, Wrana JL. SARA, a FYVE domain protein that recruits Smad2 to the TGFbeta receptor. Cell 1998;95(6) 779-791.

[2] Shi W, Chang C, Nie S, Xie S, Wan M, Cao X. Endofin acts as a Smad anchor for receptor activation in BMP signaling. J. Cell Sci. 2007;120(Pt 7) 1216-1224.

[3] Dong C, Li Z, Alvarez R, Jr., Feng XH, Goldschmidt-Clermont PJ. Microtubule binding to Smads may regulate TGF beta activity. Mol. Cell 2000;5(1) 27-34.

[4] Santibanez JF, Quintanilla M, Bernabeu C. TGF-beta/TGF-beta receptor system and its role in physiological and pathological conditions. Clin. Sci (Lond). 2011;121(6) 233-251.

[5] Shi Y, Massague J. Mechanisms of TGF-beta signaling from cell membrane to the nucleus. Cell 2003;113(6) 685-700.

[6] Jin Q, Ding W, Mulder KM. Requirement for the dynein light chain km23-1 in a Smad2-dependent transforming growth factor-beta signaling pathway. J. Biol. Chem. 2007;282(26) 19122-19132.

[7] Jin Q, Gao G, Mulder KM. Requirement of a dynein light chain in TGFbeta/Smad3 signaling. J Cell Physiol. 2009;221(3) 707-715.

[8] Miyazono K. Molecular mechanisms of transforming growth factor-beta signaling and disease: The 59th Fujihara International Seminar, 2010. Cancer Sci. 2011;102(6) 1242-1244.

[9] Kretzschmar M, Doody J, Timokhina I, Massague J. A mechanism of repression of TGFbeta/ Smad signaling by oncogenic Ras. Genes Dev. 1999;13(7) 804-816.

[10] Matsuura I, Denissova NG, Wang G, He D, Long J, Liu F. Cyclin-dependent kinases regulate the antiproliferative function of Smads. Nature 2004;430(6996) 226-231.

[11] Luo Q, Nieves E, Kzhyshkowska J, Angeletti RH. Endogenous transforming growth factor-beta receptor-mediated Smad signaling complexes analyzed by mass spectrometry. Mol. Cell Proteomics. 2006;5(7) 1245-1260.

[12] Sasaki A, Masuda Y, Ohta Y, Ikeda K, Watanabe K. Filamin associates with Smads and regulates transforming growth factor-beta signaling. J. Biol. Chem. 2001;276(21) 17871-17877.

[13] Inoue Y, Imamura T. Regulation of TGF-beta family signaling by E3 ubiquitin ligases. Cancer Sci. 2008.

[14] Alarcon C, Zaromytidou AI, Xi Q, Gao S, Yu J, Fujisawa S, et al. Nuclear CDKs drive Smad transcriptional activation and turnover in BMP and TGF-beta pathways. Cell. 2009;139(4) 757-769.

[15] Sapkota G, Alarcon C, Spagnoli FM, Brivanlou AH, Massague J. Balancing BMP signaling through integrated inputs into the Smad1 linker. Mol Cell. 2007;25(3) 441-454.

[16] Zhu H, Kavsak P, Abdollah S, Wrana JL, Thomsen GH. A SMAD ubiquitin ligase targets the BMP pathway and affects embryonic pattern formation. Nature 1999;400(6745) 687-693.

[17] Gao S, Alarcon C, Sapkota G, Rahman S, Chen PY, Goerner N, et al. Ubiquitin ligase Nedd4L targets activated Smad2/3 to limit TGF-beta signaling. Mol Cell. 2009;36(3) 457-468.

[18] Burstyn-Cohen T, Stanleigh J, Sela-Donenfeld D, Kalcheim C. Canonical Wnt activity regulates trunk neural crest delamination linking BMP/noggin signaling with G1/S transition. Development. 2004;131(21) 5327-5339.

[19] Sela-Donenfeld D, Kalcheim C. Regulation of the onset of neural crest migration by coordinated activity of BMP4 and Noggin in the dorsal neural tube. Development. 1999;126(21) 4749-4762.

[20] Alexandrova EM, Thomsen GH. Smurf1 regulates neural patterning and folding in Xenopus embryos by antagonizing the BMP/Smad1 pathway. Dev. Biol. 2006;299(2) 398-410.

[21] Stuhlmiller TJ, Garcia-Castro MI. FGF/MAPK signaling is required in the gastrula epiblast for avian neural crest induction. Development. 2012;139(2) 289-300.

[22] Makkar P, Metpally RP, Sangadala S, Reddy BV. Modeling and analysis of MH1 domain of Smads and their interaction with promoter DNA sequence motif. J Mol Graph. Model. 2009;27(7) 803-812.

[23] Eivers E, Demagny H, De Robertis EM. Integration of BMP and Wnt signaling via vertebrate Smad1/5/8 and Drosophila Mad. Cytokine Growth Factor Rev. 2009;20(5-6) 357-365.

[24] Scherer A, Graff JM. Calmodulin differentially modulates Smad1 and Smad2 signaling. J. Biol. Chem. 2000;275(52) 41430-41438.

[25] Kretzschmar M, Doody J, Massague J. Opposing BMP and EGF signalling pathways converge on the TGF-beta family mediator Smad1. Nature 1997;389(6651) 618-622.

[26] Fuentealba LC, Eivers E, Ikeda A, Hurtado C, Kuroda H, Pera EM, et al. Integrating patterning signals: Wnt/GSK3 regulates the duration of the BMP/Smad1 signal. Cell. 2007;131(5) 980-993.

[27] Kuroda H, Fuentealba L, Ikeda A, Reversade B, De Robertis EM. Default neural induction: neuralization of dissociated Xenopus cells is mediated by Ras/MAPK activation. Genes Dev. 2005;19(9) 1022-1027.

[28] Hough C, Radu M, Dore JJ. Tgf-Beta induced erk phosphorylation of smad linker region regulates smad signaling. PLoS. ONE. 2012;7(8) e42513.

[29] Luo K. Ski and SnoN: negative regulators of TGF-beta signaling. Curr. Opin. Genet. Dev. 2004;14(1) 65-70.

[30] Mizuide M, Hara T, Furuya T, Takeda M, Kusanagi K, Inada Y, et al. Two short segments of Smad3 are important for specific interaction of Smad3 with c-Ski and SnoN. J. Biol. Chem. 2003;278(1) 531-536.

[31] Wu JW, Krawitz AR, Chai J, Li W, Zhang F, Luo K, et al. Structural mechanism of Smad4 recognition by the nuclear oncoprotein Ski: insights on Ski-mediated repression of TGF-beta signaling. Cell 2002;111(3) 357-367.

[32] Deheuninck J, Luo K. Ski and SnoN, potent negative regulators of TGF-beta signaling. Cell Res. 2009;19(1) 47-57.

[33] Wang W, Mariani FV, Harland RM, Luo K. Ski represses bone morphogenic protein signaling in Xenopus and mammalian cells. Proc. Natl. Acad. Sci. U. S. A 2000;97(26) 14394-14399.

[34] Conidi A, Cazzola S, Beets K, Coddens K, Collart C, Cornelis F, et al. Few Smad proteins and many Smad-interacting proteins yield multiple functions and action modes in TGFbeta/BMP signaling in vivo. Cytokine Growth Factor Rev. 2011;22(5-6) 287-300.

[35] Chng Z, Teo A, Pedersen RA, Vallier L. SIP1 mediates cell-fate decisions between neuroectoderm and mesendoderm in human pluripotent stem cells. Cell Stem Cell. 2010;6(1) 59-70.

[36] Nitta KR, Tanegashima K, Takahashi S, Asashima M. XSIP1 is essential for early neural gene expression and neural differentiation by suppression of BMP signaling. Dev. Biol. 2004;275(1) 258-267.

[37] Nitta KR, Takahashi S, Haramoto Y, Fukuda M, Tanegashima K, Onuma Y, et al. The N-terminus zinc finger domain of Xenopus SIP1 is important for neural induction, but not for suppression of Xbra expression. Int J Dev. Biol. 2007;51(4) 321-325.

[38] Weng Q, Chen Y, Wang H, Xu X, Yang B, He Q, et al. Dual-mode modulation of Smad signaling by Smad-interacting protein Sip1 is required for myelination in the central nervous system. Neuron. 2012;73(4) 713-728.

[39] Drummond AE, Le MT, Ethier JF, Dyson M, Findlay JK. Expression and localization of activin receptors, Smads, and beta glycan to the postnatal rat ovary. Endocrinology. 2002;143(4) 1423-1433.

[40] Findlay JK, Drummond AE, Dyson M, Baillie AJ, Robertson DM, Ethier JF. Production and actions of inhibin and activin during folliculogenesis in the rat. Mol Cell Endocrinol. 2001;180(1-2) 139-144.

[41] Xu J, Oakley J, McGee EA. Stage-specific expression of Smad2 and Smad3 during folliculogenesis. Biol Reprod. 2002;66(6) 1571-1578.

[42] Tian X, Halfhill AN, Diaz FJ. Localization of phosphorylated SMAD proteins in granulosa cells, oocytes and oviduct of female mice. Gene Expr. Patterns. 2010;10(2-3) 105-112.

[43] Pangas SA, Rademaker AW, Fishman DA, Woodruff TK. Localization of the activin signal transduction components in normal human ovarian follicles: implications for autocrine and paracrine signaling in the ovary. J Clin. Endocrinol. Metab. 2002;87(6) 2644-2657.

[44] Osterlund C, Fried G. TGFbeta receptor types I and II and the substrate proteins Smad 2 and 3 are present in human oocytes. Mol Hum. Reprod. 2000;6(6) 498-503.

[45] Kuo FT, Fan K, Ambartsumyan G, Menon P, Ketefian A, tsi-Barnes IK, et al. Relative expression of genes encoding SMAD signal transduction factors in human granulosa cells is correlated with oocyte quality. J Assist. Reprod. Genet. 2011;28(10) 931-938.

[46] Li X, Tripurani SK, James R, Pangas SA. Minimal fertility defects in mice deficient in oocyte-expressed Smad4. Biol Reprod. 2012;86(1) 1-6.

[47] Tan Q, Balofsky A, Weisz K, Peng C. Role of activin, transforming growth factor-beta and bone morphogenetic protein 15 in regulating zebrafish oocyte maturation. Comp Biochem. Physiol A Mol Integr. Physiol. 2009;153(1) 18-23.

[48] Snape A, Wylie CC, Smith JC, Heasman J. Changes in states of commitment of single animal pole blastomeres of Xenopus laevis. Dev. Biol. 1987;119(2) 503-510.

[49] Dunn NR, Vincent SD, Oxburgh L, Robertson EJ, Bikoff EK. Combinatorial activities of Smad2 and Smad3 regulate mesoderm formation and patterning in the mouse embryo. Development. 2004;131(8) 1717-1728.

[50] Jia S, Ren Z, Li X, Zheng Y, Meng A. smad2 and smad3 are required for mesendoderm induction by transforming growth factor-beta/nodal signals in zebrafish. J Biol Chem. 2008;283(4) 2418-2426.

[51] Nomura M, Li E. Smad2 role in mesoderm formation, left-right patterning and craniofacial development. Nature. 1998;393(6687) 786-790.

[52] Weinstein M, Yang X, Li C, Xu X, Gotay J, Deng CX. Failure of egg cylinder elongation and mesoderm induction in mouse embryos lacking the tumor suppressor smad2. Proc Natl Acad Sci U S A. 1998;95(16) 9378-9383.

[53] Dupont S, Zacchigna L, Cordenonsi M, Soligo S, Adorno M, Rugge M, et al. Germ-layer specification and control of cell growth by Ectodermin, a Smad4 ubiquitin ligase. Cell. 2005;121(1) 87-99.

[54] Howell M, Itoh F, Pierreux CE, Valgeirsdottir S, Itoh S, ten Dijke P, et al. Xenopus Smad4beta is the co-Smad component of developmentally regulated transcription factor complexes responsible for induction of early mesodermal genes. Dev. Biol. 1999;214(2) 354-369.

[55] Hemmati-Brivanlou A, Melton D. Vertebrate neural induction. Annu. Rev Neurosci. 1997;20:43-60. 43-60.

[56] Hemmati-Brivanlou A, Melton D. Vertebrate embryonic cells will become nerve cells unless told otherwise. Cell. 1997;88(1) 13-17.

[57] Reversade B, Kuroda H, Lee H, Mays A, De Robertis EM. Depletion of Bmp2, Bmp4, Bmp7 and Spemann organizer signals induces massive brain formation in Xenopus embryos. Development. 2005;132(15) 3381-3392.

[58] Linker C, Stern CD. Neural induction requires BMP inhibition only as a late step, and involves signals other than FGF and Wnt antagonists. Development. 2004;131(22) 5671-5681.

[59] Chang C, Harland RM. Neural induction requires continued suppression of both Smad1 and Smad2 signals during gastrulation. Development. 2007;134(21) 3861-3872.

[60] Yaguchi S, Yaguchi J, Burke RD. Sp-Smad2/3 mediates patterning of neurogenic ectoderm by nodal in the sea urchin embryo. Dev. Biol. 2007;302(2) 494-503.

[61] Jia S, Wu D, Xing C, Meng A. Smad2/3 activities are required for induction and patterning of the neuroectoderm in zebrafish. Dev. Biol. 2009;333(2) 273-284.

[62] Delaune E, Lemaire P, Kodjabachian L. Neural induction in Xenopus requires early FGF signalling in addition to BMP inhibition. Development. 2005;132(2) 299-310.

[63] Streit A, Berliner AJ, Papanayotou C, Sirulnik A, Stern CD. Initiation of neural induction by FGF signalling before gastrulation. Nature. 2000;406(6791) 74-78.

[64] Wilson SI, Graziano E, Harland R, Jessell TM, Edlund T. An early requirement for FGF signalling in the acquisition of neural cell fate in the chick embryo. Curr. Biol. 2000;20;10(8) 421-429.

[65] Di-Gregorio A, Sancho M, Stuckey DW, Crompton LA, Godwin J, Mishina Y, et al. BMP signalling inhibits premature neural differentiation in the mouse embryo. Development. 2007;134(18) 3359-3369.

[66] Chambers SM, Fasano CA, Papapetrou EP, Tomishima M, Sadelain M, Studer L. Highly efficient neural conversion of human ES and iPS cells by dual inhibition of SMAD signaling. Nat Biotechnol. 2009;27(3) 275-280.

[67] Ganat YM, Calder EL, Kriks S, Nelander J, Tu EY, Jia F, et al. Identification of embryonic stem cell-derived midbrain dopaminergic neurons for engraftment. J Clin. Invest. 2012;122(8) 2928-2939.

[68] Yaguchi S, Yaguchi J, Wei Z, Jin Y, Angerer LM, Inaba K. Fez function is required to maintain the size of the animal plate in the sea urchin embryo. Development. 2011;138(19) 4233-4243.

[69] Juriloff DM, Harris MJ. Mouse models for neural tube closure defects. Hum. Mol Genet. 2000;9(6) 993-1000.

[70] Stottmann RW, Berrong M, Matta K, Choi M, Klingensmith J. The BMP antagonist Noggin promotes cranial and spinal neurulation by distinct mechanisms. Dev. Biol. 2006;295(2) 647-663.

[71] Eom DS, Amarnath S, Fogel JL, Agarwala S. Bone morphogenetic proteins regulate neural tube closure by interacting with the apicobasal polarity pathway. Development. 2011;138(15) 3179-3188.

[72] Eom DS, Amarnath S, Fogel JL, Agarwala S. Bone morphogenetic proteins regulate hinge point formation during neural tube closure by dynamic modulation of apicobasal polarity. Birth Defects Res A Clin. Mol Teratol. 2012; 10.

[73] Ybot-Gonzalez P, Gaston-Massuet C, Girdler G, Klingensmith J, Arkell R, Greene ND, et al. Neural plate morphogenesis during mouse neurulation is regulated by antagonism of Bmp signalling. Development. 2007;134(17) 3203-3211.

[74] Chizhikov VV, Millen KJ. Mechanisms of roof plate formation in the vertebrate CNS. Nat Rev Neurosci. 2004;5(10) 808-812.

[75] Caspary T, Anderson KV. Patterning cell types in the dorsal spinal cord: what the mouse mutants say. Nat Rev Neurosci. 2003;4(4) 289-297.

[76] Dessaud E, McMahon AP, Briscoe J. Pattern formation in the vertebrate neural tube: a sonic hedgehog morphogen-regulated transcriptional network. Development. 2008;135(15) 2489-2503.

[77] Perron JC, Dodd J. Inductive specification and axonal orientation of spinal neurons mediated by divergent bone morphogenetic protein signaling pathways. Neural Dev. 2011;6:36. 36.

[78] Perron JC, Dodd J. Structural distinctions in BMPs underlie divergent signaling in spinal neurons. Neural Dev. 2012;7:16. 16.

[79] Le DG, Garcia-Campmany L, Rabadan MA, Ferronha T, Tozer S, Briscoe J, et al. Canonical BMP7 activity is required for the generation of discrete neuronal populations in the dorsal spinal cord. Development. 2012;139(2) 259-268.

[80] Hu Q, Ueno N, Behringer RR. Restriction of BMP4 activity domains in the developing neural tube of the mouse embryo. EMBO Rep. 2004;5(7) 734-739.

[81] Xie Z, Chen Y, Li Z, Bai G, Zhu Y, Yan R, et al. Smad6 promotes neuronal differentiation in the intermediate zone of the dorsal neural tube by inhibition of the Wnt/beta-catenin pathway. Proc Natl Acad Sci U S A. 2011;19;108(29) 12119-12124.

[82] Hazen VM, Phan KD, Hudiburgh S, Butler SJ. Inhibitory Smads differentially regulate cell fate specification and axon dynamics in the dorsal spinal cord. Dev. Biol. 2011;356(2) 566-575.

[83] Garcia-Campmany L, Marti E. The TGF{beta} intracellular effector Smad3 regulates neuronal differentiation and cell fate specification in the developing spinal cord. Development 2007;134(1) 65-75.

[84] Heeg-Truesdell E, LaBonne C. A slug, a fox, a pair of sox: transcriptional responses to neural crest inducing signals. Birth Defects Res C. Embryo. Today. 2004;72(2) 124-139.

[85] Faure S, de Santa BP, Roberts DJ, Whitman M. Endogenous patterns of BMP signaling during early chick development. Dev. Biol. 2002;244(1) 44-65.

[86] Liem KF, Jr., Tremml G, Jessell TM. A role for the roof plate and its resident TGFbeta-related proteins in neuronal patterning in the dorsal spinal cord. Cell. 1997;91(1) 127-138.

[87] Liem KF, Jr., Tremml G, Roelink H, Jessell TM. Dorsal differentiation of neural plate cells induced by BMP-mediated signals from epidermal ectoderm. Cell. 1995;82(6) 969-979.

[88] Linker C, de A, I, Papanayotou C, Stower M, Sabado V, Ghorani E, et al. Cell communication with the neural plate is required for induction of neural markers by BMP inhibition: evidence for homeogenetic induction and implications for Xenopus animal cap and chick explant assays. Dev. Biol. 2009;327(2) 478-486.

[89] Patthey C, Edlund T, Gunhaga L. Wnt-regulated temporal control of BMP exposure directs the choice between neural plate border and epidermal fate. Development. 2009;136(1) 73-83.

[90] Patthey C, Gunhaga L. Specification and regionalisation of the neural plate border. Eur. J Neurosci. 2011;34(10) 1516-1528.

[91] Streit A, Stern CD. Establishment and maintenance of the border of the neural plate in the chick: involvement of FGF and BMP activity. Mech. Dev. 1999;82(1-2) 51-66.

[92] Chalazonitis A, D'Autreaux F, Guha U, Pham TD, Faure C, Chen JJ, et al. Bone morphogenetic protein-2 and -4 limit the number of enteric neurons but promote development of a TrkC-expressing neurotrophin-3-dependent subset. J. Neurosci. 2004;24(17) 4266-4282.

[93] Chalazonitis A, D'Autreaux F, Pham TD, Kessler JA, Gershon MD. Bone morphogenetic proteins regulate enteric gliogenesis by modulating ErbB3 signaling. Dev. Biol. 2011;350(1) 64-79.

[94] Harada J, Kokura K, Kanei-Ishii C, Nomura T, Khan MM, Kim Y, et al. Requirement of the co-repressor homeodomain-interacting protein kinase 2 for ski-mediated inhibition of bone morphogenetic protein-induced transcriptional activation. J. Biol. Chem. 2003;278(40) 38998-39005.

[95] Chalazonitis A, Tang AA, Shang Y, Pham TD, Hsieh I, Setlik W, et al. Homeodomain interacting protein kinase 2 regulates postnatal development of enteric dopaminergic neurons and glia via BMP signaling. J Neurosci. 2011;31(39) 13746-13757.

[96] Zhang J, Pho V, Bonasera SJ, Holtzman J, Tang AT, Hellmuth J, et al. Essential function of HIPK2 in TGFbeta-dependent survival of midbrain dopamine neurons. Nat Neurosci. 2007;10(1) 77-86.

[97] Anitha M, Shahnavaz N, Qayed E, Joseph I, Gossrau G, Mwangi S, et al. BMP2 promotes differentiation of nitrergic and catecholaminergic enteric neurons through a Smad1-dependent pathway. Am. J Physiol Gastrointest. Liver Physiol. 2010;298(3) G375-G383.

[98] Dore JJ, Crotty KL, Birren SJ. Inhibition of glial maturation by bone morphogenetic protein 2 in a neural crest-derived cell line. Dev. Neurosci. 2005;27(1) 37-48.

[99] Dore JJ, Dewitt JC, Setty N, Donald MD, Joo E, Chesarone MA, et al. Multiple Signaling Pathways Converge to Regulate Bone-Morphogenetic-Protein-Dependent Glial Gene Expression. Dev. Neurosci. 2009.

[100] Gross RE, Mehler MF, Mabie PC, Zang Z, Santschi L, Kessler JA. Bone morphogenetic proteins promote astroglial lineage commitment by mammalian subventricular zone progenitor cells. Neuron. 1996;17(4) 595-606.

[101] Gomes WA, Mehler MF, Kessler JA. Transgenic overexpression of BMP4 increases astroglial and decreases oligodendroglial lineage commitment. Dev. Biol. 2003;255(1) 164-177.

[102] Stipursky J, Francis D, Gomes FC. Activation of MAPK/PI3K/SMAD Pathways by TGF-beta(1) Controls Differentiation of Radial Glia into Astrocytes in vitro. Dev. Neurosci. 2012;34(1) 68-81.

[103] Malatesta P, Hack MA, Hartfuss E, Kettenmann H, Klinkert W, Kirchhoff F, et al. Neuronal or glial progeny: regional differences in radial glia fate. Neuron. 2003;37(5) 751-764.

[104] Stipursky J, Spohr TC, Sousa VO, Gomes FC. Neuron-Astroglial Interactions in Cell-Fate Commitment and Maturation in the Central Nervous System. Neurochem. Res. 2012.

[105] Stipursky J, Gomes FC. TGF-beta1/SMAD signaling induces astrocyte fate commitment in vitro: implications for radial glia development. Glia. 2007;55(10) 1023-1033.

[106] Gomes FC, Paulin D, Moura N, V. Glial fibrillary acidic protein (GFAP): modulation by growth factors and its implication in astrocyte differentiation. Braz. J. Med. Biol. Res. 1999;32(5) 619-631.

[107] Sousa VO, Romao L, Neto VM, Gomes FC. Glial fibrillary acidic protein gene promoter is differently modulated by transforming growth factor-beta 1 in astrocytes from distinct brain regions. Eur. J. Neurosci. 2004;19(7) 1721-1730.

[108] Gomes FC, Garcia-Abreu J, Galou M, Paulin D, Moura N, V. Neurons induce GFAP gene promoter of cultured astrocytes from transgenic mice. Glia. 1999;26(2) 97-108.

[109] de Sampaio e Spohr T, Martinez R, da Silva EF, Neto VM, Gomes FC. Neuro-glia interaction effects on GFAP gene: a novel role for transforming growth factor-beta1. Eur. J. Neurosci. 2002;16(11) 2059-2069.

[110] Imura T, Tane K, Toyoda N, Fushiki S. Endothelial cell-derived bone morphogenetic proteins regulate glial differentiation of cortical progenitors. Eur. J Neurosci. 2008;27(7) 1596-1606.

[111] Mekki-Dauriac S, Agius E, Kan P, Cochard P. Bone morphogenetic proteins negatively control oligodendrocyte precursor specification in the chick spinal cord. Development. 2002;129(22) 5117-5130.

[112] Voumvourakis KI, Antonelou RC, Kitsos DK, Stamboulis E, Tsiodras S. TGF-beta/BMPs: crucial crossroad in neural autoimmune disorders. Neurochem. Int. 2011;59(5) 542-550.

[113] Hampton DW, Asher RA, Kondo T, Steeves JD, Ramer MS, Fawcett JW. A potential role for bone morphogenetic protein signalling in glial cell fate determination following adult central nervous system injury in vivo. Eur. J Neurosci. 2007;26(11) 3024-3035.

[114] Bilican B, Fiore-Heriche C, Compston A, Allen ND, Chandran S. Induction of Olig2 precursors by FGF involves BMP signalling blockade at the Smad level. PLoS. ONE. 2008;3(8) e2863.

[115] Agius E, Decker Y, Soukkarieh C, Soula C, Cochard P. Role of BMPs in controlling the spatial and temporal origin of GFAP astrocytes in the embryonic spinal cord. Dev. Biol. 2010;344(2) 611-620.

[116] Buckwalter MS, Yamane M, Coleman BS, Ormerod BK, Chin JT, Palmer T, et al. Chronically Increased Transforming Growth Factor-{beta}1 Strongly Inhibits Hippocampal Neurogenesis in Aged Mice. Am. J. Pathol. 2006;169(1) 154-164.

[117] Wachs FP, Winner B, Couillard-Despres S, Schiller T, Aigner R, Winkler J, et al. Transforming growth factor-beta1 is a negative modulator of adult neurogenesis. J. Neuropathol. Exp. Neurol. 2006;65(4) 358-370.

[118] Vogel T, Ahrens S, Buttner N, Krieglstein K. Transforming growth factor beta promotes neuronal cell fate of mouse cortical and hippocampal progenitors in vitro and in vivo: identification of Nedd9 as an essential signaling component. Cereb. Cortex. 2010;20(3) 661-671.

[119] Garcia-Campmany L, Marti E. The TGFbeta intracellular effector Smad3 regulates neuronal differentiation and cell fate specification in the developing spinal cord. Development. 2007;134(1) 65-75.

[120] Lu J, Wu Y, Sousa N, Almeida OF. SMAD pathway mediation of BDNF and TGF beta 2 regulation of proliferation and differentiation of hippocampal granule neurons. Development. 2005;132(14) 3231-3242.

[121] Battista D, Ferrari CC, Gage FH, Pitossi FJ. Neurogenic niche modulation by activated microglia: transforming growth factor beta increases neurogenesis in the adult dentate gyrus. Eur. J. Neurosci. 2006;23(1) 83-93.

[122] Ma M, Ma Y, Yi X, Guo R, Zhu W, Fan X, et al. Intranasal delivery of transforming growth factor-beta1 in mice after stroke reduces infarct volume and increases neurogenesis in the subventricular zone. BMC. Neurosci. 2008;9:117. 117.

[123] Wang Y, Symes AJ. Smad3 deficiency reduces neurogenesis in adult mice. J Mol Neurosci. 2010;41(3) 383-396.

[124] Yang X, Letterio JJ, Lechleider RJ, Chen L, Hayman R, Gu H, et al. Targeted disruption of SMAD3 results in impaired mucosal immunity and diminished T cell responsiveness to TGF-beta. EMBO J. 1999;18(5) 1280-1291.

[125] Roussa E, Wiehle M, Dunker N, Becker-Katins S, Oehlke O, Krieglstein K. Transforming growth factor beta is required for differentiation of mouse mesencephalic progenitors into dopaminergic neurons in vitro and in vivo: ectopic induction in dorsal mesencephalon. Stem Cells. 2006;24(9) 2120-2129.

[126] Kendall SE, Battelli C, Irwin S, Mitchell JG, Glackin CA, Verdi JM. NRAGE mediates p38 activation and neural progenitor apoptosis via the bone morphogenetic protein signaling cascade. Mol Cell Biol. 2005;25(17) 7711-7724.

[127] Gambaro K, Aberdam E, Virolle T, Aberdam D, Rouleau M. BMP-4 induces a Smad-dependent apoptotic cell death of mouse embryonic stem cell-derived neural precursors. Cell Death. Differ. 2006;13(7) 1075-1087.

[128] Brederlau A, Faigle R, Kaplan P, Odin P, Funa K. Bone morphogenetic proteins but not growth differentiation factors induce dopaminergic differentiation in mesencephalic precursors. Mol Cell Neurosci. 2002;21(3) 367-378.

[129] Toulouse A, Collins GC, Sullivan AM. Neurotrophic effects of growth/differentiation factor 5 in a neuronal cell line. Neurotox. Res. 2012;21(3) 256-265.

[130] Lindvall O. Dopaminergic neurons for Parkinson's therapy. Nat Biotechnol. 2012;30(1) 56-58.

[131] Rios I, Alvarez-Rodriguez R, Marti E, Pons S. Bmp2 antagonizes sonic hedgehog-mediated proliferation of cerebellar granule neurones through Smad5 signalling. Development. 2004;131(13) 3159-3168.

[132] Zhou YX, Zhao M, Li D, Shimazu K, Sakata K, Deng CX, et al. Cerebellar deficits and hyperactivity in mice lacking Smad4. J Biol Chem. 2003;278(43) 42313-42320.

[133] Morikawa Y, Zehir A, Maska E, Deng C, Schneider MD, Mishina Y, et al. BMP signaling regulates sympathetic nervous system development through Smad4-dependent and -independent pathways. Development. 2009;136(21) 3575-3584.

[134] Lopez-Coviella I, Mellott TM, Kovacheva VP, Berse B, Slack BE, Zemelko V, et al. Developmental pattern of expression of BMP receptors and Smads and activation of Smad1 and Smad5 by BMP9 in mouse basal forebrain. Brain Res. 2006;1088(1) 49-56.

[135] Williams S, Souchelnytskyi S, Danik M. TGFbeta2 mediates rapid inhibition of calcium influx in identified cholinergic basal forebrain neurons. Biochem. Biophys. Res Commun. 2002;290(4) 1321-1327.

[136] George O, Parducz A, Dupret D, Kharouby M, Le MM, Piazza PV, et al. Smad-dependent alterations of PPT cholinergic neurons as a pathophysiological mechanism of age-related sleep-dependent memory impairments. Neurobiol Aging. 2006;27(12) 1848-1858.

[137] Lopez-Coviella I, Berse B, Krauss R, Thies RS, Blusztajn JK. Induction and maintenance of the neuronal cholinergic phenotype in the central nervous system by BMP-9. Science. 2000;289(5477) 313-316.

[138] Schnitzler AC, Mellott TJ, Lopez-Coviella I, Tallini YN, Kotlikoff MI, Follettie MT, et al. BMP9 (bone morphogenetic protein 9) induces NGF as an autocrine/paracrine cholinergic trophic factor in developing basal forebrain neurons. J Neurosci. 2010;30(24) 8221-8228.

[139] Lopez-Coviella I, Mellott TJ, Schnitzler AC, Blusztajn JK. BMP9 protects septal neurons from axotomy-evoked loss of cholinergic phenotype. PLoS. ONE. 2011;6(6) e21166.

[140] Cho G, Lim Y, Golden JA. XLMR candidate mouse gene, Zcchc12 (Sizn1) is a novel marker of Cajal-Retzius cells. Gene Expr. Patterns. 2011;11(3-4) 216-220.

[141] Cho G, Lim Y, Zand D, Golden JA. Sizn1 is a novel protein that functions as a transcriptional coactivator of bone morphogenic protein signaling. Mol Cell Biol. 2008;28(5) 1565-1572.

[142] Yanagisawa M, Nakashima K, Takeda K, Ochiai W, Takizawa T, Ueno M, et al. Inhibition of BMP2-induced, TAK1 kinase-mediated neurite outgrowth by Smad6 and Smad7. Genes Cells. 2001;6(12) 1091-1099.

[143] Iwasaki S, Hattori A, Sato M, Tsujimoto M, Kohno M. Characterization of the bone morphogenetic protein-2 as a neurotrophic factor. Induction of neuronal differentiation of PC12 cells in the absence of mitogen-activated protein kinase activation. J Biol Chem. 1996;19;271(29) 17360-17365.

[144] Iwasaki S, Iguchi M, Watanabe K, Hoshino R, Tsujimoto M, Kohno M. Specific activation of the p38 mitogen-activated protein kinase signaling pathway and induction of neurite outgrowth in PC12 cells by bone morphogenetic protein-2. J Biol Chem. 1999;274(37) 26503-26510.

[145] Ebisawa T, Fukuchi M, Murakami G, Chiba T, Tanaka K, Imamura T, et al. Smurf1 interacts with transforming growth factor-beta type I receptor through Smad7 and induces receptor degradation. J. Biol. Chem. 2001;276(16) 12477-12480.

[146] Althini S, Usoskin D, Kylberg A, Kaplan PL, Ebendal T. Blocked MAP kinase activity selectively enhances neurotrophic growth responses. Mol Cell Neurosci. 2004;25(2) 345-354.

[147] Benavente F, Pinto C, Parada M, Henriquez JP, Osses N. Bone morphogenetic protein 2 inhibits neurite outgrowth of motor neuron-like NSC-34 cells and up-regulates its type II receptor. J Neurochem. 2012;122(3) 594-604.

[148] Ueberham U, Ueberham E, Gruschka H, Arendt T. Altered subcellular location of phosphorylated Smads in Alzheimer's disease. Eur. J Neurosci. 2006;24(8) 2327-2334.

[149] Ueberham U, Lange P, Ueberham E, Bruckner MK, Hartlage-Rubsamen M, Pannicke T, et al. Smad2 isoforms are differentially expressed during mouse brain development and aging. Int J Dev. Neurosci. 2009;27(5) 501-510.

[150] Stegmuller J, Huynh MA, Yuan Z, Konishi Y, Bonni A. TGFbeta-Smad2 signaling regulates the Cdh1-APC/SnoN pathway of axonal morphogenesis. J Neurosci. 2008;20;28(8) 1961-1969.

[151] Stegmuller J, Konishi Y, Huynh MA, Yuan Z, Dibacco S, Bonni A. Cell-intrinsic regulation of axonal morphogenesis by the Cdh1-APC target SnoN. Neuron. 2006;50(3) 389-400.

[152] Huynh MA, Ikeuchi Y, Netherton S, de lT-U, Kanadia R, Stegmuller J, et al. An isoform-specific SnoN1-FOXO1 repressor complex controls neuronal morphogenesis and positioning in the mammalian brain. Neuron. 2011;69(5) 930-944.

[153] Ikeuchi Y, Stegmuller J, Netherton S, Huynh MA, Masu M, Frank D, et al. A SnoN-Ccd1 pathway promotes axonal morphogenesis in the mammalian brain. J Neurosci. 2009;29(13) 4312-4321.

[154] Stegmuller J, Bonni A. Moving past proliferation: new roles for Cdh1-APC in postmitotic neurons. Trends Neurosci. 2005;28(11) 596-601.

[155] Konishi Y, Stegmuller J, Matsuda T, Bonni S, Bonni A. Cdh1-APC controls axonal growth and patterning in the mammalian brain. Science 2004;303(5660) 1026-1030.

[156] Makwana M, Raivich G. Molecular mechanisms in successful peripheral regeneration. FEBS J. 2005;272(11) 2628-2638.

[157] Goldberg JL, Klassen MP, Hua Y, Barres BA. Amacrine-signaled loss of intrinsic axon growth ability by retinal ganglion cells. Science. 2002;296(5574) 1860-1864.

[158] Zou H, Ho C, Wong K, Tessier-Lavigne M. Axotomy-induced Smad1 activation promotes axonal growth in adult sensory neurons. J Neurosci. 2009;29(22) 7116-7123.

[159] Parikh P, Hao Y, Hosseinkhani M, Patil SB, Huntley GW, Tessier-Lavigne M, et al. Regeneration of axons in injured spinal cord by activation of bone morphogenetic protein/Smad1 signaling pathway in adult neurons. Proc Natl Acad Sci U S A. 2011;108(19) E99-107.

[160] Zhu S, Wang W, Clarke DC, Liu X. Activation of Mps1 promotes transforming growth factor-beta-independent Smad signaling. J Biol Chem. 2007;282(25) 18327-18338.

[161] Ma CH, Brenner GJ, Omura T, Samad OA, Costigan M, Inquimbert P, et al. The BMP coreceptor RGMb promotes while the endogenous BMP antagonist noggin reduces

neurite outgrowth and peripheral nerve regeneration by modulating BMP signaling. J Neurosci. 2011;31(50) 18391-18400.

[162] Serpe M, O'Connor MB. The metalloprotease tolloid-related and its TGF-beta-like substrate Dawdle regulate Drosophila motoneuron axon guidance. Development. 2006;133(24) 4969-4979.

[163] Hodge LK, Klassen MP, Han BX, Yiu G, Hurrell J, Howell A, et al. Retrograde BMP signaling regulates trigeminal sensory neuron identities and the formation of precise face maps. Neuron 2007;55(4) 572-586.

[164] Ting CY, Herman T, Yonekura S, Gao S, Wang J, Serpe M, et al. Tiling of r7 axons in the Drosophila visual system is mediated both by transduction of an activin signal to the nucleus and by mutual repulsion. Neuron. 2007;56(5) 793-806.

[165] McCabe BD, Marques G, Haghighi AP, Fetter RD, Crotty ML, Haerry TE, et al. The BMP homolog Gbb provides a retrograde signal that regulates synaptic growth at the Drosophila neuromuscular junction. Neuron. 2003;39(2) 241-254.

[166] Ji SJ, Jaffrey SR. Intra-axonal translation of SMAD1/5/8 mediates retrograde regulation of trigeminal ganglia subtype specification. Neuron. 2012;74(1) 95-107.

[167] Takatoh J, Wang F. Axonally translated SMADs link up BDNF and retrograde BMP signaling. Neuron. 2012;74(1) 3-5.

[168] Jiang Y, McLennan IS, Koishi K, Hendry IA. Transforming growth factor-beta 2 is anterogradely and retrogradely transported in motoneurons and up-regulated after nerve injury. Neuroscience 2000;97(4) 735-742.

[169] Batut J, Howell M, Hill CS. Kinesin-mediated transport of Smad2 is required for signaling in response to TGF-beta ligands. Dev. Cell 2007;12(2) 261-274.

[170] Jin Q, Gao G, Mulder KM. Requirement of a dynein light chain in TGFbeta/Smad3 signaling. J. Cell Physiol 2009;221(3) 707-715.

[171] Eaton BA, Fetter RD, Davis GW. Dynactin is necessary for synapse stabilization. Neuron. 2002;34(5) 729-741.

[172] Allan DW, St Pierre SE, Miguel-Aliaga I, Thor S. Specification of neuropeptide cell identity by the integration of retrograde BMP signaling and a combinatorial transcription factor code. Cell 2003;113(1) 73-86.

[173] Goold CP, Davis GW. The BMP ligand Gbb gates the expression of synaptic homeostasis independent of synaptic growth control. Neuron. 2007;56(1) 109-123.

[174] Romao LF, Sousa VO, Neto VM, Gomes FC. Glutamate activates GFAP gene promoter from cultured astrocytes through TGF-beta1 pathways. J Neurochem. 2008;106(2) 746-756.

[175] Susarla BT, Laing ED, Yu P, Katagiri Y, Geller HM, Symes AJ. Smad proteins differentially regulate transforming growth factor-beta-mediated induction of chondroitin sulfate proteoglycans. J Neurochem. 2011;119(4) 868-878.

[176] Schachtrup C, Ryu JK, Helmrick MJ, Vagena E, Galanakis DK, Degen JL, et al. Fibrinogen triggers astrocyte scar formation by promoting the availability of active TGF-beta after vascular damage. J Neurosci. 2010;30(17) 5843-5854.

[177] Hellal F, Hurtado A, Ruschel J, Flynn KC, Laskowski CJ, Umlauf M, et al. Microtubule stabilization reduces scarring and causes axon regeneration after spinal cord injury. Science. 2011;331(6019) 928-931.

[178] Dummula K, Vinukonda G, Chu P, Xing Y, Hu F, Mailk S, et al. Bone morphogenetic protein inhibition promotes neurological recovery after intraventricular hemorrhage. J Neurosci. 2011;31(34) 12068-12082.

[179] Sweeney ST, Davis GW. Unrestricted synaptic growth in spinster-a late endosomal protein implicated in TGF-beta-mediated synaptic growth regulation. Neuron. 2002;36(3) 403-416.

[180] Rawson JM, Lee M, Kennedy EL, Selleck SB. Drosophila neuromuscular synapse assembly and function require the TGF-beta type I receptor saxophone and the transcription factor Mad. J Neurobiol. 2003;55(2) 134-150.

[181] Aberle H, Haghighi AP, Fetter RD, McCabe BD, Magalhaes TR, Goodman CS. wishful thinking encodes a BMP type II receptor that regulates synaptic growth in Drosophila. Neuron. 2002;33(4) 545-558.

[182] Marques G, Bao H, Haerry TE, Shimell MJ, Duchek P, Zhang B, et al. The Drosophila BMP type II receptor Wishful Thinking regulates neuromuscular synapse morphology and function. Neuron. 2002;33(4) 529-543.

[183] McCabe BD, Hom S, Aberle H, Fetter RD, Marques G, Haerry TE, et al. Highwire regulates presynaptic BMP signaling essential for synaptic growth. Neuron. 2004;41(6) 891-905.

[184] Wan HI, DiAntonio A, Fetter RD, Bergstrom K, Strauss R, Goodman CS. Highwire regulates synaptic growth in Drosophila. Neuron. 2000;26(2) 313-329.

[185] Dudu V, Bittig T, Entchev E, Kicheva A, Julicher F, Gonzalez-Gaitan M. Postsynaptic mad signaling at the Drosophila neuromuscular junction. Curr. Biol. 2006;16(7) 625-635.

[186] Ellis JE, Parker L, Cho J, Arora K. Activin signaling functions upstream of Gbb to regulate synaptic growth at the Drosophila neuromuscular junction. Dev. Biol. 2010;342(2) 121-133.

[187] Nahm M, Kim S, Paik SK, Lee M, Lee S, Lee ZH, et al. dCIP4 (Drosophila Cdc42-interacting protein 4) restrains synaptic growth by inhibiting the secretion of the retrograde Glass bottom boat signal. J Neurosci. 2010;30(24) 8138-8150.

[188] Dickson DW. Neuropathology of non-Alzheimer degenerative disorders. Int. J. Clin. Exp. Pathol. 2009;3(1) 1-23.

[189] Arendt T. Synaptic plasticity and cell cycle activation in neurons are alternative effector pathways: the 'Dr. Jekyll and Mr. Hyde concept' of Alzheimer's disease or the yin and yang of neuroplasticity. Prog. Neurobiol. 2003;71(2-3) 83-248.

[190] Lee HG, Ueda M, Zhu X, Perry G, Smith MA. Ectopic expression of phospho-Smad2 in Alzheimer's disease: uncoupling of the transforming growth factor-beta pathway? J Neurosci Res. 2006;84(8) 1856-1861.

[191] Chalmers KA, Love S. Neurofibrillary tangles may interfere with Smad 2/3 signaling in neurons. J Neuropathol. Exp. Neurol. 2007;66(2) 158-167.

[192] Ueberham U, Hilbrich I, Ueberham E, Rohn S, Glockner P, Dietrich K, et al. Transcriptional control of cell cycle-dependent kinase 4 by Smad proteins-implications for Alzheimer's disease. Neurobiol. Aging 2012;33(12) 2827-2840.

[193] Lee MH, Lin SR, Chang JY, Schultz L, Heath J, Hsu LJ, et al. TGF-beta induces TIAF1 self-aggregation via type II receptor-independent signaling that leads to generation of amyloid beta plaques in Alzheimer's disease. Cell Death. Dis. 2010;1:e110. e110.

[194] Metuzals J, Robitaille Y, Houghton S, Gauthier S, Leblanc R. Paired helical filaments and the cytoplasmic-nuclear interface in Alzheimer's disease. J. Neurocytol. 1988;17(6) 827-833.

[195] Sheffield LG, Miskiewicz HB, Tannenbaum LB, Mirra SS. Nuclear pore complex proteins in Alzheimer disease. J. Neuropathol. Exp. Neurol. 2006;65(1) 45-54.

[196] Worman HJ. Inner nuclear membrane and regulation of Smad-mediated signaling. Biochim. Biophys. Acta 2006;1761(5-6) 626-631.

[197] Xu L, Kang Y, Col S, Massague J. Smad2 nucleocytoplasmic shuttling by nucleoporins CAN/Nup214 and Nup153 feeds TGFbeta signaling complexes in the cytoplasm and nucleus. Mol. Cell 2002;10(2) 271-282.

[198] Ellgaard L, Ruddock LW. The human protein disulphide isomerase family: substrate interactions and functional properties. EMBO Rep. 2005;6(1) 28-32.

[199] Cataldo AM, Petanceska S, Terio NB, Peterhoff CM, Durham R, Mercken M, et al. Abeta localization in abnormal endosomes: association with earliest Abeta elevations in AD and Down syndrome. Neurobiol. Aging 2004;25(10) 1263-1272.

[200] Walter J, Fluhrer R, Hartung B, Willem M, Kaether C, Capell A, et al. Phosphorylation regulates intracellular trafficking of beta-secretase. J. Biol. Chem. 2001;276(18) 14634-14641.

[201] Hayes S, Chawla A, Corvera S. TGF beta receptor internalization into EEA1-enriched early endosomes: role in signaling to Smad2. J. Cell Biol. 2002;158(7) 1239-1249.

[202] Penheiter SG, Mitchell H, Garamszegi N, Edens M, Dore JJ, Jr., Leof EB. Internalization-dependent and -independent requirements for transforming growth factor beta receptor signaling via the Smad pathway. Mol. Cell Biol. 2002;22(13) 4750-4759.

[203] Runyan CE, Schnaper HW, Poncelet AC. The role of internalization in transforming growth factor beta1-induced Smad2 association with Smad anchor for receptor activation (SARA) and Smad2-dependent signaling in human mesangial cells. J. Biol. Chem. 2005;280(9) 8300-8308.

[204] Gagnon E, Duclos S, Rondeau C, Chevet E, Cameron PH, Steele-Mortimer O, et al. Endoplasmic reticulum-mediated phagocytosis is a mechanism of entry into macrophages. Cell 2002;110(1) 119-131.

[205] Touret N, Paroutis P, Grinstein S. The nature of the phagosomal membrane: endoplasmic reticulum versus plasmalemma. J. Leukoc. Biol. 2005;77(6) 878-885.

[206] Ueberham U, Arendt T. The expression of cell cycle proteins in neurons and its relevance for Alzheimer's disease. Curr. Drug Targets. CNS. Neurol. Disord. 2005;4(3) 293-306.

[207] Baig S, van HZ, Love S. Tau hyperphosphorylation affects Smad 2/3 translocation. Neuroscience. 2009;163(2) 561-570.

[208] Cowan CM, Bossing T, Page A, Shepherd D, Mudher A. Soluble hyper-phosphorylated tau causes microtubule breakdown and functionally compromises normal tau in vivo. Acta Neuropathol. 2010;120(5) 593-604.

[209] Connor B, Young D, Lawlor P, Gai W, Waldvogel H, Faull RL, et al. Trk receptor alterations in Alzheimer's disease. Brain Res. Mol. Brain Res. 1996;42(1) 1-17.

[210] Hock C, Heese K, Hulette C, Rosenberg C, Otten U. Region-specific neurotrophin imbalances in Alzheimer disease: decreased levels of brain-derived neurotrophic factor and increased levels of nerve growth factor in hippocampus and cortical areas. Arch. Neurol. 2000;57(6) 846-851.

[211] Arendt T, Holzer M, Stobe A, Gartner U, Luth HJ, Bruckner MK, et al. Activated mitogenic signaling induces a process of dedifferentiation in Alzheimer's disease that eventually results in cell death. Ann. N. Y. Acad. Sci. 2000;920 249-255.

[212] Moustakas A, Pardali K, Gaal A, Heldin CH. Mechanisms of TGF-beta signaling in regulation of cell growth and differentiation. Immunol. Lett. 2002;82(1-2) 85-91.

[213] Bachman KE, Park BH. Duel nature of TGF-beta signaling: tumor suppressor vs. tumor promoter. Curr. Opin. Oncol. 2005;17(1) 49-54.

[214] Peng B, Fleming JB, Breslin T, Grau AM, Fojioka S, Abbruzzese JL, et al. Suppression of tumorigenesis and induction of p15(ink4b) by Smad4/DPC4 in human pancreatic cancer cells. Clin. Cancer Res. 2002;8(11) 3628-3638.

[215] Motta M, Imbesi R, Di RM, Stivala F, Malaguarnera L. Altered plasma cytokine levels in Alzheimer's disease: correlation with the disease progression. Immunol. Lett. 2007;114(1) 46-51.

[216] Ueberham U, Ueberham E, Gruschka H, Arendt T. Connective tissue growth factor in Alzheimer's disease. Neuroscience 2003;116(1) 1-6.

[217] Docagne F, Gabriel C, Lebeurrier N, Lesne S, Hommet Y, Plawinski L, et al. Sp1 and Smad transcription factors co-operate to mediate TGF-beta-dependent activation of amyloid-beta precursor protein gene transcription. Biochem. J. 2004;383(Pt 2) 393-399.

[218] Burton T, Liang B, Dibrov A, Amara F. Transforming growth factor-beta-induced transcription of the Alzheimer beta-amyloid precursor protein gene involves interaction between the CTCF-complex and Smads. Biochem. Biophys. Res Commun. 2002;19;295(3) 713-723.

[219] Lee EO, Kang JL, Chong YH. The amyloid-beta peptide suppresses transforming growth factor-beta1-induced matrix metalloproteinase-2 production via Smad7 expression in human monocytic THP-1 cells. J Biol Chem. 2005;280(9) 7845-7853.

[220] Wyss-Coray T, Lin C, Yan F, Yu GQ, Rohde M, McConlogue L, et al. TGF-beta1 promotes microglial amyloid-beta clearance and reduces plaque burden in transgenic mice. Nat. Med. 2001;7(5) 612-618.

[221] Tichauer JE, von Bernhardi R. Transforming growth factor-beta stimulates beta amyloid uptake by microglia through Smad3-dependent mechanisms. J Neurosci Res. 2012;90(10) 1970-1980.

[222] Wisniewski HM, Wegiel J, Wang KC, Kujawa M, Lach B. Ultrastructural studies of the cells forming amyloid fibers in classical plaques. Can. J Neurol Sci. 1989;16(4 Suppl) 535-542.

[223] Town T, Laouar Y, Pittenger C, Mori T, Szekely CA, Tan J, et al. Blocking TGF-beta-Smad2/3 innate immune signaling mitigates Alzheimer-like pathology. Nat Med. 2008;14(6) 681-687.

[224] Chalmers KA, Love S. Phosphorylated Smad 2/3 colocalizes with phospho-tau inclusions in Pick disease, progressive supranuclear palsy, and corticobasal degeneration but not with alpha-synuclein inclusions in multiple system atrophy or dementia with Lewy bodies. J Neuropathol. Exp. Neurol. 2007;66(11) 1019-1026.

[225] Iravani MM, McCreary AC, Jenner P. Striatal plasticity in Parkinson's disease and L-dopa induced dyskinesia. Parkinsonism. Relat Disord. 2012;18 Suppl 1:S123-5. S123-S125.

[226] Wise RA. Roles for nigrostriatal--not just mesocorticolimbic--dopamine in reward and addiction. Trends Neurosci. 2009;32(10) 517-524.

[227] Lee CS, Samii A, Sossi V, Ruth TJ, Schulzer M, Holden JE, et al. In vivo positron emission tomographic evidence for compensatory changes in presynaptic dopaminergic nerve terminals in Parkinson's disease. Ann. Neurol. 2000;47(4) 493-503.

[228] Sossi V, de lF-F, Holden JE, Schulzer M, Ruth TJ, Stoessl J. Changes of dopamine turnover in the progression of Parkinson's disease as measured by positron emission tomography: their relation to disease-compensatory mechanisms. J Cereb. Blood Flow Metab. 2004;24(8) 869-876.

[229] Braithwaite SP, Stock JB, Mouradian MM. alpha-Synuclein phosphorylation as a therapeutic target in Parkinson's disease. Rev Neurosci. 2012;23(2) 191-198.

[230] Krieglstein K, Richter S, Farkas L, Schuster N, Dunker N, Oppenheim RW, et al. Reduction of endogenous transforming growth factors beta prevents ontogenetic neuron death. Nat. Neurosci. 2000;3(11) 1085-1090.

[231] Tapia-Gonzalez S, Giraldez-Perez RM, Cuartero MI, Casarejos MJ, Mena MA, Wang XF, et al. Dopamine and alpha-synuclein dysfunction in Smad3 null mice. Mol Neurodegener. 2011;6:72. 72.

[232] Hoy SM, Keating GM. Rasagiline: a review of its use in the treatment of idiopathic Parkinson's disease. Drugs. 2012;72(5) 643-669.

[233] Kriks S, Shim JW, Piao J, Ganat YM, Wakeman DR, Xie Z, et al. Dopamine neurons derived from human ES cells efficiently engraft in animal models of Parkinson's disease. Nature. 2011;480(7378) 547-551.

[234] Tsang HT, Edwards TL, Wang X, Connell JW, Davies RJ, Durrington HJ, et al. The hereditary spastic paraplegia proteins NIPA1, spastin and spartin are inhibitors of mammalian BMP signalling. Hum. Mol Genet. 2009;18(20) 3805-3821.

[235] Katsuno M, Adachi H, Minamiyama M, Waza M, Doi H, Kondo N, et al. Disrupted transforming growth factor-beta signaling in spinal and bulbar muscular atrophy. J Neurosci. 2010;30(16) 5702-5712.

[236] Mitchell JD, Borasio GD. Amyotrophic lateral sclerosis. Lancet. 2007;369(9578) 2031-2041.

[237] Strong MJ, Kesavapany S, Pant HC. The pathobiology of amyotrophic lateral sclerosis: a proteinopathy? J Neuropathol. Exp. Neurol. 2005;64(8) 649-664.

[238] Redler RL, Dokholyan NV. The complex molecular biology of amyotrophic lateral sclerosis (ALS). Prog. Mol Biol Transl. Sci. 2012;107:215-62. 215-262.

[239] Nakamura M, Ito H, Wate R, Nakano S, Hirano A, Kusaka H. Phosphorylated Smad2/3 immunoreactivity in sporadic and familial amyotrophic lateral sclerosis and its mouse model. Acta Neuropathol. 2008;115(3) 327-334.

[240] Nakamura M, Kaneko S, Wate R, Asayama S, Nakamura Y, Fujita K, et al. Regionally different immunoreactivity for Smurf2 and pSmad2/3 in TDP-43-positive inclusions of amyotrophic lateral sclerosis. Neuropathol. Appl. Neurobiol. 2012; 10-2990.

[241] Day WA, Koishi K, Nukuda H, McLennan IS. Transforming growth factor-beta 2 causes an acute improvement in the motor performance of transgenic ALS mice. Neurobiol. Dis. 2005;19(1-2) 323-330.

[242] Nakamura M, Kaneko S, Ito H, Jiang S, Fujita K, Wate R, et al. Activation of Transforming Growth Factor-beta/Smad Signaling Reduces Aggregate Formation of Mislocalized TAR DNA-Binding Protein-43. Neurodegener. Dis. 2012.

Section 2

Wnt Signaling and Neuronal Fate Decision

Chapter 4

Wnt Signaling Roles on the Structure and Function of the Central Synapses: Involvement in Alzheimer's Disease

Nibaldo C. Inestrosa and Lorena Varela-Nallar

Additional information is available at the end of the chapter

1. Introduction

Wnts compromise a large family of secreted glycoproteins that have shown to be part of the signaling molecules that regulate several aspects of development such as axis formation and midbrain development [1, 2]. In mammals at least 19 Wnt members have been found. The interaction of a Wnt protein with members of the Frizzled (Fz) family of seven-pass transmembrane cell-surface receptors triggers the activation of the Wnt signaling pathway [3-5]. In human and mice, 10 members of the Fz family have been identified. In addition, receptor-like tyrosine kinase (Ryk) and receptor tyrosine kinase-like orphan receptor (Ror2) have been identified as alternative Wnt receptors [6-8]. Different Wnt signaling cascades are activated downstream the Wnt receptors, identified as Wnt/β-catenin or canonical pathway, and β-catenin-independent or non-canonical pathways. The canonical pathway involves the transcription of Wnt target genes, while activation of non-canonical Wnt pathways may induce either an increase in intracellular calcium concentration or activation of the c-Jun-N-terminal kinase (JNK) cascade [3, 9, 10].

The Wnt pathway participates in the development of the central nervous system (CNS) and growing evidence indicate that Wnts also regulates the function of the adult nervous system [11, 12]. In fact, most of the key components including Wnts and Fz receptors are expressed in the adult brain [13, 14]. Wnt ligands have shown to regulate synaptic assembly as well synaptic plasticity and neurotransmission [15-20], and more recently it has also been involved in the adult neurogenesis [21-25].

Deregulation of the Wnt signaling has been associated to several pathologies, been cancer the most widely documented [26-28]. More recently, altered Wnt signaling have been related to mental disorders, mood disorders and neurodegenerative diseases [12, 29-32].

In the first part of this chapter we will address what is currently known about the signaling cascades of canonical and non-canonical pathways. Then, we will review recent findings from our and other labs on the specific effects of different Wnt ligands on the structure of pre- and postsynaptic regions and on glutamatergic neurotransmission in hippocampal neurons. The synaptic role of some Fz receptors will also be reviewed. Finally, the neuroprotective effect of the Wnt signaling activation will be discussed mainly focused on the protection against the toxicity of Aβ-peptide aggregates associated to the pathogenesis of Alzheimer's disease.

2. The Wnt signaling pathway: Canonical and non–canonical signaling cascades

The binding of Wnt ligands to Fz receptors can trigger the activation of different signaling cascades. In addition to Fz, other proteins have been described as alternative receptors or co-receptors, such as the low-density lipoprotein receptor-related protein 5 (LRP5), LRP6, Ror1, Ror2 and Ryk [3, 33-36], increasing the complexity of the Wnt signaling activation. It has been suggested that the binding of Wnts to specific receptors/co-receptors may selectively activate distinct signaling pathways.

The first Wnt signaling pathway identified was the canonical Wnt/β-catenin pathway (Figure 1). In the absence of Wnt stimulation, the levels of cytoplasmic β-catenin are low since it is ubiquitinated and constantly degraded in the proteasome [37]. β-catenin is phosphorylated by casein kinase 1α (CK1α) and glycogen synthase kinase-3β (GSK-3β) in a multiprotein complex composed also of the scaffold protein axin and adenomatous polyposis coli (APC) [38-42]. Phosphorylated β-catenin is recognized by β-TrCP, which is part of an E3 ubiquitin ligase complex, and is ubiquitinated and subsequently degraded [43]. Activation of the Wnt/β-catenin pathway initiated by the binding of a Wnt ligand to a Fz receptor and coreceptors LRP5/6 activates the protein Dishevelled (Dvl) usually by phosphorylation, and triggers the recruitment of axin to the phosphorylated tail of LRP, inhibiting the degradation pathway consequently inducing the cytoplasmic stabilization of β-catenin which enters the nucleus and regulates the transcription of Wnt target genes [28]. Recently, it was shown that when the destruction complex is associated with phosphorylated LRP, it may still capture and phosphorylates β-catenin, but ubiquitination is blocked (Figure 1, right panel) [44].

In the nucleus, β-catenin binds to members of the family of T-cell factor (Tcf) and lymphoid enhancer factor (Lef) [45-47]; this binding displaces Groucho, which is bound to Tcf/Lef and recruits histone deacetylases (HDAC) to repress the transcription of Wnt target genes [48-51]. Several Wnt target genes have been identified including *c-Myc, cyclin D1, Axin2, Calcium/ calmodulin-dependent protein kinase type IV* (CamKIV) [52-55]. In addition, by using an *in silico* analysis based on multiple Classification and Regression Tree (CART), 89 new genes were predicted to be targets of the Wnt/β-catenin pathway [56].

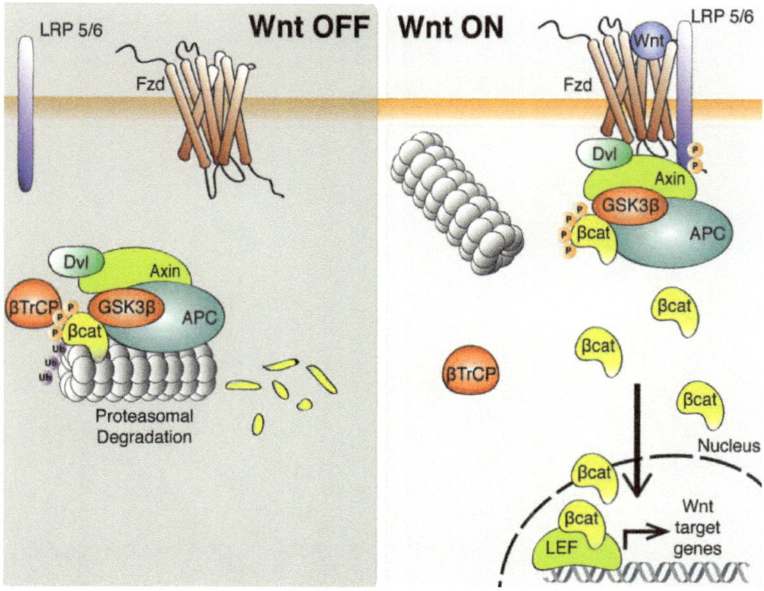

Figure 1. Canonical Wnt/β-catenin signaling pathway. (Left panel) In the absence of a Wnt protein, GSK-3β phosphorylates β-catenin which targets it for ubiquitination by β-TrCP and degradation in the proteasome. (Right panel) Activation of the signaling pathway by the binding of a Wnt ligand to Fz receptor and coreceptors LRP5/6 triggers the association of the destruction complex with phosphorylated LRP. In this condition, the complex may still capture and phosphorylate β-catenin, however the ubiquitination is blocked and it is stabilized in the cytoplasm and enters the nucleus to regulate the transcription of Wnt target genes.

There are at least two β-catenin-independent pathways: the planar cell polarity (PCP) pathway and the Ca^{2+} pathway (Figure 2). The PCP pathway was originally identified in *Drosophila* where it regulates tissue polarity and cell migration [10, 57]. This signaling pathway requires Fz receptors and Dvl and activates small GTPases including Rho and Rac and the protein kinase JNK. This pathway is also known as the Wnt/JNK pathway. The activation of the Wnt/Ca^{2+} pathway triggers the increase in intracellular Ca^{2+} levels and activates the protein kinases CamKII and protein kinase C (PKC) [10, 58]. It has been suggested that Wnt-mediated Ca^{2+} release involves heterotrimeric G proteins since it is inhibited by pertussis toxin [59]. As mentioned 10 Fz receptors are known in mammals. Fz receptors are seven-transmembrane-spanning receptors that belong to the G protein-coupled receptor (GPCR) list as a separate class [60]. Fz receptors have an extracellular amino-terminal region that contains a cysteine-rich domain (CRD) consisting of 120 to 125 residues with 10 conserved cysteines that is relevant for the binding of Wnt proteins [61]. Growing evidence indicate the involvement of G protein in the Wnt/Fz signaling. The first evidence came from inhibition of non-canonical Wnt effects by pertussis toxin [62]. Later on, many reports have indicated that heterotrimeric G protein participates of canonical and non-canonical Wnt signaling in *Drosophila, Xenopus* and mammals [63-69].

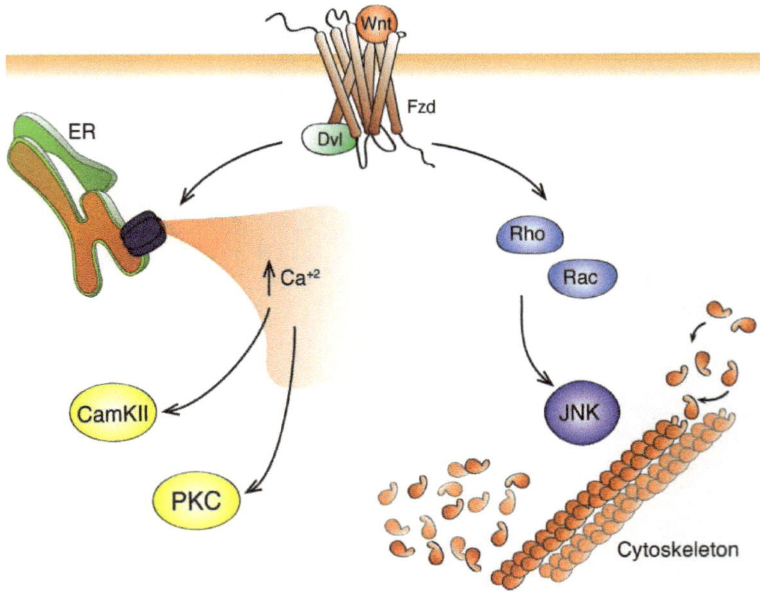

Figure 2. β-catenin-independent Wnt signaling pathways. In the Wnt/JNK pathway or PCP pathway, a Wnt ligand through a Fz receptors and Dvl activates small GTPases including Rho and Rac and JNK, which in turns modulate cytoskeletal organization. The activation of the Wnt/Ca^{2+} pathway triggers an increase in intracellular Ca^{2+} levels which activates CamKII and PKC.

3. Roles of the Wnt signaling pathway at central synapses

The Wnt signaling pathway has different roles during development linked to neurite patterning and synaptogenesis. Different Wnt ligands have been linked to the presynaptic assembly. In 1997, Salinas and co-workers demonstrated in cerebellar neurons that Wnt-7a increases the levels of synapsin I, a protein associated to synaptic vesicles [70]. Moreover, Wnt-7a mutant mice show a delay in the accumulation of synapsin I [71]. In hippocampal neurons Wnt-7a as well as Wnt-3a and Wnt-7b increases the number of pre-synaptic puncta suggesting a role for these ligands in presynaptic assembly [18, 72, 73]. In addition, Wnt-7a was found to stimulate recycling and endocytosis of synaptic vesicles using FM dyes [74]. In hippocampal neurons, Wnt-7a was also able to increase the expression as well as the clustering of the α7- nicotinic acetylcholine receptor (α7-nAChR), indicating that the Wnt signaling regulates the clustering of presynaptic receptors [75]. Interestingly, all these ligands are able to modulate presynaptic differentiation by activation of the Wnt/β-catenin signaling pathway, suggesting that some of the components associated with this pathway may be involved in the presynaptic effect. On the other hand, the non-canonical ligand Wnt-5a decreases the number of presynaptic terminals [72], indicating that canonical and non-canonical signaling pathways may have promoting and inhibitory effects on presynaptic differentiation respectively. In accordance, electrophysiological recordings on adult rat hippocampal slices showed that Wnt-7a, but not Wnt-5a, increased neurotransmitter release in CA3-CA1 synapses by decreasing paired pulse facilitation and increasing the frequency of miniature excitatory postsynaptic currents (mEPSC) [73]. Also, Wnt-7a/Dvl1 double mutant mice exhibit decreased mEPSC frequency at the mossy fiber-granule cell synapse revealing a defect in neurotransmitter release [18].

The Wnt signaling also plays relevant roles in the postsynaptic structure. Wnt-5a, which activates non-canonical Wnt signaling cascades in hippocampal neurons [19, 76], modulates postsynaptic assembly by increasing the clustering of the postsynaptic density protein-95 (PSD-95) and increases spine morphogenesis in cultured hippocampal neurons [15, 19]. PSD-95 is a scaffold protein of the postsynaptic density (PSD), which is a multiprotein complex that interacts with key molecules involved in the regulation of glutamate receptor targeting and trafficking and regulatory proteins relevant for neurotransmission [77, 78]. In hippocampal neurons, Wnt-5a induces a fast increase in the number of clusters of PSD-95 without affecting total levels of PSD-95 protein or presynaptic protein clustering [19]. This postsynaptic effect is dependent on Wnt/JNK signaling pathway as demonstrated by using JNK inhibitors. In long-term experiments, we observed that Wnt-5a is also able to increase the total number of synapses [79]. When hippocampal neurons were incubated with the formylated hexapeptide Foxy-5, which is derived from the sequence of Wnt-5a and mimics the full Wnt-5a molecule action in neurons and other systems [19, 80], there was an increase in PSD-95 since 1 hour, but after 24 hours an increase in the synaptic vesicle protein 2 (SV2) clustering was also observed. In consequence, there was an increase in the total number of synaptic contacts [79].

Also, we determined that Wnt-5a induced a transient formation of dendrite protrusions that resulted in a net increase of mature dendrite spines. Videomicroscopy revealed that Wnt-5a induced *de novo* formation of dendritic spines and also increased the size of the preexisting ones [15]. Interestingly, treatment with the soluble CRD region of Fz2, acting as a Wnt scavenger, decreased spine density in cultured neurons, supporting the physiological relevance of this finding and supporting the implication of Wnt ligands in dendrite spine morphogenesis. Wnt-7a is also able to increase the density and maturity of dendritic spines through a CamKII-dependent mechanism [81]. Wnt-7a rapidly activates CaMKII in spines and inhibition of this kinase abolishes the effects of Wnt-7a on spine growth and excitatory synaptic strength. This finding implicates the Wnt/Ca^{2+} signaling cascade in synaptic effects of Wnt ligands. Interestingly, Wnt-5a and Wnt-7a induces an increase in intracellular Ca^{2+} concentration [15, 81], supporting the activation of this non-canonical Wnt pathway.

In addition to the structural effects of Wnt ligands at the excitatory synapse, different Wnts have shown modulatory effects on glutamatergic neurotransmission. Wnt-3a modulates the recycling of synaptic vesicles in hippocampal synapses [73, 82] and is able to induce an increase in the frequency of mEPSC [20]. In hippocampal slices, blockade of Wnt signaling impairs long-term potentiation (LTP), whereas activation of Wnt signaling facilitates LTP [17]. In the case of Wnt-5a, acute application of this ligand in hippocampal slices increases the amplitude of field excitatory postsynaptic potentials (fEPSP) and upregulates synaptic NMDA receptor currents facilitating induction of LTP [15, 16]. Interestingly, Wnt-5a produced a two-step increase in the amplitude of NMDAR responses [16]. The mechanisms involved in this two-step effect of Wnt-5a were investigated by the delivery of specific protein kinase inhibitors via the recording pipette. Specifically, the role of PKC and JNK was investigated, since these are two known downstream kinases of the non-canonical pathway. Inhibition of $Ca2^{2+}$-dependent PKC isoforms with Go6976 or the more general PKC inhibitor calphostin C eliminated the first step of potentiation of NMDAR currents and did not affect the second one. On the contrary, the slower developing increase in NMDAR currents was blocked by the JNK inhibitors TI-JIP153-163 and SP600125. This indicate that there are two mechanisms involved in in the potentiation of NMDAR by Wnt-5a. There is a fast PKC-dependent potentiation and a slower JNK-dependent potentiation that does not require previous activation of PKC [16].

Wnt-5a also regulates postsynaptically the hippocampal inhibitory synapses [76]. *Wnt-5a* induces surface expression and maintenance of $GABA_A$ receptor in the membrane of hippocampal neurons, increases the amplitude of GABA-currents due to a postsynaptic mechanisms, and induces the recycling of functional $GABA_A$ receptors through activation of CaMKII [76]. Therefore Wnt-5a is able to modulate both, excitatory and inhibitory synapses which must be relevant for neurotransmission.

The novel role for Wnt ligands in synaptic transmission provides a mechanism for Wnt signaling to acutely modulate synaptic plasticity and brain function in later stages of development and in the mature organism. Importantly, neuronal activity modulates the release and expression of Wnt ligands which may be relevant for the function of these ligands during neurotransmission. Activation of NMDA receptors increases the expression of Wnt-2 in hippocampal neurons which then stimulates dendritic arborization [83]. On the other hand, tetanic stimulation induce NMDA receptor-dependent synaptic Wnt3a release [17]. The role for endogenous Wnts was supported by incubation of hippocampal slices with secreted Wnt inhibitors, such as secreted Frizzled-related protein-2 (sFRP-2), which showed that endogenous Wnt ligands are modulators of glutamatergic neurotransmission being necessary to maintain basal NMDA receptor synaptic transmission [15, 16].

The *in vivo* relevance for the role of Wnt signaling in activity-mediated synaptic connectivity was revealed in mice exposed to an enriched environment (EE). These animals showed increased complexity and number of large mossy fiber terminals in the CA3 region [84]. EE increased Wnt7a/b levels in CA3 pyramidal neurons and inhibiting Wnt signaling through locally applied sFRP-1, suppressed the effects of EE on synapse numbers and further reduced synapse numbers in control mice.

These findings show that Wnt ligands are important regulators of the synaptic structure during development and in adult neurons, and that the Wnt pathway is one of the signaling cascades regulated by neuronal activity that is involved in the regulation of neurotransmission in adult nervous system.

In addition to the role of Wnts, Fz receptor have also been involved in synaptic structure and function. In the hippocampus, we have determined that different Fz receptors have very different patterns of expression during development, being some of them highly expressed in adulthood and others during early development [85]. In addition, the distribution of Fzs in hippocampal neurons is also very specific. Some receptors, are located in the synaptic region, while others are mainly located in the soma or in the growth cones of young neurons [85]. These findings suggest that these receptors could be important regulators for the specific activation of the Wnt signaling cascades during the development of hippocampal circuits. In fact, we determined an association of the distribution with specific functions. In hippocampal neurons, Fz1 is located in the synaptic region co-localizing with presynaptic proteins and with active synaptic vesicle recycling sites [82]. Interestingly, overexpression of Fz1 increased the number of clusters of Bassoon, a component of the active zone involved in the structural organization of neurotransmitter release sites that is recruited early during synapse formation [86], suggesting that Fz1 regulates synaptic differentiation. In agreement, treatment with the extracellular CRD of Fz1 decreased Bassoon clustering which was not observed with the CRD of Fz2, indicating a receptor specificity for the synaptic effect [82]. Fz5 also has a role in mature neurons where it modulates the synaptogenic effect of Wnt7a [87]. As well as Fz1, Fz5 is present in synaptosomes and colocalizes with synaptic markers, and changes in the expression of this receptor modulates the density of synaptic sites [87]. In addition to its function in mature neurons, Fz5 was shown to be in high levels in the growth cones of developing hippocampal neurons [85], and we have recently determined that this receptor is involved in neural polarization (unpublished results). We determined that overexpression of Fz5 triggers a mislocalization of axonal proteins such as Tau-1 and phosphorylated MAP1B (MAP1BP), which change their distribution to the whole cell suggesting altered polarization. When the expression of Fz5 is knocked-down by shRNA, MAP1BP is not polarized and is almost completely lost. These findings suggest that in developing hippocampal neurons Fz5 is relevant for neural polarization. These studies indicate that Fz receptors are relevant players in both the developing and the adult nervous system and support the notion that the Wnt signaling pathway is crucial for different aspects of the development and function of the CNS.

4. Role of Wnt signaling in adult neurogenesis

In the adult brain, there are two regions where there is a continuous generation of new neurons (Figure 3A), the subventricular zone (SVZ) of the lateral ventricles [88] and the subgranular zone (SGZ) in the hippocampal dentate gyrus [89]. In the SVZ, astrocyte-like neural stem cells (NSCs), called type B1 cells, generate type C cells that rapidly proliferate and give rise to type A neuroblasts (Figure 3B). These cells migrate through the rostral migratory stream to the olfactory bulb where they became interneurons [88] (Figure 3A). In the SGZ, radial and non-radial neural precursor cells give rise to transient amplifying progenitors that generate neuroblasts and then became immature neurons that extend dendrites toward the molecular layer and project their axons through the hilus toward the CA3 region [90] (Figure 3C). Newborn neurons then mature and fully integrate into the preexisting hippocampal circuitry.

Adult neurogenesis is highly regulated by intrinsic and extrinsic mechanisms. Many signaling pathways have been identified as regulators of different aspects of neurogenesis. Notch, Shh,

BMPs, and Wnts are part of the signaling molecules of the niche that regulate the maintenance, activation and fate specification of neural precursor cells [91, 92].

In Wnt/β-catenin reporter mice (BATGAL) it was shown that this pathway is active in the SGZ and the dentate granule cell layer [23]. In that study, authors determined that Wnt3 is expressed in adult hippocampal astrocytes and that adult hippocampal progenitor (AHP) cells express key components of the Wnt/β-catenin signaling pathway. These findings suggested that the Wnt pathway may be involved in the regulation of adult neurogenesis. *In vitro* analysis in cultured cells revealed that Wnts derived from hippocampal astrocytes stimulate Wnt/β-catenin signaling in isolated AHPs inducing their neuronal commitment [23]. The effect of the Wnt signaling was supported *in vivo* using lentiviral vectors expressing Wnt3a or a secreted mutant Wnt1 protein that blocks Wnt signaling. Lentiviruses were stereotactically injected into the dentate gyrus of rats. As assessed by the incorporation of the nucleotide analog BrdU and immunodetection of the immature neuron protein doublecortin (DCX), blocking the Wnt signaling decreases adult hippocampal neurogenesis while stimulating this pathway has the opposite effect [23]. More recently, and by using the same lentiviral approach to block Wnt signaling in the dentate gyrus of adult rats it was shown that Wnt-mediated adult hippocampal neurogenesis contributes to learning and memory [93]. In the SVZ, β-catenin signaling also plays a role in the proliferation of progenitor cells in the adult mouse brain [94]. Retrovirus-mediated expression of a stabilized β-catenin promoted the proliferation of type C cells and inhibited their differentiation into neuroblasts. Also in the SVZ, transduction of the β-catenin inhibitor axin by intracranial lentiviral delivery decreased cell proliferation as revealed by decreased BrdU labeling [95], further supporting a role for Wnt/β-catenin signaling in neural stem cell proliferation in the neurogenic areas of adult brain.

The Wnt-mediated effects in neurogenesis may be caused by the transcriptional activation of NeuroD1 which is dependent on the Wnt/β-catenin signaling activation [25]. NeuroD1 is a basic helix-loop-helix transcription factor important for the generation of granule cell and olfactory neuron in the embryonic and adult brain [96]. NeuroD1 gene promoter has overlapping DNA-binding site for Sox2 and TCF/LEF, then the activation of this gene implies activation of the canonical Wnt pathway and removal of Sox2 repression from the NeuroD1 gene promoter [25]. More recently, Prox1 was also determined as a target of the Wnt/β-catenin pathway relevant for neurogenesis [22]. Prox1 is expressed in newborn and mature granule cells and is required for the proper differentiation and survival of newborn granule cells, but not for the maintenance of granule cells after they have fully matured [22].

In addition, Wnts could indirectly modulate adult neurogenesis thorough their effects on neuronal activity. As previously described, different Wnts regulate glutamatergic neurotransmission, and evidence indicates that neural progenitor cells respond to neuronal activity as part of their differentiation program [97]. GABA is an important modulator of adult hippocampal neurogenesis being critical for the proper development and maturation of adult-born neurons [98-100]. Interestingly, Wnt-5a through activation of CaMKII, induces the recycling of functional $GABA_A$ receptors on hippocampal neurons and modulates inhibitory synapses [76].

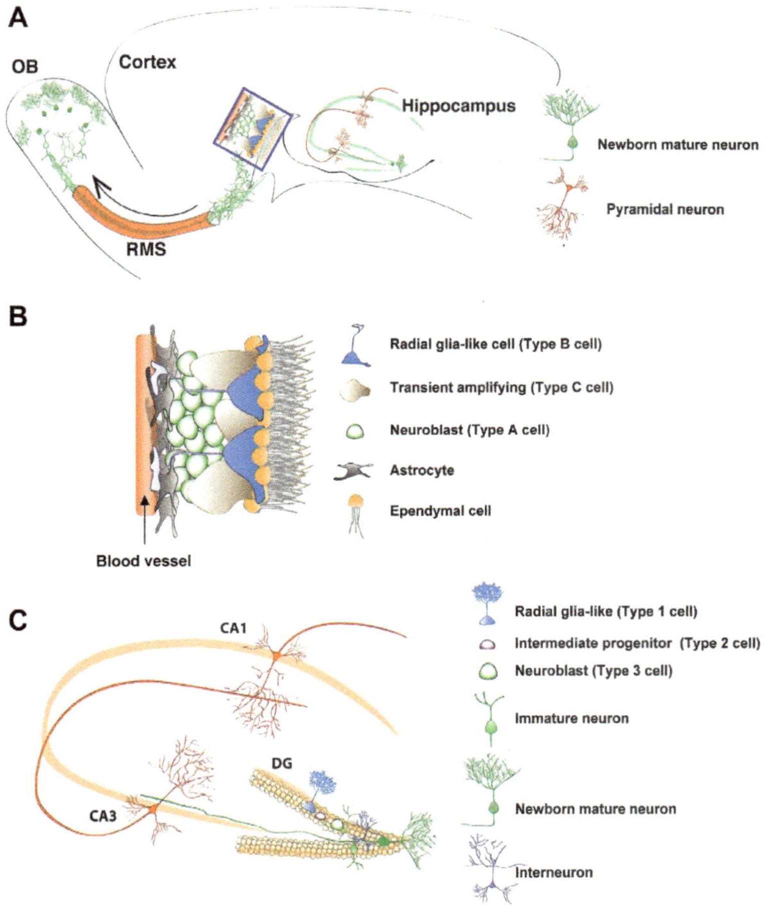

Figure 3. Neurogenesis in the adult brain. (A) Schematic representation of adult rodent brain highlighting the two neurogenic regions. The hippocampus and the SVZ (boxed). (B) Schematic of the SVZ in the wall of the lateral ventricles. Distinct stem/progenitor cell types (types B, C, and A) are shown. (C) Neurogenesis in the SGZ of the hippocampal dentate gyrus. The progression of radial type 1 cells to mature newborn granule neurons is schematized.

As mentioned, in neurogenic niches Wnts are provided by astrocytes [23], and during aging it was reported that the levels of Wnt3 protein and the number of Wnt3-secreting astrocytes declines [101], which may be one of the factors underlying the impairment of neurogenesis that is observed in aging [102, 103]. On the contrary, running, that is a potent stimulator of adult neurogenesis in the SGZ [104] was found to significantly increase *de novo* expression of Wnt-3 [101], pointing to the Wnt pathway as one of the factors involved in running-mediated increase in neurogenesis. In addition to astrocytes-derived Wnts, an autocrine Wnt signaling activity has been observed in adult hippocampal progenitors (AHPs) derived from adult rat brains. Inhibiting this autocrine Wnt signaling increases the number of neurons formed and leads to a loss of multipotency among AHPs indicating that this autocrine pathway may preserve the balance between neural stem cell maintenance and differentiation [105].

The Wnt signaling has also been involved in the mechanism of the orphan nuclear receptor TLX (also known as NR2E1), which is an important regulator of neural stem cell maintenance and self-renewal in embryonic and adult brains [106, 107] and is involved in neurogenesis in the SVZ [108] and hippocampus [109]. To stimulate neural stem cell proliferation and self-renewal TLX activates the Wnt/β-catenin pathway in adult mouse neural stem cells by activating the expression of Wnt-7a, which expression was found to be downregulated in TLX-null mice, through binding to two TLX binding sites present in the Wnt-7a gene promoter [95]. Wnt-7a is important for adult neural stem cell proliferation *in vivo* since there is a decreased BrdU labeling in the SGZ and SVZ of adult Wnt7a knockout mice. In $TLX^{-/-}$ mice, intracranial lentiviral transduction of active β-catenin led to a considerable rescue of cell proliferation in the SVZ, suggesting that Wnt/β-catenin acts downstream of TLX to regulate neural stem cell proliferation *in vivo* [95].

It has been shown that low oxygen is associated with increased levels of β-catenin *in vivo*, and that hypoxia inducible factor-1α (HIF-1α) modulates the Wnt/β-catenin signaling in embryonic stem cells exposed to low oxygen [110]. Recently, we determined *in vivo* that hypoxia stimulates the activation of the Wnt/β-catenin signaling pathway in the hippocampus of adult mice (our unpublished results), and stimulates cell proliferation in the SGZ of 2 month old wild-type mice.

Altogether, these findings indicate that the Wnt pathway is relevant not only for the development of the nervous system but also for the development of new neurons in the adult brain, being important for the maintenance and self-renewal of the stem cell pool and for the commitment and proliferation of new neurons.

5. Wnt signaling in Alzheimer's disease

Alzheimer's disease (AD) is a neurodegenerative disorder characterized by a progressive deterioration of cognitive abilities, cerebral accumulation of extracellular amyloid plaques composed mainly of amyloid-β peptide (Aβ), and synaptic alterations [111]. In addition to the accumulation of Aβ aggregates, which is a product of the processing of the amyloid precursor protein (APP), cytoskeletal alterations associated to the abnormal phosphorylation of the microtubule associated protein tau [112, 113] are early manifestations that lead to aberrant remodeling of dendrites and axons, the appearance of dystrophic neurites, synaptic loss [114], and eventually progressive loss of neuronal populations [112].

During more than a decade, a strong relationship between an impaired Wnt signaling pathway activity and neuronal damage in AD has been raised [31, 115-118]. Different studies have shown that Wnt signaling components are altered in AD [119-124], and in addition, the Wnt signaling pathway has been related to other neurodegenerative disorders such as autism and schizophrenia [30, 125]. Among the Wnt components that are affected in AD, it was shown that β-catenin levels are reduced in AD patients carrying presenilin-1 (PS-1)-inherited mutations [124], while the secreted Wnt antagonist Dickkopf-1 (Dkk1) is elevated in postmortem AD brains and brains from transgenic mouse models for AD [121, 126]. A variant of the LRP6 has been associated with late-onset AD, which confers low levels of Wnt signaling [119]. In addition, genetic studies show a link between Wnt signaling and AD. Epidemiological data show an increased risk for AD in populations where the allele 4 of apo-lipoprotein E (apoE4) is present. Interestingly apoE4 causes inhibition of the canonical Wnt signaling in PC12 cells upon stimulation with Wnt-7a as determined by luciferase activities and nuclear β-catenin levels [127]. Aβ directly binds to the extracellular CRD of Fz5 at or in close proximity to the Wnt-binding site inhibiting the canonical Wnt signaling pathway [128], linking directly Aβ to Wnt impairment. Moreover, the exposure of cultured rat hippocampal neurons to Aβ results in inhibition of canonical Wnt signaling as determined by destabilization of endogenous levels of β-catenin, increase in GSK-3β activity, and a decrease in the expression of some Wnt target genes [129]. Moreover, acute exposure to Aβ increases Dkk1 mRNA levels in hippocampal brain slices, which seems to be associated to synaptic loss induced by Aβ [130].

As mentioned, one of the hallmarks of AD brains is the abnormal phosphorylation of the tau protein which accumulates as intraneuronal neurofibrillary tangles [131]. Several kinases can phosphorylate tau *in vitro*; however, the bulk of the information supports that Cdk5, extracellular signal-related kinase 2, microtubule affinity-regulating kinase and GSK-3β, a key component of the Wnt cascade, are the most relevant kinases for tau phosphorylation *in vivo* [132, 133]. Cultured neurons exposed to Aβ show an increased GSK-3β activity [134, 135], and active GSK-3β has been found in brains staged for AD neurofibrillary changes, with a concomitant decrease in β-catenin levels and an increase in *tau* hyperphosphorylation [136]. Also, neurodegeneration and spatial learning deficits have been observed in GSK-3β conditional transgenic mice [137, 138]. Interestingly, a study shows that the phosphorylation of tau antagonizes apoptosis by stabilizing β-catenin; therefore, up-regulation of β-catenin during tau phosphorylation prevents the cell from going into apoptosis. Increasing levels of phosphorylated tau was correlated with increased levels of nuclear β-catenin, and the knockdown of β-catenin antagonizes the anti-apoptotic effects of *tau* [139]. These findings support a role of β-catenin as a survival element in AD.

Several studies have shown neuroprotective properties of the Wnt signaling activation against the toxicity of Aβ peptide. In cultured hippocampal neurons, exposure to Aβ aggregates causes a decrease in endogenous β-catenin levels, and this effect was overcome by direct activation of the pathway with Wnt-3a conditioned media [117, 129]. The protective effect of Wnt-3a against the toxicity of Aβ oligomers was shown to be mediated by Fz1 receptor, since this effect is modulated by the expression levels of Fz1 in both, PC12 cells and hippocampal neurons [14]. Overexpression of Fz1 significantly increased cell survival induced by Wnt-3a and diminished caspase-3 activation, while knocking-down the expression of the receptor by antisense oligonucleotides decreased the stabilization of β-catenin induced by Wnt-3a and decreased the neuroprotive effect elicited by this Wnt ligand [14].

In agreement with the effect of Wnt-3a, inhibition of GSK-3β by lithium protects hippocampal neurons from Aβ-induced damage. More importantly, *in vivo* lithium treatment of double transgenic APPswe/PSEN1ΔE9 mice, which is a well characterized *in vivo* model of AD that shows most hallmarks of the disease [140], reduced spatial memory impairment, decreased Aβ oligomers and the activation of astrocytes and microglia [141]. *In vivo*, lithium treatment activated the Wnt signaling as shown by the increase in β-catenin and by the inhibition of GSK-3β [141]. These studies suggest that the loss of normal Wnt/β-catenin signaling activity may be involved in the Aβ-dependent neurodegeneration observed in AD and that the activation of the pathway might have beneficial effects for the treatment of the disease [12].

APPswe/PSEN1ΔE9 mice show decreased levels of adult neurogenesis [142]. In these mice, we evaluated the effect of hypoxia on the generation of new neurons in the hippocampus. As previously mentioned hypoxia induces the activation of the Wnt/β-catenin signaling pathway in the hippocampus of wild-type mice. Mice were exposed to low oxygen and neurogenesis was evaluated by incorporation of BrdU and double staining with DCX. It was determined that hypoxia is a strong stimulator of neurogenesis in AD mice (our unpublished results). Currently we are evaluating whether this effect is related to the activation of the canonical Wnt pathway. Also, we have observed that voluntary wheel running strongly increased neurogenesis in APPswe/PSEN1ΔE9 mice and also decreased Aβ burden and tau phosphorylation (our unpublished results). As previously mentioned, voluntary running was found to increase *de novo* expression of Wnt-3 [101], suggesting that the effects observed in runner AD mice could involve the activation of the Wnt signaling pathway.

In addition to the role of the canonical Wnt signaling, we have studied whether Wnt-5a is able to protect neurons against Aβ oligomers synaptotoxicity [143]. Synaptic failure is an early event in AD, and soluble Aβ oligomers are proposed to be responsible for the synaptic pathology that occurs before the plaque deposition and neuronal death [74, 144]. Electrophysiological analysis of Schaffer collaterals-CA1 glutamatergic transmission in hippocampal slices demonstrated that Wnt-5a prevents the decrease in the amplitude of fEPSP and EPSCs induced by Aβ oligomers, indicating that Wnt-5a prevents the synaptic damage triggered by Aβ [143]. Moreover, Wnt-5a prevented the decrease in the postsynaptic density scaffold protein PSD-95 and synaptic loss in cultured hippocampal neurons [143], supporting that Wnt-5a improves synaptic function in the presence of Aβ.

Additionally, the activation of several signaling pathways that crosstalk with the Wnt pathway also supports the neuroprotective potential of the Wnt cascades in AD [12].

6. Conclusions

As we have discussed throughout this Chapter, the Wnt signaling pathway has fundamental roles in the development and function of the CNS. As discussed, the canonical and non-canonical Wnt signaling cascades have shown to be important for the formation and structure of central synapses, and in addition to the structural effects, Wnt ligands acutely modulate synaptic transmission and plasticity. Also, in the adult brain the Wnt pathway is one of the signaling cascades that regulates the generation of new neurons in neurogenic niches. Importantly, different stimuli that regulate neurogenesis involve the regulation of the Wnt signaling, implicating this pathway as a relevant player in the modulation of this physiological process.

Considering all the discussed roles of Wnts, it was expected that alterations in the Wnt cascades leads to diseases associated to the nervous system. In fact, deregulation of the Wnt pathway has been related to mental disorders, mood disorders and neurodegenerative diseases. As we have discussed, a bulk of evidence associate Wnt dysfunction to AD, and strongly point to a neuroprotective potential of the Wnt cascades as a therapeutic approach. Future work should focus on explore the therapeutic benefits of stimulating the Wnt signaling pathway *in vivo*.

Acknowledgements

We thank to Felipe G. Serrano for his contribution in the artwork. This work was supported by Grants from FONDECYT (N°1120156) and the Basal Center of Excellence in Science and Technology (CONICYT-PFB12/2007) to NCI and FONDECYT (N°11110012) and Insertion of Postdoctoral Researchers in the Academy (CONICYT-79090027) to LV-N.

Author details

Nibaldo C. Inestrosa and Lorena Varela-Nallar

Center for Aging and Regeneration (CARE), Department of Cell and Molecular Biology, Faculty of Biological Sciences, Pontifical Catholic University of Chile, Santiago, Chile

References

[1] Nusse, R, & Varmus, H. Three decades of Wnts: a personal perspective on how a scientific field developed. EMBO J (2012)., 31(12), 2670-84.

[2] Van Amerongen, R, & Nusse, R. Towards an integrated view of Wnt signaling in development. Development (Cambridge, England) (2009)., 136(19), 3205-14.

[3] Gordon, M. D, & Nusse, R. Wnt signaling: multiple pathways, multiple receptors, and multiple transcription factors. J Biol Chem (2006)., 281(32), 22429-33.

[4] Schulte, G. International Union of Basic and Clinical Pharmacology. LXXX. The class Frizzled receptors. Pharmacol Rev (2010)., 62(4), 632-67.

[5] Wang, H. Y, Liu, T, & Malbon, C. C. Structure-function analysis of Frizzleds. Cell Signal (2006). , 18(7), 934-41.

[6] Keeble, T. R, Halford, M. M, Seaman, C, Kee, N, Macheda, M, Anderson, R. B, Stacker, S. A, & Cooper, H. M. The Wnt receptor Ryk is required for Wnt5a-mediated axon guidance on the contralateral side of the corpus callosum. J Neurosci (2006). , 26(21), 5840-8.

[7] Oishi, I, Suzuki, H, Onishi, N, Takada, R, Kani, S, Ohkawara, B, Koshida, I, Suzuki, K, Yamada, G, Schwabe, G. C, Mundlos, S, Shibuya, H, Takada, S, & Minami, Y. The receptor tyrosine kinase Ror2 is involved in non-canonical Wnt5a/JNK signalling pathway. Genes Cells (2003). , 8(7), 645-54.

[8] Ho, H. Y, Susman, M. W, Bikoff, J. B, Ryu, Y. K, Jonas, A. M, Hu, L, Kuruvilla, R, & Greenberg, M. E. Wnt5a-Ror-Dishevelled signaling constitutes a core developmental pathway that controls tissue morphogenesis. Proc Natl Acad Sci U S A (2012). , 109(11), 4044-51.

[9] Angers, S, & Moon, R. T. Proximal events in Wnt signal transduction. Nat Rev Mol Cell Biol (2009). , 10(7), 468-77.

[10] Veeman, M. T, Axelrod, J. D, & Moon, R. T. A second canon. Functions and mechanisms of beta-catenin-independent Wnt signaling. Developmental cell (2003). , 5(3), 367-77.

[11] Salinas, P. C, & Zou, Y. Wnt signaling in neural circuit assembly. Annu Rev Neurosci (2008). , 31-339.

[12] Inestrosa, N. C, & Arenas, E. Emerging roles of Wnts in the adult nervous system. Nature reviews (2010). , 11(2), 77-86.

[13] Shimogori, T, Vansant, J, Paik, E, & Grove, E. A. Members of the Wnt, Fz, and Frp gene families expressed in postnatal mouse cerebral cortex. J Comp Neurol (2004). , 473(4), 496-510.

[14] Chacon, M. A, Varela-Nallar, L, & Inestrosa, N. C. Frizzled-1 is involved in the neuroprotective effect of Wnt3a against Abeta oligomers. J Cell Physiol (2008). , 217(1), 215-27.

[15] Varela-Nallar, L, Alfaro, I. E, Serrano, F. G, Parodi, J, & Inestrosa, N. C. Wingless-type family member 5A (Wnt-5a) stimulates synaptic differentiation and function of glutamatergic synapses. Proc Natl Acad Sci U S A (2010). , 107(49), 21164-9.

[16] Cerpa, W, Gambrill, A, Inestrosa, N. C, & Barria, A. Regulation of NMDA-receptor synaptic transmission by Wnt signaling. J Neurosci (2011). , 31(26), 9466-71.

[17] Chen, J, Park, C. S, & Tang, S. J. Activity-dependent synaptic Wnt release regulates hippocampal long term potentiation. J Biol Chem (2006). , 281(17), 11910-6.

[18] Ahmad-Annuar, A, Ciani, L, Simeonidis, I, Herreros, J, Fredj, N. B, Rosso, S. B, Hall, A, Brickley, S, & Salinas, P. C. Signaling across the synapse: a role for Wnt and Dish-

evelled in presynaptic assembly and neurotransmitter release. J Cell Biol (2006). , 174(1), 127-39.

[19] Farias, G. G, Alfaro, I. E, Cerpa, W, Grabowski, C. P, Godoy, J. A, Bonansco, C, & Inestrosa, N. C. Wnt-5a/JNK signaling promotes the clustering of PSD-95 in hippocampal neurons. J Biol Chem (2009). , 284(23), 15857-66.

[20] Avila, M. E, Sepulveda, F. J, Burgos, C. F, Moraga-Cid, G, Parodi, J, Moon, R. T, Aguayo, L. G, Opazo, C, & De Ferrari, G. V. Canonical Wnt3a modulates intracellular calcium and enhances excitatory neurotransmission in hippocampal neurons. J Biol Chem (2010). , 285(24), 18939-47.

[21] Clevers, H, & Nusse, R. Wnt/beta-catenin signaling and disease. Cell (2012). , 149(6), 1192-205.

[22] Karalay, O, Doberauer, K, Vadodaria, K. C, Knobloch, M, Berti, L, Miquelajauregui, A, Schwark, M, Jagasia, R, Taketo, M. M, Tarabykin, V, Lie, D. C, & Jessberger, S. Prospero-related homeobox 1 gene (Prox1) is regulated by canonical Wnt signaling and has a stage-specific role in adult hippocampal neurogenesis. Proc Natl Acad Sci U S A (2011). , 108(14), 5807-12.

[23] Lie, D. C, Colamarino, S. A, Song, H. J, Desire, L, Mira, H, Consiglio, A, Lein, E. S, Jessberger, S, Lansford, H, Dearie, A. R, & Gage, F. H. Wnt signalling regulates adult hippocampal neurogenesis. Nature (2005). , 437(7063), 1370-5.

[24] Zhang, L, Yang, X, Yang, S, & Zhang, J. The Wnt /beta-catenin signaling pathway in the adult neurogenesis. Eur J Neurosci (2011). , 33(1), 1-8.

[25] Kuwabara, T, Hsieh, J, Muotri, A, Yeo, G, Warashina, M, Lie, D. C, Moore, L, Nakashima, K, Asashima, M, & Gage, F. H. Wnt-mediated activation of NeuroD1 and retro-elements during adult neurogenesis. Nat Neurosci (2009). , 12(9), 1097-105.

[26] Polakis, P. The many ways of Wnt in cancer. Curr Opin Genet Dev (2007). , 17(1), 45-51.

[27] Klaus, A, & Birchmeier, W. Wnt signalling and its impact on development and cancer. Nat Rev Cancer (2008). , 8(5), 387-98.

[28] Logan, C. Y, & Nusse, R. The Wnt signaling pathway in development and disease. Annu Rev Cell Dev Biol (2004). , 20, 781-810.

[29] De Ferrari, G. V, & Moon, R. T. The ups and downs of Wnt signaling in prevalent neurological disorders. Oncogene (2006). , 25(57), 7545-53.

[30] Lovestone, S, & Killick, R. Di Forti M,Murray R. Schizophrenia as a GSK-3 dysregulation disorder. Trends Neurosci (2007). , 30(4), 142-9.

[31] De Ferrari, G. V, & Inestrosa, N. C. Wnt signaling function in Alzheimer's disease. Brain Res Brain Res Rev (2000). , 33(1), 1-12.

[32] Williams, R. S, & Harwood, A. J. Lithium therapy and signal transduction. Trends Pharmacol Sci (2000). , 21(2), 61-4.

[33] Fradkin, L. G, Dura, J. M, & Noordermeer, J. N. Ryks: new partners for Wnts in the developing and regenerating nervous system. Trends Neurosci (2009). , 33(2), 84-92.

[34] Green, J. L, Kuntz, S. G, & Sternberg, P. W. Ror receptor tyrosine kinases: orphans no more. Trends Cell Biol (2008). , 18(11), 536-44.

[35] Kikuchi, A, Yamamoto, H, & Kishida, S. Multiplicity of the interactions of Wnt proteins and their receptors. Cell Signal (2007). , 19(4), 659-71.

[36] Cadigan, K. M, & Liu, Y. I. Wnt signaling: complexity at the surface. J Cell Sci (2006). Pt 3) 395-402.

[37] Aberle, H, Bauer, A, Stappert, J, Kispert, A, & Kemler, R. beta-catenin is a target for the ubiquitin-proteasome pathway. EMBO J (1997). , 16(13), 3797-804.

[38] Ikeda, S, Kishida, S, Yamamoto, H, Murai, H, Koyama, S, & Kikuchi, A. Axin, a negative regulator of the Wnt signaling pathway, forms a complex with GSK-3beta and beta-catenin and promotes GSK-3beta-dependent phosphorylation of beta-catenin. EMBO J (1998). , 17(5), 1371-84.

[39] Kishida, S, Yamamoto, H, Ikeda, S, Kishida, M, Sakamoto, I, Koyama, S, & Kikuchi, A. Axin, a negative regulator of the wnt signaling pathway, directly interacts with adenomatous polyposis coli and regulates the stabilization of beta-catenin. J Biol Chem (1998). , 273(18), 10823-6.

[40] Hart, M. J. de los Santos R, Albert IN, Rubinfeld B,Polakis P. Downregulation of beta-catenin by human Axin and its association with the APC tumor suppressor, beta-catenin and GSK3 beta. Curr Biol (1998). , 8(10), 573-81.

[41] Itoh, K, Krupnik, V. E, & Sokol, S. Y. Axis determination in Xenopus involves biochemical interactions of axin, glycogen synthase kinase 3 and beta-catenin. Curr Biol (1998). , 8(10), 591-4.

[42] Sakanaka, C, Weiss, J. B, & Williams, L. T. Bridging of beta-catenin and glycogen synthase kinase-3beta by axin and inhibition of beta-catenin-mediated transcription. Proc Natl Acad Sci U S A (1998). , 95(6), 3020-3.

[43] Liu, C, Li, Y, Semenov, M, Han, C, Baeg, G. H, Tan, Y, Zhang, Z, Lin, X, & He, X. Control of beta-catenin phosphorylation/degradation by a dual-kinase mechanism. Cell (2002). , 108(6), 837-47.

[44] Li, V. S, Ng, S. S, Boersema, P. J, Low, T. Y, Karthaus, W. R, Gerlach, J. P, Mohammed, S, Heck, A. J, Maurice, M. M, Mahmoudi, T, & Clevers, H. Wnt signaling through inhibition of beta-catenin degradation in an intact Axin1 complex. Cell (2012). , 149(6), 1245-56.

[45] Behrens, J, Von Kries, J. P, Kuhl, M, Bruhn, L, Wedlich, D, Grosschedl, R, & Birchmeier, W. Functional interaction of beta-catenin with the transcription factor LEF-1. Nature (1996)., 382(6592), 638-42.

[46] Eastman, Q, & Grosschedl, R. Regulation of LEF-1/TCF transcription factors by Wnt and other signals. Curr Opin Cell Biol (1999)., 11(2), 233-40.

[47] Huber, O, Korn, R, Mclaughlin, J, Ohsugi, M, Herrmann, B. G, & Kemler, R. Nuclear localization of beta-catenin by interaction with transcription factor LEF-1. Mech Dev (1996)., 59(1), 3-10.

[48] Roose, J, Molenaar, M, Peterson, J, Hurenkamp, J, Brantjes, H, & Moerer, P. van de Wetering M, Destree O,Clevers H. The Xenopus Wnt effector XTcf-3 interacts with Groucho-related transcriptional repressors. Nature (1998)., 395(6702), 608-12.

[49] Cavallo, R. A, Cox, R. T, Moline, M. M, Roose, J, Polevoy, G. A, Clevers, H, Peifer, M, & Bejsovec, A. Drosophila Tcf and Groucho interact to repress Wingless signalling activity. Nature (1998)., 395(6702), 604-8.

[50] Hurlstone, A. Clevers H. T-cell factors: turn-ons and turn-offs. EMBO J (2002)., 21(10), 2303-11.

[51] Chen, G, Fernandez, J, Mische, S, & Courey, A. J. A functional interaction between the histone deacetylase Rpd3 and the corepressor groucho in Drosophila development. Genes Dev (1999)., 13(17), 2218-30.

[52] Arrazola, M. S, Varela-Nallar, L, Colombres, M, Toledo, E. M, Cruzat, F, Pavez, L, Assar, R, Aravena, A, Gonzalez, M, Montecino, M, Maass, A, Martinez, S, & Inestrosa, N. C. Calcium/calmodulin-dependent protein kinase type IV is a target gene of the Wnt/beta-catenin signaling pathway. J Cell Physiol (2009)., 221(3), 658-67.

[53] Jho, E. H, Zhang, T, Domon, C, Joo, C. K, Freund, J. N, & Costantini, F. Wnt/beta-catenin/Tcf signaling induces the transcription of Axin2, a negative regulator of the signaling pathway. Mol Cell Biol (2002)., 22(4), 1172-83.

[54] Jung, H. C, & Kim, K. Identification of MYCBP as a beta-catenin/LEF-1 target using DNA microarray analysis. Life Sci (2005)., 77(11), 1249-62.

[55] Tetsu, O, & Mccormick, F. Beta-catenin regulates expression of cyclin D1 in colon carcinoma cells. Nature (1999)., 398(6726), 422-6.

[56] Hodar, C, Assar, R, Colombres, M, Aravena, A, Pavez, L, Gonzalez, M, Martinez, S, Inestrosa, N. C, & Maass, A. Genome-wide identification of new Wnt/beta-catenin target genes in the human genome using CART method. BMC Genomics (2010)., 11:348

[57] Adler, P. N. Planar signaling and morphogenesis in Drosophila. Developmental cell (2002)., 2(5), 525-35.

[58] Kohn, A. D, & Moon, R. T. Wnt and calcium signaling: beta-catenin-independent pathways. Cell Calcium (2005). , 38(3-4), 439-46

[59] Slusarski, D. C, Yang-snyder, J, Busa, W. B, & Moon, R. T. Modulation of embryonic intracellular Ca2+ signaling by Wnt-5A. Dev Biol (1997). , 182(1), 114-20.

[60] Foord, S. M, Bonner, T. I, Neubig, R. R, Rosser, E. M, Pin, J. P, Davenport, A. P, Spedding, M, & Harmar, A. J. International Union of Pharmacology. XLVI. G protein-coupled receptor list. Pharmacol Rev (2005). , 57(2), 279-88.

[61] Dann, C. E, Hsieh, J. C, Rattner, A, Sharma, D, Nathans, J, & Leahy, D. J. Insights into Wnt binding and signalling from the structures of two Frizzled cysteine-rich domains. Nature (2001). , 412(6842), 86-90.

[62] Slusarski, D. C, Corces, V. G, & Moon, R. T. Interaction of Wnt and a Frizzled homologue triggers G-protein-linked phosphatidylinositol signalling. Nature (1997). , 390(6658), 410-3.

[63] Liu, X, Rubin, J. S, & Kimmel, A. R. Rapid, Wnt-induced changes in GSK3beta associations that regulate beta-catenin stabilization are mediated by Galpha proteins. Curr Biol (2005). , 15(22), 1989-97.

[64] Salmanian, S, Najafi, S. M, Rafipour, M, Arjomand, M. R, Shahheydari, H, Ansari, S, Kashkooli, L, Rasouli, S. J, Jazi, M. S, & Minaei, T. Regulation of GSK-3beta and beta-Catenin by Galphaq in HEK293T cells. Biochem Biophys Res Commun (2010). , 395(4), 577-82.

[65] Najafi, S. M. Activators of G proteins inhibit GSK-3beta and stabilize beta-Catenin in Xenopus oocytes. Biochem Biophys Res Commun (2009). , 382(2), 365-9.

[66] Katanaev, V. L, Ponzielli, R, Semeriva, M, & Tomlinson, A. Trimeric G protein-dependent frizzled signaling in Drosophila. Cell (2005). , 120(1), 111-22.

[67] Katanaev, V. L, & Tomlinson, A. Dual roles for the trimeric G protein Go in asymmetric cell division in Drosophila. Proc Natl Acad Sci U S A (2006). , 103(17), 6524-9.

[68] Jernigan, K. K, Cselenyi, C. S, Thorne, C. A, Hanson, A. J, Tahinci, E, Hajicek, N, Oldham, W. M, Lee, L. A, Hamm, H. E, Hepler, J. R, Kozasa, T, Linder, M. E, & Lee, E. Gbetagamma activates GSK3 to promote LRP6-mediated beta-catenin transcriptional activity. Sci Signal (2010). ra37.

[69] Liu, X, Liu, T, Slusarski, D. C, Yang-snyder, J, Malbon, C. C, Moon, R. T, & Wang, H. Activation of a frizzled-2/beta-adrenergic receptor chimera promotes Wnt signaling and differentiation of mouse F9 teratocarcinoma cells via Galphao and Galphat. Proc Natl Acad Sci U S A (1999). , 96(25), 14383-8.

[70] Lucas, F. R, & Salinas, P. C. WNT-7a induces axonal remodeling and increases synapsin I levels in cerebellar neurons. Dev Biol (1997). , 192(1), 31-44.

[71] Hall, A. C, Lucas, F. R, & Salinas, P. C. Axonal remodeling and synaptic differentiation in the cerebellum is regulated by WNT-7a signaling. Cell (2000)., 100(5), 525-35.

[72] Davis, E. K, Zou, Y, & Ghosh, A. Wnts acting through canonical and noncanonical signaling pathways exert opposite effects on hippocampal synapse formation. Neural Dev (2008)., 3, 32.

[73] Cerpa, W, Godoy, J. A, Alfaro, I, Farias, G. G, Metcalfe, M. J, Fuentealba, R, Bonansco, C, & Inestrosa, N. C. Wnt-7a modulates the synaptic vesicle cycle and synaptic transmission in hippocampal neurons. J Biol Chem (2008)., 283(9), 5918-27.

[74] Cerpa, W, Dinamarca, M. C, & Inestrosa, N. C. Structure-function implications in Alzheimer's disease: effect of Abeta oligomers at central synapses. Curr Alzheimer Res (2008)., 5(3), 233-43.

[75] Farias, G. G, Valles, A. S, Colombres, M, Godoy, J. A, Toledo, E. M, Lukas, R. J, Barrantes, F. J, & Inestrosa, N. C. Wnt-7a induces presynaptic colocalization of alpha 7-nicotinic acetylcholine receptors and adenomatous polyposis coli in hippocampal neurons. J Neurosci (2007)., 27(20), 5313-25.

[76] Cuitino, L, Godoy, J. A, Farias, G. G, Couve, A, Bonansco, C, Fuenzalida, M, & Inestrosa, N. C. Wnt-5a modulates recycling of functional GABAA receptors on hippocampal neurons. J Neurosci (2010)., 30(25), 8411-20.

[77] Han, K, & Kim, E. Synaptic adhesion molecules and PSD-95. Progress in neurobiology (2008)., 84(3), 263-83.

[78] Li, Z, & Sheng, M. Some assembly required: the development of neuronal synapses. Nat Rev Mol Cell Biol (2003)., 4(11), 833-41.

[79] Varela-Nallar, L, Parodi, J, Farias, G. G, & Inestrosa, N. C. Wnt-5a is a synaptogenic factor with neuroprotective properties against Abeta toxicity. Neurodegener Dis (2012)., 10(1-4), 23-6.

[80] Safholm, A, Leandersson, K, Dejmek, J, Nielsen, C. K, Villoutreix, B. O, & Andersson, T. A formylated hexapeptide ligand mimics the ability of Wnt-5a to impair migration of human breast epithelial cells. J Biol Chem (2006)., 281(5), 2740-9.

[81] Ciani, L, Boyle, K. A, Dickins, E, Sahores, M, Anane, D, Lopes, D. M, Gibb, A. J, & Salinas, P. C. Wnt7a signaling promotes dendritic spine growth and synaptic strength through Ca2+/Calmodulin-dependent protein kinase II. Proc Natl Acad Sci U S A (2011)., 108(26), 10732-7.

[82] Varela-Nallar, L, Grabowski, C. P, Alfaro, I. E, Alvarez, A. R, & Inestrosa, N. C. Role of the Wnt receptor Frizzled-1 in presynaptic differentiation and function. Neural Dev (2009)., 4, 41.

[83] Wayman, G. A, Impey, S, Marks, D, Saneyoshi, T, Grant, W. F, Derkach, V, & Soderling, T. R. Activity-dependent dendritic arborization mediated by CaM-kinase I acti-

vation and enhanced CREB-dependent transcription of Wnt-2. Neuron (2006)., 50(6), 897-909.

[84] Gogolla, N, Galimberti, I, Deguchi, Y, & Caroni, P. Wnt signaling mediates experience-related regulation of synapse numbers and mossy fiber connectivities in the adult hippocampus. Neuron (2009)., 62(4), 510-25.

[85] Varela-Nallar, L, Ramirez, V. T, Gonzalez-billault, C, & Inestrosa, N. C. Frizzled receptors in neurons: From growth cones to the synapse. Cytoskeleton (Hoboken) (2012)., 69(7), 528-34.

[86] Zhai, R, Olias, G, Chung, W. J, Lester R. A, tom Dieck, S, Langnaese, K, Kreutz, M. R, Kindler, S, Gundelfinger, E. D, & Garner C. C. Temporal appearance of the presynaptic cytomatrix protein bassoon during synaptogenesis. Mol Cell Neurosci (2000)., 15(5), 417-28.

[87] Sahores, M, Gibb, A, & Salinas, P. C. Frizzled-5, a receptor for the synaptic organizer Wnt7a, regulates activity-mediated synaptogenesis. Development (Cambridge, England) (2010)., 137(13), 2215-25.

[88] Alvarez-Buylla, A, & Garcia-Verdugo, J. M. Neurogenesis in adult subventricular zone. J Neurosci (2002)., 22(3), 629-34.

[89] Gage, F. H. Mammalian neural stem cells. Science (New York, N.Y.) (2000)., 287(5457), 1433-8.

[90] Zhao, C, Teng, E. M, Summers, R. G Jr, Ming, G. L, & Gage, F. H. Distinct morphological stages of dentate granule neuron maturation in the adult mouse hippocampus. J Neurosci (2006)., 26(1), 3-11.

[91] Suh, H, Deng, W, & Gage, F. H. Signaling in adult neurogenesis. Annu Rev Cell Dev Biol (2009)., 25, 253-75.

[92] Ming, G. L, & Song, H. Adult neurogenesis in the mammalian brain: significant answers and significant questions. Neuron (2011)., 70(4), 687-702.

[93] Jessberger, S, Clark, R. E, Broadbent, N. J, Clemenson, G. D Jr, Consiglio, A, Lie, D. C, Squire, L. R, & Gage, F. H. Dentate gyrus-specific knockdown of adult neurogenesis impairs spatial and object recognition memory in adult rats. Learn Mem (2009)., 16(2), 147-54.

[94] Adachi, K, Mirzadeh, Z, Sakaguchi, M, Yamashita, T, Nikolcheva, T, Gotoh, Y, Peltz, G, Gong, L, Kawase, T, Alvarez-Buylla, A, Okano, H, & Sawamoto, K. Beta-catenin signaling promotes proliferation of progenitor cells in the adult mouse subventricular zone. Stem Cells (2007)., 25(11), 2827-36.

[95] Qu, Q, Sun, G, Li, W, Yang, S, Ye, P, Zhao, C, Yu, R. T, Gage, F. H, Evans, R. M, & Shi, Y. Orphan nuclear receptor TLX activates Wnt/beta-catenin signalling to stimulate neural stem cell proliferation and self-renewal. Nat Cell Biol (2010). sup , 1-9.

[96] Gao, Z, Ure, K, Ables, J. L, Lagace, D. C, Nave, K. A, Goebbels, S, Eisch, A. J, & Hsieh, J. Neurod1 is essential for the survival and maturation of adult-born neurons. Nat Neurosci (2009)., 12(9), 1090-2.

[97] Deisseroth, K, Singla, S, Toda, H, Monje, M, Palmer, T. D, & Malenka, R. C. Excitation-neurogenesis coupling in adult neural stem/progenitor cells. Neuron (2004)., 42(4), 535-52.

[98] Ge, S, Goh, E. L, Sailor, K. A, Kitabatake, Y, Ming, G. L, & Song, H. GABA regulates synaptic integration of newly generated neurons in the adult brain. Nature (2006)., 439(7076), 589-93.

[99] Jagasia, R, Steib, K, Englberger, E, Herold, S, Faus-kessler, T, Saxe, M, Gage, F. H, Song, H, & Lie, D. C. GABA-cAMP response element-binding protein signaling regulates maturation and survival of newly generated neurons in the adult hippocampus. J Neurosci (2009)., 29(25), 7966-77.

[100] Tozuka, Y, Fukuda, S, Namba, T, Seki, T, & Hisatsune, T. GABAergic excitation promotes neuronal differentiation in adult hippocampal progenitor cells. Neuron (2005)., 47(6), 803-15.

[101] Okamoto, M, Inoue, K, Iwamura, H, Terashima, K, Soya, H, Asashima, M, & Kuwabara, T. Reduction in paracrine Wnt3 factors during aging causes impaired adult neurogenesis. Faseb J (2011)., 25(10), 3570-82.

[102] Kuhn, H. G, Dickinson-anson, H, & Gage, F. H. Neurogenesis in the dentate gyrus of the adult rat: age-related decrease of neuronal progenitor proliferation. J Neurosci (1996)., 16(6), 2027-33.

[103] Varela-Nallar, L, Aranguiz, F. C, Abbott, A. C, Slater, P. G, & Inestrosa, N. C. Adult hippocampal neurogenesis in aging and Alzheimer's disease. Birth Defects Res C Embryo Today (2010)., 90(4), 284-96.

[104] Van Praag, H, Kempermann, G, & Gage, F. H. Running increases cell proliferation and neurogenesis in the adult mouse dentate gyrus. Nat Neurosci (1999)., 2(3), 266-70.

[105] Wexler, E. M, Paucer, A, Kornblum, H. I, Palmer, T. D, & Geschwind, D. H. Endogenous Wnt signaling maintains neural progenitor cell potency. Stem Cells (2009)., 27(5), 1130-41.

[106] Shi, Y. Chichung Lie, D, Taupin, P, Nakashima, K, Ray, J, Yu, R. T, Gage, F. H, & Evans, R. M. Expression and function of orphan nuclear receptor TLX in adult neural stem cells. Nature (2004)., 427(6969), 78-83.

[107] Li, W, Sun, G, Yang, S, Qu, Q, Nakashima, K, & Shi, Y. Nuclear receptor TLX regulates cell cycle progression in neural stem cells of the developing brain. Mol Endocrinol (2008)., 22(1), 56-64.

[108] Liu, H. K, Belz, T, Bock, D, Takacs, A, Wu, H, Lichter, P, Chai, M, & Schutz, G. The nuclear receptor tailless is required for neurogenesis in the adult subventricular zone. Genes Dev (2008). , 22(18), 2473-8.

[109] Zhang, C. L, Zou, Y, He, W, Gage, F. H, & Evans, R. M. A role for adult TLX-positive neural stem cells in learning and behaviour. Nature (2008). , 451(7181), 1004-7.

[110] Mazumdar , J, O'Brien, W. T, Johnson, R. S, LaManna, J. C, Chavez, J. C, Klein, P. S, & Simon, M. C. O2 regulates stem cells through Wnt/beta-catenin signalling. Nat Cell Biol (2010). , 12(10), 1007-13.

[111] Toledo, E. M, Colombres, M, & Inestrosa, N. C. Wnt signaling in neuroprotection and stem cell differentiation. Progress in neurobiology (2008). , 86(3), 281-96.

[112] Dickson, D. W. Apoptotic mechanisms in Alzheimer neurofibrillary degeneration: cause or effect? J Clin Invest (2004). , 114(1), 23-7.

[113] Takashima, A, Noguchi, K, Sato, K, Hoshino, T, & Imahori, K. Tau protein kinase I is essential for amyloid beta-protein-induced neurotoxicity. Proc Natl Acad Sci U S A (1993). , 90(16), 7789-93.

[114] Tsai, L. H, Lee, M. S, & Cruz, J. Cdk5, a therapeutic target for Alzheimer's disease? Biochim Biophys Acta (2004). , 1697(1-2), 137-42

[115] Garrido, J. L, Godoy, J. A, Alvarez, A, Bronfman, M, & Inestrosa, N. C. Protein kinase C inhibits amyloid beta peptide neurotoxicity by acting on members of the Wnt pathway. Faseb J (2002). , 16(14), 1982-4.

[116] Inestrosa, N. C, Alvarez, A, Godoy, J, Reyes, A, & De Ferrari, G. V. Acetylcholinesterase-amyloid-beta-peptide interaction and Wnt signaling involvement in Abeta neurotoxicity. Acta Neurol Scand Suppl (2000). , 53-9.

[117] De Ferrari, G. V, Chacon, M. A, Barria, M. I, Garrido, J. L, Godoy, J. A, Olivares, G, Reyes, A. E, Alvarez, A, Bronfman, M, & Inestrosa, N. C. Activation of Wnt signaling rescues neurodegeneration and behavioral impairments induced by beta-amyloid fibrils. Mol Psychiatry (2003). , 8(2), 195-208.

[118] Inestrosa, N, De Ferrari, G. V, Garrido, J. L, Alvarez, A, Olivares, G. H, Barria, M. I, Bronfman, M, & Chacon, M. A. Wnt signaling involvement in beta-amyloid-dependent neurodegeneration. Neurochem Int (2002). , 41(5), 341-4.

[119] De Ferrari, G. V, Papassotiropoulos, A, Biechele, T, Wavrant De-Vrieze, F, Avila, M. E, Major, M. B, Myers, A, Sáez, K, Henríquez, J. P, Zhao, A, Wollmer, M. A, Nitsch, R. M, Hock, C, Morris, C. M, Hardy, J, & Moon, R. T. Common genetic variation within the low-density lipoprotein receptor-related protein 6 and late-onset Alzheimer's disease. Proc Natl Acad Sci U S A (2007). , 104(22), 9434-9.

[120] Alvarez, G, Munoz-montano, J. R, Satrustegui, J, Avila, J, Bogonez, E, & Diaz-nido, J. Regulation of tau phosphorylation and protection against beta-amyloid-induced neu-

rodegeneration by lithium. Possible implications for Alzheimer's disease. Bipolar Disord (2002)., 4(3), 153-65.

[121] Caricasole, A, Copani, A, Caraci, F, Aronica, E, Rozemuller, A. J, Caruso, A, Storto, M, Gaviraghi, G, Terstappen, G. C, & Nicoletti, F. Induction of Dickkopf-1, a negative modulator of the Wnt pathway, is associated with neuronal degeneration in Alzheimer's brain. J Neurosci (2004)., 24(26), 6021-7.

[122] Ghanevati, M, & Miller, C. A. Phospho-beta-catenin accumulation in Alzheimer's disease and in aggresomes attributable to proteasome dysfunction. J Mol Neurosci (2005)., 25(1), 79-94.

[123] Takashima, A, Murayama, M, Murayama, O, Kohno, T, Honda, T, Yasutake, K, Nihonmatsu, N, Mercken, M, Yamaguchi, H, Sugihara, S, & Wolozin, B. Presenilin 1 associates with glycogen synthase kinase-3beta and its substrate tau. Proc Natl Acad Sci U S A (1998)., 95(16), 9637-41.

[124] Zhang, Z, Hartmann, H, Do, V. M, Abramowski, D, Sturchler-Pierrat, C, Staufenbiel, M, Sommer, B, van de Wetering, M, Clevers, H, Saftig, P, De Strooper, B, He, X, & Yankner B. A. Destabilization of beta-catenin by mutations in presenilin-1 potentiates neuronal apoptosis. Nature (1998)., 395(6703), 698-702.

[125] Moon, R. T, Kohn, A. D, De Ferrari, G. V, & Kaykas, A. WNT and beta-catenin signalling: diseases and therapies. Nat Rev Genet (2004)., 5(9), 691-701.

[126] Rosi, M. C, Luccarini, I, Grossi, C, Fiorentini, A, Spillantini, M. G, Prisco, A, Scali, C, Gianfriddo, M, Caricasole, A, Terstappen, G. C, & Casamenti, F. Increased Dickkopf-1 expression in transgenic mouse models of neurodegenerative disease. J Neurochem (2010)., 112(6), 1539-51.

[127] Caruso, A, Motolese, M, Iacovelli, L, Caraci, F, Copani, A, Nicoletti, F, Terstappen, G. C, Gaviraghi, G, & Caricasole, A. Inhibition of the canonical Wnt signaling pathway by apolipoprotein E4 in PC12 cells. J Neurochem (2006)., 98(2), 364-71.

[128] Magdesian, M. H, Carvalho, M. M, Mendes, F. A, Saraiva, L. M, Juliano, M. A, Juliano, L, Garcia-abreu, J, & Ferreira, S. T. Amyloid-beta binds to the extracellular cysteine-rich domain of Frizzled and inhibits Wnt/beta-catenin signaling. J Biol Chem (2008)., 283(14), 9359-68.

[129] Alvarez, A. R, Godoy, J. A, Mullendorff, K, Olivares, G. H, Bronfman, M, & Inestrosa, N. C. Wnt-3a overcomes beta-amyloid toxicity in rat hippocampal neurons. Exp Cell Res (2004)., 297(1), 186-96.

[130] Purro, S. A, Dickins, E. M, & Salinas, P. C. The secreted Wnt antagonist Dickkopf-1 is required for amyloid beta-mediated synaptic loss. J Neurosci (2010)., 32(10), 3492-8.

[131] Ballard, C, Gauthier, S, Corbett, A, Brayne, C, Aarsland, D, & Jones, E. Alzheimer's disease. Lancet (2011)., 377(9770), 1019-31.

[132] Churcher, I. Tau therapeutic strategies for the treatment of Alzheimer's disease. Curr Top Med Chem (2006). , 6(6), 579-95.

[133] Hooper, C, Killick, R, & Lovestone, S. The GSK3 hypothesis of Alzheimer's disease. J Neurochem (2008). , 104(6), 1433-9.

[134] Takashima, A, Noguchi, K, Michel, G, Mercken, M, Hoshi, M, Ishiguro, K, & Imahori, K. Exposure of rat hippocampal neurons to amyloid beta peptide (25-35) induces the inactivation of phosphatidyl inositol-3 kinase and the activation of tau protein kinase I/glycogen synthase kinase-3 beta. Neurosci Lett (1996). , 203(1), 33-6.

[135] Takashima, A, Honda, T, Yasutake, K, Michel, G, Murayama, O, Murayama, M, Ishiguro, K, & Yamaguchi, H. Activation of tau protein kinase I/glycogen synthase kinase-3beta by amyloid beta peptide (25-35) enhances phosphorylation of tau in hippocampal neurons. Neurosci Res (1998). , 31(4), 317-23.

[136] Pei, J. J, Braak, E, Braak, H, Grundke-iqbal, I, Iqbal, K, Winblad, B, & Cowburn, R. F. Distribution of active glycogen synthase kinase 3beta (GSK-3beta) in brains staged for Alzheimer disease neurofibrillary changes. J Neuropathol Exp Neurol (1999). , 58(9), 1010-9.

[137] Hernandez, F, Borrell, J, Guaza, C, Avila, J, & Lucas, J. J. Spatial learning deficit in transgenic mice that conditionally over-express GSK-3beta in the brain but do not form tau filaments. J Neurochem (2002). , 83(6), 1529-33.

[138] Lucas, J. J, Hernandez, F, Gomez-Ramos, P, Moran, M. A, Hen, R, & Avila, J. Decreased nuclear beta-catenin, tau hyperphosphorylation and neurodegeneration in GSK-3beta conditional transgenic mice. EMBO J (2001). , 20(1-2), 27-39.

[139] Li, H. L, Wang, H. H, Liu, S. J, Deng, Y. Q, Zhang, Y. J, Tian, Q, Wang, X. C, Chen, X. Q, Yang, Y, Zhang, J. Y, Wang, Q, Xu, H, Liao, F. F, & Wang, J. Z. Phosphorylation of tau antagonizes apoptosis by stabilizing beta-catenin, a mechanism involved in Alzheimer's neurodegeneration. Proc Natl Acad Sci U S A (2007). , 104(9), 3591-6.

[140] Garcia-Alloza, M, Robbins, E. M, Zhang-nunes, S. X, Purcell, S. M, Betensky, R. A, Raju, S, Prada, C, Greenberg, S. M, Bacskai, B. J, & Frosch, M. P. Characterization of amyloid deposition in the APPswe/PS1dE9 mouse model of Alzheimer disease. Neurobiol Dis (2006). , 24(3), 516-24.

[141] Toledo, E. M, & Inestrosa, N. C. Activation of Wnt signaling by lithium and rosiglitazone reduced spatial memory impairment and neurodegeneration in brains of an APPswe/PSEN1DeltaE9 mouse model of Alzheimer's disease. Molecular psychiatry (2010). , 15(3), 272-85.

[142] Hu, Y. S, Xu, P, Pigino, G, Brady, S. T, Larson, J, & Lazarov, O. Complex environment experience rescues impaired neurogenesis, enhances synaptic plasticity, and attenuates neuropathology in familial Alzheimer's disease-linked APPswe/PS1DeltaE9 mice. FASEB J (2010). , 24(6), 1667-81.

[143] Cerpa, W, Farias, G. G, Godoy, J. A, Fuenzalida, M, Bonansco, C, & Inestrosa, N. C. Wnt-5a occludes Abeta oligomer-induced depression of glutamatergic transmission in hippocampal neurons. Mol Neurodegener (2010). , 5, 3.

[144] Selkoe, D. J. Alzheimer's disease is a synaptic failure. Science (New York, N.Y.) (2002). , 298(5594), 789-91.

Chapter 5

Regulation of Cell Fate in the Brain by GSK3

Adam R. Cole

Additional information is available at the end of the chapter

1. Introduction

The human brain is the most complex object in the known universe. It contains ~100 billion neurons, each forming between 1,000 and 10,000 connections with other neurons to form interconnecting circuits containing up to 1,000 trillion connections. This extreme complexity arises from a single cell at conception. Therefore, brain development needs to be tightly controlled to ensure proper patterning and circuit formation. Defects in this process lead to debilitating neurodevelopmental disorders, including autism and microcephaly. Until recently, it was assumed that once an adult brain had matured, it was 'fixed' or 'hard-wired' and no new neurons were generated. However, research over the last 15-20 years has demonstrated the existence of neural precursor cells (NPC's) that produce and incorporate new neurons into existing circuits of the adult brain, a process known as neurogenesis [1]. Adult neurogenesis is similar in organisation and mechanism to early brain development [2]. The ability to control neurogenesis could enable the brain to repair itself following injury (e.g. stroke, spinal chord injury, head trauma) and to enhance mental functioning (e.g. delay or prevent age-related cognitive decline and neurodegenerative diseases). Therefore, there is a clear and urgent need to understand the mechanisms controlling neurogenesis in the developing and adult brain.

NPC's give rise to all cell types in the brain by undergoing asymmetric cell division, generating one daughter cell that retains pluripotency and another daughter cell that is committed to a neuronal or glial fate. In adults, this predominantly occurs in the dentate gyrus of the hippocampus and the subventricular zone/olfactory system. Thousands of new cells are generated every day in the hippocampus, although less than half survive beyond a few weeks to permanently integrate into adult brain circuits [3]. This process is an important component of neuroplasticity in the hippocampus, facilitating learning and memory. Other brain regions are thought to have limited neurogenic potential that might be induced following injury. The fate of NPC's is controlled by extracellular stimuli (e.g. growth factors, Wnt, Notch, Hedgehog) that trigger intracellular signalling pathways and changes in gene transcription, although the transcriptional regulators targeted by these signalling pathways and their target genes are yet to be fully clarified.

2. GSK3 and neurogenesis

In 1980, Hammond and Dale noticed that lithium treatment of grey collie dogs increased their blood cell counts, which they suggested was due to increased proliferation of haematopoetic stem cells [4]. This was confirmed shortly afterwards [5], although the mechanism for lithium's action was not understood. In 1996, GSK3 was identified as a key target of lithium in cells [6], although it was another 8 years before a key role for GSK3 in regulating stem cell pluripotency was elucidated [7, 8]. Pharmacological inhibition of GSK3 activity was shown to maintain the undifferentiated phenotype in mouse and human embryonic stem (ES) cells, while its withdrawal promoted differentiation into multiple cell lineages [7]. More recently, it was demonstrated that the complex mixture of cytokines, growth factors, hormones, serum and feeder cells traditionally used to maintain self-renewal of ES cells can be replaced with two pharmacological inhibitors; a MAPK inhibitor and a GSK3 inhibitor [8], thus emphasizing the importance of GSK3 for regulating pluripotency. The GSK3 substrates c-myc [9] and Klf5 [10] are among several transcription factors that have been used to induce pluripotency (iPS system). Thus, GSK3 is a key regulator of neurogenesis, although the precise molecular mechanisms are not yet fully understood. This review provides an overview of the extracellular stimuli and intracellular signalling pathways controlling GSK3 activity, as well as the downstream targets of GSK3 directly linking it to cellular proliferation and differentiation in the brain. GSK3 inhibitors are currently in clinical trials for several neurological disorders associated with impaired neurogenesis, therefore it is timely that cell fate pathways involving GSK3 are delineated.

3. GSK3

GSK3 is a Ser/Thr kinase of the CMGC family of proline-directed kinases that is highly conserved in all eukaryotes. In mammals, it is ubiquitously expressed in all tissues and subcellular organelles, most highly in the brain [11]. There are 2 isoforms encoded by separate genes (chromosome 19q13.2 for GSK3α and chromosome 3q13.3 for GSK3β) [11]. Their kinase domains are 98% homologous and their substrate specificities are similar, but not identical [12]. A splice variant of GSK3β containing a 13 amino acid insert in the catalytic domain is specifically expressed in the brain [13], although its function is only just beginning to be investigated [12]. Interestingly, GSK3 is one of the most unusual kinases in the human genome for 3 main reasons; 1) Most (if not all) substrates require 'priming' phosphorylation 4 or 5 residues C-terminal to the GSK3 target site by another kinase *before* they can be efficiently phosphorylated by GSK3 [14]. 2) GSK3 is highly active in cells under basal conditions, opposite to most other kinases. 3) Phosphorylation of GSK3 at an N-terminal serine residue *inhibits* its kinase activity

(Ser21 in GSK3α, Ser9 in GSK3β) [15, 16]. This phosphoserine acts as a pseudo-substrate and binds to the phosphate-binding pocket on GSK3, preventing interaction with primed substrates [17]. Phosphorylation is mediated by members of the AGC family of kinases (e.g. Akt) and commonly occurs downstream of growth factor and PI3K signaling [15]. Activation of the canonical Wnt signaling pathway also inhibits GSK3 activity, preventing phosphorylation of β-catenin, although this is not mediated by N-terminal phosphorylation, but by protein-protein interactions [18, 19]. GSK3 is also modified by phosphorylation at a tyrosine residue on the activation loop of the kinase domain (Tyr279 for GSK3α and Tyr216 for GSK3β). Phosphorylation at these sites is absolutely required for kinase activity and is most likely constitutively modified (i.e. not regulatable) [20, 21].

4. Neurogenesis in GSK3 mutant mice

Valuable information on the role of GSK3 in cell fate determination has been obtained from mice genetically modified to either increase or decrease expression of GSK3α and β. While GSK3β-knockout mice die in late development due to defects in heart development and/or hepatic apoptosis [22, 23], GSK3β-heterozygous mice and GSK3α-knockout (homozygous) mice are viable and display several behavioural defects, including increased anxiety, decreased aggression and memory defects [24-28]. Also, GSK3α-null mice exhibit decreased numbers and size of Purkinje cells in the cerebellum [24]. Conditional overexpression of GSK3β in the forebrain using the doxycycline/Tet system impaired memory and spatial learning in mice [29]. At the cellular level, GSK3β overexpression increased neuronal cell death, astrocytosis, gliosis and reduced LTP induction. These effects could be restored by reducing GSK3 activity to normal levels by silencing the transgene or by treatment with lithium [30, 31]. In another report, overexpression of GSK3β-S9A in post-natal neurons (Thy-1 promoter) reduced brain size in adult mice, especially in the cerebral cortex, predominantly caused by reduced size of neuronal cell bodies and the somatodendritic compartment [32]. Together, these observations clearly demonstrate that GSK3 is important for healthy development and function of the brain.

In addition to conventional under/over-expression mouse models, GSK3-knockin mice were developed that are insensitive to growth factor inhibition (Ser21/9 mutated to Ala in GSK3α and β, respectively), but remain sensitive to Wnt-induced inhibition [33]. These mice are viable and display no overt developmental or growth defects, but do exhibit increased susceptibility to hyperactivity, stress-induced depression and mild anxiety, as well as abnormal LTP and memory functions [34, 35]. NPC's isolated from GSK3-knockin mice exhibit reduced neurogenesis, despite normal proliferation [36], suggesting defective differentiation/maturation or survival of NPC's. In contrast, mice with double homozygous deletion of GSK3α and β isoforms (i.e. all GSK3 isoforms deleted) display a dramatic increase in proliferation of NPC's and decreased differentiation into post-mitotic neurons [37]. This is accompanied by deregulation of Wnt, Notch, Hedgehog and FGF signalling pathways. In another mouse model, mice expressing a mutant form of the scaffolding protein Disrupted in Schizophrenia (DISC1), which is mutated in schizophrenia and mood disorder patients, display increased GSK3 activity, causing inhibition of the Wnt signaling pathway and decreased NPC proliferation

[38]. Together, these observations suggest that inhibition of GSK3 by the Wnt signalling pathway promotes NPC proliferation, while inhibition of GSK3 by growth factor signalling promotes differentiation of NPC's into post-mitotic neurons.

5. GSK3 and Wnt signaling

Wnt signaling is amongst the most important signaling pathways controlling neurogenesis in the developing and adult brain. Several studies have shown that attenuation of this pathway reduces the number of granule neurons and size of the hippocampus, as well as a reduction in the number of radial glial cells due to proliferation and patterning defects [39-41]. It is well accepted that Wnt's help to maintain the proliferative capacity of ES cells and keep them in an undifferentiated state [7], however there is also evidence for Wnt's being required to promote neural differentiation [42, 43]. These seemingly contradictory views are united in a model whereby Wnt signaling promotes proliferation and inhibits differentiation of pluripotent cells. Inhibition of this pathway promotes initial stages of differentiation into neural progenitors, but reactivation of Wnt signaling is required at later stages of the differentiation program to generate mature neurons [44, 45]. Indeed, in adult neurogenesis in the dentate gyrus of the hippocampus, Wnt's are secreted by local astrocytes where they predominantly regulate differentiation into mature neurons (mostly inhibitory GABAergic interneurons), rather than proliferation of NPC's [46-48].

GSK3 is a key component of the Wnt signaling pathway. In unstimulated cells, GSK3 is part of a multi-protein complex with APC, Axin and other proteins that facilitates phosphorylation of β-catenin by CK1 at Ser45, followed by phosphorylation of Ser33/37/41 by GSK3. This creates a recognition site for the E3 ubiquitin ligase βTrCP, which ubiquitinates β-catenin and targets it for degradation via the proteasome. In Wnt-stimulated cells, this multi-protein complex is disrupted, preventing phosphorylation and subsequent ubiquination of β-catenin, thus stabilizing the protein and increasing its cellular abundance. This leads to translocation to the nucleus, where β-catenin binds to several transcription factors facilitating transcription of target genes involved in cell fate regulation, including c-myc [49], NeuroD1 [48, 50, 51], Prox1 [52] and LINE-1 [50]. In adult neurogenesis, Wnt-induced expression of NeuroD1 is required for survival and maturation of adult-born neurons [48, 50, 51]. The prototypcial binding partners of β-catenin in the nucleus are members of the TCF/LEF family, which have been shown to be central mediators of tumourigenesis in the colon, breast and other tissues. In NPC's, activation of the Wnt pathway and elevated transcriptional activity of β-catenin has been shown to promote proliferation and inhibit neuronal differentiation [53, 54], while inhibition of Wnt signaling promotes neuronal differentiation [55, 56]. Accordingly, deletion of GSK3 isoforms promotes proliferation and inhibits differentiation of stem cells [57], consistent with pharmacological GSK3 inhibitors and Wnt-induced inhibition of GSK3 activity [7, 8]. This is dependent on elevated levels of transcriptionally active β-catenin [58], but surprisingly not by members of the TCF/LEF family. Instead, β-catenin was shown to bind to another transcription factor called Oct4, which increased expression of the pluripotency regulator and stem cell marker Nanog [58, 59].

Some transcriptional targets of the Wnt pathway are also targeted by GSK3 post-translationally. For example, *c-myc* is an established target of the Wnt pathway that promotes cell cycle progression and proliferation [49]. Meanwhile, its protein product is directly phosphorylated by GSK3 at Thr58, which targets it for ubiquitination by the E3 ligase Fbw7, followed by proteasome-mediated degradation [60, 61]. Thus, Wnt-induced inhibition of GSK3 activity could promote high c-myc activity both transcriptionally and post-translationally. However, it has not yet been proven that Wnt-mediated inhibition of GSK3 reduces phosphorylation of c-myc, or any protein other than β-catenin for that matter. Alternatively, simultaneous stimulation of cells by Wnt and growth factors would activate c-myc transcription and reduce its phosphorylation and degradation, respectively, thus combining to increase c-myc abundance. This would promote proliferation and inhibit differentiation of NPC's. Interestingly, a viral oncogenic form of c-myc is mutated at the GSK3 target site (Thr58) [60]. This mutation prevents phosphorylation of c-myc by GSK3 and subsequent ubiquitination, thus stabilizing the protein and driving uncontrolled proliferation in tumourigenesis. Thus, emphasizing the importance of phosphorylation of c-myc by GSK3 in the regulation of cell fate.

Other isoforms of c-myc are also phosphorylated and targeted for degradation by GSK3 (i.e. L-myc, N-myc). In NPC's, deletion of c- and L-myc does not affect proliferation/differentiation, while deletion of N-myc significantly decreases NPC proliferation and impairs differentiation into mature neurons [62], suggesting that N-myc is the critical member of this family regulating neurogenesis and brain development [63, 64]. Like c-myc, GSK3 phosphorylates N-myc at Thr58 to promote ubiquitination by Fbw7 and degradation by the lysosome [65]. This is antagonized by growth factor-mediated inhibition of GSK3 activity (e.g. IGF1). Phosphorylation of N-myc by GSK3 requires prior 'priming' phosphorylation at Ser62 by Cdk1, which is increased during mitosis, causing increased N-myc degradation [65]. This was shown to be important for exiting the cell cycle – the first step along the differentiation pathway. Cdk1 activity is dependent on binding to its co-factors cyclin A and B1 [66], whose transcription is controlled by the Hedgehog pathway, as is the transcription of N-myc [67, 68]. Therefore, N-myc appears to be a point at which multiple signaling pathways involving GSK3 intersect in NPC's to control cell fate.

Some substrates of GSK3 are upstream of the Wnt pathway and can regulate its activity. For example, hypoxia-inducible factor 1 α (HIF1α) is a basic helix-loop-helix (bHLH)-structured transcription factor that is induced by low oxygen conditions to activate transcription of genes that provide protection and adaption of cells to oxidative stress and hypoxic conditions. HIF1α is phosphorylated by GSK3, promoting its degradation by the proteasome [69, 70]. Recently, it was shown that HIF1α promotes Wnt activation and transcription of TCF/LEF members in undifferentiated, but not differentiated cells [71]. Low GSK3 activity in undifferentiated cells would reduce GSK3-mediated phosphorylation and degradation of HIF1α, thus stabilizing the protein and leading to activation of the Wnt pathway. Simultaneously, low GSK3 activity (downstream of Wnt) would prevent β-catenin phosphorylation/degradation, increasing its transcriptional activity with TCF/LEF. Interestingly, the authors show that the subgranular zone of the dentate gyrus containing NPC's is hypoxic due to fewer blood vessels in the region and contains relatively high levels of HIF1α and transcriptionally active β-catenin.

Thus, decreased oxygen levels could be important for maintaining the NPC niche in the hippocampus via GSK3, HIF1α and the Wnt pathway. It be should be noted that other groups have found that prolonged hypoxia increases the activity of GSK3 in cultured cells and *in vivo* [69, 72]. This might reflect differences between GSK3-mediated phosphorylation and degradation of HIF1α in undifferentiated versus differentiated cells.

6. GSK3, DISC1 and mood disorders

GSK3's involvement in the Wnt pathway is also regulated by the scaffolding protein DISC1. This protein directly binds to GSK3 to inhibit phosphorylation of β-catenin, preventing its degradation and activating its transcriptional activity [38]. This promotes NPC proliferation during embryonic development and in the adult brain. Depletion of DISC1 or expression of DISC1 mutants associated with mood disorders and schizophrenia reduced NPC proliferation and induced schizophrenia and depression-like symptoms in mice [38, 73]. These defects were normalized by administration of pharmacological inhibitors of GSK3. These studies demonstrate that DISC1 is a negative regulator of the Wnt pathway and NPC proliferation by directly inhibiting GSK3-mediated phosphorylation of β-catenin. Interestingly, one schizophrenia-associated mutant of DISC1 (S704C) did not affect GSK3 activity, Wnt signaling or NPC proliferation, but instead impaired neuronal migration in the developing cortex via reduced binding to cytoskeletal proteins (Dixdc1) [73]. Elsewhere, it was shown that DISC1 acts as a molecular switch between proliferation and migration in NPC's, whereby DISC1 inhibits GSK3-mediated phosphorylation of β-catenin and activates its transcriptional activity to drive proliferation of NPC's, while in committed, post-mitotic neurons, DISC1 regulates neuronal migration via another protein called BBS1 and the centrosome [74]. Together, these studies demonstrate that DISC1 regulates NPC proliferation and neuronal migration through GSK3-dependent and independent pathways, respectively.

As well as DISC1, other upstream regulators of GSK3 are genetically linked to mood disorders and schizophrenia, including Akt [75], Neuregulin [76] and the dopamine/β-arrestin signaling complex [77, 78]. GSK3 kinase activity is also inhibited by several mood-stabilizers, anti-depressants and anti-psychotic drugs [6, 79, 80], while genetic manipulation of GSK3 activity in mice produces behaviours correlating with mood disorders [24-28]. A single nucleotide polymorphism in the promoter region of GSK3β has also been correlated with onset of Bipolar disorder [81]. Together, these observations strongly implicate elevated GSK3 activity in the etiology of mood disorders and schizophrenia. Neurogenesis is decreased in these disorders [82, 83], but is promoted by mood stabilizing drugs, such as lithium [84, 85]. Therefore, mood-stabilizing drugs may act (at least in part) by promoting neurogenesis via inhibition of GSK3. If so, promoting neurogenesis using GSK3 inhibitors could also be beneficial to other mental disorders, including neurodegenerative diseases such as Alzheimer's disease and age-related cognitive decline, as well repair following brain injury, such as stroke and spinal chord injuries.

7. GSK3 and Notch signaling

A role for the Notch signaling pathway in regulating development was discovered almost a century ago by pioneering work in fruit flies by John Dexter and Thomas Hunt Morgan [86]. It was later found that absence of Notch in flies caused neuronal hyperplasia and a decrease in glial cells in the brain [87]. Generally, Notch signaling promotes proliferation of NPCs and inhibits their differentiation, but has also been linked with glial cell specification [88, 89], neurite outgrowth [90] and learning and memory [91]. Notch is a family of 4 single-pass transmembrane proteins (Notch1-4) that are expressed at the cell surface of ES cells and NPCs (especially Notch1). Ligand-mediated activation of Notch leads to its proteolytic cleavage by Presenillin-g, releasing the Notch intracellular domain (NICD) for translocation to the nucleus where it binds with the transcription factor RBP-Jk to activate transcription of target genes including the bHLH transcriptional repressors *Hes1* and *Hes5*. These proteins repress transcription of pro-neural genes, thus inhibiting differentiation into neurons and maintaining proliferation of NPC's. Ligands that activate Notch, such as Delta-like 1 (Dll1) and Jagged1 (Jag1) are themselves transmembrane proteins. These are typically located at the cell surface of differentiated neurons that bind and stimulate activation of Notch on neighbouring NPC's. Thus, Notch signaling functions in a localized fashion, whereby a differentiating neuron expressing the ligands Dll1 or Jag1 binds Notch on a neighbouring cell to activate downstream signaling that inhibits differentiation and maintains proliferation of NPC's, thus establishing a stem cell niche in the brain. In other words, Notch signaling prevents equipotent cells from acquiring the same fate.

GSK3 was originally found to be associated with the Notch signaling pathway in *Drosophila* development [92]. Since then, it has been shown to bind and phosphorylate the intracellular domain of Notch, stabilizing the protein by reducing its degradation by the proteasome [93]. However, other studies report that phosphorylation *de*stabilizes Notch and promotes its degradation [94, 95]. The reason for these contradictory observations are not clear, although considering that low GSK3 activity and high Notch signaling correlate with the highly proliferative, undifferentiated nature of ES cells/NPC's, it is likely that GSK3-mediated phosphorylation targets Notch for degradation by the proteasome. That is, low GSK3-mediated phosphorylation and degradation of NICD increases its abundance and transcriptional activity to promote proliferation/suppress differentiation. This is consistent with many other proteins that are destabilized by GSK3 phosphorylation, such as c-myc, HIF1α, β-catenin, etc. It is possible that prior phosphorylation by the cyclin C:Cdk8 complex could prime NICD for subsequent phosphorylation by GSK3 [96], although this remains to be proven.

Cross-talk between the Notch and Wnt signaling pathways has been suggested by several studies, although the reports are contradictory. One study shows that Notch binds to the unphosphorylated, transcriptionally-active form of β-catenin, targeting it for degradation by the lysosome, thus suppressing expression of Wnt target genes [97]. At first glance, this is surprising, since both pathways are pro-proliferation/anti-differentiation. However, it should be noted that Notch-mediated degradation of β-catenin does not require ligand activation. Therefore, this mechanism might be more relevant to differentiated cells, such that in the absence of ligand stimulation, Notch reduces β-catenin levels to antagonize Wnt signaling. Thus, both pathways are suppressed, consistent with a differentiated phenotype. Another report has shown that FGF2-mediated inhibition of GSK3 activity leads to an increase in transcriptionally-active β-catenin in the cell nucleus, which simultaneously activates TCF/LEF and Notch/RBP-Jk transcriptional complexes, promoting proliferation and inhibiting differentiation, respectively [98]. Although both pathways promote maintenance of stem cells as expected, FGF2-mediated inhibition of GSK3 is unexpected, since it is commonly assumed that growth factors do not influence β-catenin levels in the Wnt pathway [19], although this observation has been confirmed by several other groups [99, 100]. It is possible that FGF signaling is an exception to the growth factor rule. All together, it seems clear that there are interactions between Notch and other cell fate pathways involving GSK3, although the precise mechanisms are yet to be fully clarified.

8. GSK3 and Hedgehog signalling

The Hedgehog signaling pathway is a critical regulator of cell fate during development and for maintaining proliferation of cell stem niches in adults, including NPC's in the brain. In mammals, there are 3 Hedgehog proteins, with Sonic hedgehog being the most widely studied. These are secreted proteins that bind to a receptor at the surface of target cells called patched. When Hedgehog binds to patched, patched is released from another receptor protein at the cell surface called smoothened, allowing smoothened levels to increase. Smoothened inhibits the proteolytic cleavage of the zinc-finger proteins Gli (*cubitus interruptus* in flies), which are critical effectors of the Hedgehog pathway. Gli1 and Gli2 are transcriptional activators, while Gli3 is a repressor. These proteins regulate the transcription of cell cycle-related genes, such as cyclins D and E, N-myc, Bcl2, POU3F1, Runx2 and Tbx2, as well as patched in a negative feedback loop. In the absence of Hedgehog ligands, Gli associates with a scaffolding complex containing Cos2 and Fused that facilitates phosphorylation by GSK3 and CK1 (following priming by PKA). This phosphorylation targets Gli for ubiquitination and proteolysis, generating a truncated repressor form lacking the C-terminal activation domains [101-105]. But in the presence of Hedgehog, this signaling complex is disrupted, inhibiting phosphorylation and processing of Gli, leading to accumulation of transcriptionally active full-length protein in the nucleus. Thus, GSK3 antagonises Hedgehog signaling by mediating the degradation of Gli proteins. The scaffolding protein Sufu, a negative regulator of Hedgehog signaling, is also phosphorylated by GSK3, which stabilizes the protein and increases degradation of Gli proteins [106]. Thus, GSK3 promotes Gli degradation directly and via stabilization of Sufu.

The Hedgehog pathway is similar to the Wnt pathway, in that it utilizes the constitutive activity of GSK3 to negatively regulate the key transcriptional effector of each pathway (β-catenin for Wnt, Gli for Hedgehog). Ligand-mediated activation of both pathways reduces phosphorylation of these key effectors by disrupting their respective signaling/scaffolding complexes without directly inhibiting GSK3 activity (i.e. they exclusively reduce phosphorylation of a specific substrate). In contrast, growth factor signaling directly inhibits GSK3 kinase activity via phosphorylation of the N-terminal serine residues. Therefore, it seems that the Wnt and Hedgehog pathways regulate specific substrates within their respective signaling complexes, while growth factor stimulation affects a wider range of GSK3 substrates (Fig.1). It should also be mentioned that signaling complexes containing the scaffolding protein AKAP220 have been shown to promote inhibitory Ser21/9 phosphorylation of GSK3 [107, 108]. Hence, the number of scaffolding/signal complex-associated proteins reported to bind and regulate GSK3 activity is increasing, suggesting that this mechanism might be common, rather than an exception, although this remains to be proven. Nevertheless, it is highly likely that other signaling complexes regulating GSK3 are likely to be discovered.

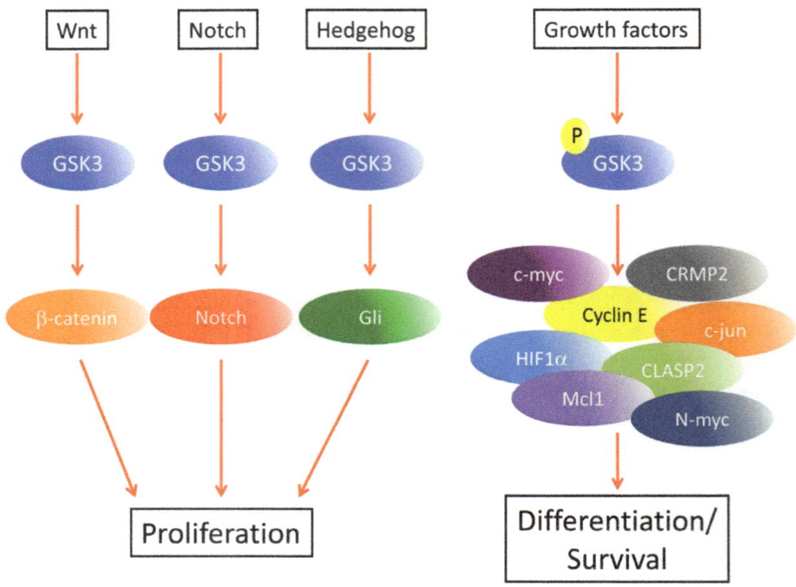

Figure 1. Signalling pathways regulating cell fate target different subsets of GSK3 substrates. Ligand-stimulated activation of the Wnt, Notch and Hedgehog pathways prevents phosphorylation of a single substrate by disrupting multi-subunit signalling complexes required to mediate their phosphorylation, driving proliferation. In contrast, growth factor-mediated inhibition of GSK3 via phosphorylation of N-terminal serine residues reduces phosphorylation of many substrates, promoting survival and differentiation of newly generated neurons.

9. GSK3 and growth factor signaling

In general, growth factors positively influence neurogenesis in the developing and adult brain by supporting differentiation and survival of newly generated neurons. Direct injection of many growth factors into the subventricular zone of mice increases neurogenesis, including

FGF [109], EGF [110], TGF [110], CNTF [111]. Among the most potent growth factors are the neurotrophins (BDNF, NGF, NT-3, NT-4), whereby direct administration [112] or genetic deletion [113] increases and reduces neurogenesis, respectively. Accordingly, their receptor molecules, called Trk receptors, are predominantly expressed by post-mitotic neurons, but not NPC's or neural crest cells [114]. BDNF signaling, in particular, has been shown to promote survival of newly-generated neurons [115], while defects in BDNF signaling have been linked to decreased neurogenesis and neuronal survival in several neurological disorders, including Alzheimer's disease, age-related cognitive decline, Bipolar disorder and Schizophrenia (for reviews, see [116, 117]).

GSK3 is an established target of many growth factor signaling pathways. Ligand-binding to their respective receptors at the cell surface induces dimerisation/oligomerisation, activating their intrinsic kinase activities and autophosphorylation of key tyrosine residues. This provides binding sites for SH2 and SH3-domain-containing adaptor proteins, such as IRS and Grb proteins, promoting recruitment and activation of phosphatidylinositol 3 kinase (PI3K). This lipid kinase converts phosphatidylinositol 4,5 bisphosphate (PIP2) to PIP3, recruiting members of the AGC family of kinases (e.g. PKB/Akt), where they are phosphorylated and activated by PDK1. These AGC kinases phosphorylate an N-terminal serine on GSK3 (Ser21 on GSK3α, Ser9 on GSK3β) that binds to the substrate binding site on GSK3, thus acting as a pseudo-substrate to inhibit phosphorylation of primed substrates [17].

Numerous studies have demonstrated that pharmacological inhibitors of GSK3 promote survival of neurons subjected to a range of toxic stimuli (for a review, see [118]), while over-expression of GSK3 promotes neuronal apoptosis *in vitro* and *in vivo* [29, 119, 120]. Importantly, GSK3α/β -knockin mice (S21/9A) that are insensitive to growth factor inhibition exhibit reduced neurogenesis, despite normal proliferation of NPC's [36]. As noted previously, this could suggest defective differentiation patterns in the NPC's, but could equally represent decreased survival of newly generated neurons. In addition, several substrates of GSK3 are associated with cell survival (discussed below). Together, these observations strongly suggest that growth factor-mediated inhibition of GSK3 appears to be a key mechanism by which growth factors promote survival of newly generated neurons during neurogenesis.

A key downstream target of GSK3 promoting survival is Mcl1. This anti-apoptotic, pro-survival member of the Bcl2 family is directly phosphorylated by GSK3 at Ser155 and Ser159, targeting it for ubiquitination by E3 ligases (Fbw7, βTrCP and/or Trim17) and degradation by the proteasome [121, 122]. Upon growth factor stimulation, GSK3 is inhibited, reducing GSK3-mediated phosphorylation of Mcl1, thus stabilizing the protein and promoting neuronal survival. The Notch signaling pathway has also been shown to promote survival of neurons via Mcl-1, although the role of GSK3 was not investigated [123]. NPC's and newly-committed neurons in the subventricular zone and surrounding areas of mice express high levels of Mcl-1, while Mcl-1 deficiency caused widespread apoptosis, especially in newly-committed neurons as they migrate away from this region [124]. This suggests that a key target of growth factor and GSK3-mediated protection of neurons is via Mcl-1. Indeed, nutrient deprivation correlates with decreased levels of Mcl-1 and induction of apoptosis in neurons, which was dependent on phosphorylation by GSK3 [125, 126]. In contrast, Bax is a pro-apoptotic member of the Bcl2 family. Phosphorylation by GSK3 at Ser163 promotes its translocation to the mitochondrial outer membrane, where it oligomerizes to form a pore promoting cytochrome c release and cell death [127, 128]. Inhibition of GSK3 via growth factor signaling or therapeutics (e.g. lithium) antagonizes Bax translocation and cytochrome c release, promoting cell survival.

Other downstream targets of GSK3 that promote neuronal survival include the transcription factors HIF1α, HSF1 [129], Mef2D [130] and Bcl3 [131] by activating transcription of pro-survival genes. For example, increased activity of GSK3 during potassium withdrawal from cerebellar granule neurons leads to increased phosphorylation and degradation of Mef2D, which could be blocked by a GSK3-resistant form of Mef2D [130]. The neurotrophins NGF and BDNF promote Mef2D stability by reducing GSK3-mediated degradation, leading to increased transcription of its target gene Bcl-w, an anti-apoptotic member of the Bcl-2 family [132].

10. GSK3, ubiquitin ligases and proteasome-mediated degradation

It is noticeable that many substrates of GSK3 are targeted for ubiquitination and proteasome-mediated degradation following phosphorylation by GSK3. Most of these are transcription factors that are phosphorylated by GSK3 within an [ST]PPx[ST]P motif, including c-myc [61, 133, 134], c-jun [135], Klf5 [136, 137], cyclin E1 [138], Gli3 [101, 102] and snail [139]. These transcription factors have short half-lives, largely due to the actions of GSK3, which is highly active under basal conditions in mature, differentiated cells. However, GSK3 activity levels are comparatively lower in undifferentiated cells, induced by persistent Wnt, Notch, Hedgehog and/or growth factor signaling to maintain the proliferative capacity of these cells [140]. Here, phosphorylation and ubiquitination of transcription factors by GSK3 is reduced, thus stabilizing the proteins (prolonging their half-lives) and contributing to stem/precursor cell proliferation. A common E3 ligase targeting GSK3 substrates is Fbw7. In fact, most of the reported targets of Fbw7 are established GSK3 substrates (see [141]). Genetic studies in mice indicate that Fbw7 is required for differentiation and survival of NPC's. For example, brain-specific deletion of Fbw7 increased apoptosis of NPC's, which could be rescued by concomitant deletion of c-jun [142]. Similar results were observed for cerebellar development in mice [143]. NPC differentiation was also impaired, particularly a decrease in the number of mature neurons and increased glial progenitors (although no change in mature astrocytes). This was alleviated by inhibition of Notch signaling. Supporting this, a separate study showed that brain-specific deletion of Fbw7 skewed the differentiation of NPC's towards astrocytes, rather than neurons, which could be restored with a pharmacological inhibitor of the Notch pathway [144]. Meanwhile, the maintenance/proliferation of the NPC's was not affected. Together, these observations show that GSK3 and Fbw7 share common substrates that regulate the differentiation and survival of neurons.

11. GSK3 and NPC migration and polarization

Correct positioning of newly generated neurons is crucial during development and for healthy function of the adult brain. Neuronal migration is tightly regulated by extracellular cues, including Wnts and growth factors. Accordingly, there is emerging evidence that their common downstream target, GSK3, may be involved in this process, primarily via regulation of cytoskeleton-associated proteins. Migration requires cellular polarization and extension at the leading edge of the cell. This involves dynamic reorganization of microtubules by a variety of microtubule-binding proteins. Several of these are directly phosphorylated and regulated by GSK3, including Tau, CRMP2, MAP1B, MAP2C, CLASP2, pVHL and APC (for reviews, see [145, 146]). Phosphorylation of many of these substrates by GSK3 reduces their ability to bind microtubules, thus making them less stable. Interestingly, GSK3 activity is typically low at the leading edge of migrating cells or at the tips of growing neurites in neuronal polarization [147-149]. This would promote substrate binding and stabilization of microtubules, facilitating forward movement of the cell's leading edge or growing neurite. Similarly, local inhibition of GSK3 activity is essential for polarization of newly generated neurons and growth of the nascent axon [150, 151]. Meanwhile, global inhibition of GSK3 induces formation of multiple axons [150, 152]. Several upstream inhibitors of GSK3 have been implicated in this process, including Cdc42 [149], ILK [153], LKB1 [147] and Akt [150]. Apart from the latter, these signaling proteins are not established regulators of GSK3 activity, so the precise molecular mechanisms by which they inhibit GSK3 activity await clarification.

12. Conclusions

It is clear that GSK3 is an important target of several signaling pathways controlling cell fate in the brain. It is also clear that many of these pathways can be activated simultaneously in the same cells/tissues. One possibility is that GSK3 acts as an integrator of these simultaneous inputs to determine the cellular outcome. That is, GSK3 acts as a node for multiple signaling pathways and the sum of these inhibitory signals dictates cell fate. This is unlikely, since although each of these pathways target GSK3, their downstream targets are different. For example, growth factor signaling inhibits phosphorylation of CRMP2, but not β-catenin, and *vice versa* for Wnt [19, 154, 155]. An alternative explanation is that different subsets of GSK3 substrates are selectively affected by particular stimuli. That is, ligand-stimulated activation of the Wnt, Notch and Hedgehog pathways prevents phosphorylation of a single substrate (β-catenin, Notch and Gli, respectively) by disrupting multi-subunit signaling complexes required to mediate their phosphorylation. This increases the stability of these proteins, translocation to the cell nucleus and regulation of gene transcription programs that promote proliferation of ES cells/NPC's. In contrast, growth factor-mediated inhibition of GSK3 via phosphorylation of N-terminal serine residues reduces phosphorylation of many substrates (although not β-catenin), promoting survival and differentiation of newly generated neurons. It is possible that signaling complexes associated with β-catenin (and perhaps Notch and Gli) are able to surmount the inhibitory N-terminal serine phosphorylation induced by growth factor signaling. Indeed, the protein phosphatase PP2A is a known component of the β-catenin/APC/Axin signaling complex [156] and PP2A is able to activate GSK3 by dephosphorylating its N-terminal serine residue [157]. If this is true, these signaling complexes could be seen to *activate* GSK3 activity (at least phosphorylation of a particular substrate e.g. β-catenin). It might be more accurate to say that GSK3 is *not* inhibited by these pathways, but rather GSK3 *antagonizes* them. Then upon ligand stimulation, this function of GSK3 is alleviated by disruption of the signaling complex, activating the pathway. It is important to catalogue the pathway-specific targets of GSK3 and their effects on cell fate and survival, since this knowledge could identify novel therapeutic targets for artificially controlling neurogenesis and promoting recovery in diseased or damaged brains.

Author details

Adam R. Cole

Neurosignalling Group, Garvan Institute of Medical Research, Darlinghurst, Sydney, Australia

References

[1] Altman J, Das GD (1965) Autoradiographic and histological evidence of postnatal hippocampal neurogenesis in rats. *J Comp Neurol* 124, 319-335.

[2] Duan X, Kang E, Liu CY, Ming GL, Song H (2008) Development of neural stem cell in the adult brain. *Curr Opin Neurobiol* 18, 108-115.

[3] Cameron HA, McKay RD (2001) Adult neurogenesis produces a large pool of new granule cells in the dentate gyrus. *J Comp Neurol* 435, 406-417.

[4] Hammond WP, Dale DC (1980) Lithium therapy of canine cyclic hematopoiesis. *Blood* 55, 26-28.

[5] Levitt LJ, Quesenberry PJ (1980) The effect of lithium on murine hematopoiesis in a liquid culture system. *N Engl J Med* 302, 713-719.

[6] Klein PS, Melton DA (1996) A molecular mechanism for the effect of lithium on development. *Proc Natl Acad Sci U S A* 93, 8455-8459.

[7] Sato N, Meijer L, Skaltsounis L, Greengard P, Brivanlou AH (2004) Maintenance of pluripotency in human and mouse embryonic stem cells through activation of Wnt signaling by a pharmacological GSK-3-specific inhibitor. *Nat Med* 10, 55-63.

[8] Ying QL, Wray J, Nichols J, Batlle-Morera L, Doble B, Woodgett J, Cohen P, Smith A (2008) The ground state of embryonic stem cell self-renewal. *Nature* 453, 519-523.

[9] Hall J, Guo G, Wray J, Eyres I, Nichols J, Grotewold L, Morfopoulou S, Humphreys P, Mansfield W, Walker R, Tomlinson S, Smith A (2009) Oct4 and LIF/Stat3 additively induce Kruppel factors to sustain embryonic stem cell self-renewal. *Cell Stem Cell* 5, 597-609.

[10] Jiang J, Chan YS, Loh YH, Cai J, Tong GQ, Lim CA, Robson P, Zhong S, Ng HH (2008) A core Klf circuitry regulates self-renewal of embryonic stem cells. *Nat Cell Biol* 10, 353-360.

[11] Woodgett JR (1990) Molecular cloning and expression of glycogen synthase kinase-3/factor A. *EMBO J* 9, 2431-2438.

[12] Soutar MP, Kim WY, Williamson R, Peggie M, Hastie CJ, McLauchlan H, Snider WD, Gordon-Weeks PR, Sutherland C (2010) Evidence that glycogen synthase kinase-3 isoforms have distinct substrate preference in the brain. *J Neurochem* 115, 974-983.

[13] Mukai F, Ishiguro K, Sano Y, Fujita SC (2002) Alternative splicing isoform of tau protein kinase I/glycogen synthase kinase 3beta. *J Neurochem* 81, 1073-1083.

[14] Kennelly PJ, Krebs EG (1991) Consensus sequences as substrate specificity determinants for protein kinases and protein phosphatases. *J Biol Chem* 266, 15555-15558.

[15] Cross DA, Alessi DR, Cohen P, Andjelkovich M, Hemmings BA (1995) Inhibition of glycogen synthase kinase-3 by insulin mediated by protein kinase B. *Nature* 378, 785-789.

[16] Sutherland C, Leighton IA, Cohen P (1993) Inactivation of glycogen synthase kinase-3 beta by phosphorylation: new kinase connections in insulin and growth-factor signalling. *Biochem J* 296 (Pt 1), 15-19.

[17] Frame S, Cohen P, Biondi RM (2001) A common phosphate binding site explains the unique substrate specificity of GSK3 and its inactivation by phosphorylation. *Mol Cell* 7, 1321-1327.

[18] Thomas GM, Frame S, Goedert M, Nathke I, Polakis P, Cohen P (1999) A GSK3-binding peptide from FRAT1 selectively inhibits the GSK3-catalysed phosphorylation of axin and beta-catenin. *FEBS Lett* 458, 247-251.

[19] Ding VW, Chen RH, McCormick F (2000) Differential regulation of glycogen synthase kinase 3beta by insulin and Wnt signaling. *J Biol Chem* 275, 32475-32481.

[20] Cole A, Frame S, Cohen P (2004) Further evidence that the tyrosine phosphorylation of glycogen synthase kinase-3 (GSK3) in mammalian cells is an autophosphorylation event. *Biochem J* 377, 249-255.

[21] Lochhead PA, Kinstrie R, Sibbet G, Rawjee T, Morrice N, Cleghon V (2006) A chaperone-dependent GSK3beta transitional intermediate mediates activation-loop autophosphorylation. *Mol Cell* 24, 627-633.

[22] Hoeflich KP, Luo J, Rubie EA, Tsao MS, Jin O, Woodgett JR (2000) Requirement for glycogen synthase kinase-3beta in cell survival and NF-kappaB activation. *Nature* 406, 86-90.

[23] Kerkela R, Kockeritz L, Macaulay K, Zhou J, Doble BW, Beahm C, Greytak S, Woulfe K, Trivedi CM, Woodgett JR, Epstein JA, Force T, Huggins GS (2008) Deletion of GSK-3beta in mice leads to hypertrophic cardiomyopathy secondary to cardiomyoblast hyperproliferation. *J Clin Invest* 118, 3609-3618.

[24] Kaidanovich-Beilin O, Lipina TV, Takao K, van Eede M, Hattori S, Laliberte C, Khan M, Okamoto K, Chambers JW, Fletcher PJ, Macaulay K, Doble BW, Henkelman M, Miyakawa T, Roder J, Woodgett JR (2009) Abnormalities in brain structure and behavior in GSK-3alpha mutant mice. *Mol Brain* 2, 35.

[25] O'Brien WT, Harper AD, Jove F, Woodgett JR, Maretto S, Piccolo S, Klein PS (2004) Glycogen synthase kinase-3beta haploinsufficiency mimics the behavioral and molecular effects of lithium. *J Neurosci* 24, 6791-6798.

[26] Kimura T, Yamashita S, Nakao S, Park JM, Murayama M, Mizoroki T, Yoshiike Y, Sahara N, Takashima A (2008) GSK-3beta is required for memory reconsolidation in adult brain. *PLoS One* 3, e3540.

[27] Beaulieu JM, Zhang X, Rodriguiz RM, Sotnikova TD, Cools MJ, Wetsel WC, Gainetdinov RR, Caron MG (2008) Role of GSK3 beta in behavioral abnormalities induced by serotonin deficiency. *Proc Natl Acad Sci U S A* 105, 1333-1338.

[28] Prickaerts J, Moechars D, Cryns K, Lenaerts I, van Craenendonck H, Goris I, Daneels G, Bouwknecht JA, Steckler T (2006) Transgenic mice overexpressing glycogen synthase kinase 3beta: a putative model of hyperactivity and mania. *J Neurosci* 26, 9022-9029.

[29] Lucas JJ, Hernandez F, Gomez-Ramos P, Moran MA, Hen R, Avila J (2001) Decreased nuclear beta-catenin, tau hyperphosphorylation and neurodegeneration in GSK-3beta conditional transgenic mice. *EMBO J* 20, 27-39.

[30] Hedgepeth CM, Conrad LJ, Zhang J, Huang HC, Lee VM, Klein PS (1997) Activation of the Wnt signaling pathway: a molecular mechanism for lithium action. *Dev Biol* 185, 82-91.

[31] Hooper C, Markevich V, Plattner F, Killick R, Schofield E, Engel T, Hernandez F, Anderton B, Rosenblum K, Bliss T, Cooke SF, Avila J, Lucas JJ, Giese KP, Stephenson J, Lovestone S (2007) Glycogen synthase kinase-3 inhibition is integral to long-term potentiation. *Eur J Neurosci* 25, 81-86.

[32] Spittaels K, Van den Haute C, Van Dorpe J, Terwel D, Vandezande K, Lasrado R, Bruynseels K, Irizarry M, Verhoye M, Van Lint J, Vandenheede JR, Ashton D, Mercken M, Loos R, Hyman B, Van der Linden A, Geerts H, Van Leuven F (2002) Neonatal

neuronal overexpression of glycogen synthase kinase-3 beta reduces brain size in transgenic mice. *Neuroscience* 113, 797-808.

[33] McManus EJ, Sakamoto K, Armit LJ, Ronaldson L, Shpiro N, Marquez R, Alessi DR (2005) Role that phosphorylation of GSK3 plays in insulin and Wnt signalling defined by knockin analysis. *EMBO J* 24, 1571-1583.

[34] Polter A, Beurel E, Yang S, Garner R, Song L, Miller CA, Sweatt JD, McMahon L, Bartolucci AA, Li X, Jope RS (2010) Deficiency in the inhibitory serine-phosphorylation of glycogen synthase kinase-3 increases sensitivity to mood disturbances. *Neuropsychopharmacology* 35, 1761-1774.

[35] Ackermann TF, Kempe DS, Lang F, Lang UE (2010) Hyperactivity and enhanced curiosity of mice expressing PKB/SGK-resistant glycogen synthase kinase-3 (GSK-3). *Cell Physiol Biochem* 25, 775-786.

[36] Eom TY, Jope RS (2009) Blocked inhibitory serine-phosphorylation of glycogen synthase kinase-3alpha/beta impairs in vivo neural precursor cell proliferation. *Biol Psychiatry* 66, 494-502.

[37] Kim WY, Wang X, Wu Y, Doble BW, Patel S, Woodgett JR, Snider WD (2009) GSK-3 is a master regulator of neural progenitor homeostasis. *Nat Neurosci* 12, 1390-1397.

[38] Mao Y, Ge X, Frank CL, Madison JM, Koehler AN, Doud MK, Tassa C, Berry EM, Soda T, Singh KK, Biechele T, Petryshen TL, Moon RT, Haggarty SJ, Tsai LH (2009) Disrupted in schizophrenia 1 regulates neuronal progenitor proliferation via modulation of GSK3beta/beta-catenin signaling. *Cell* 136, 1017-1031.

[39] Lee SM, Tole S, Grove E, McMahon AP (2000) A local Wnt-3a signal is required for development of the mammalian hippocampus. *Development* 127, 457-467.

[40] Zhou CJ, Zhao C, Pleasure SJ (2004) Wnt signaling mutants have decreased dentate granule cell production and radial glial scaffolding abnormalities. *J Neurosci* 24, 121-126.

[41] Galceran J, Miyashita-Lin EM, Devaney E, Rubenstein JL, Grosschedl R (2000) Hippocampus development and generation of dentate gyrus granule cells is regulated by LEF1. *Development* 127, 469-482.

[42] Otero JJ, Fu W, Kan L, Cuadra AE, Kessler JA (2004) Beta-catenin signaling is required for neural differentiation of embryonic stem cells. *Development* 131, 3545-3557.

[43] Muroyama Y, Fujihara M, Ikeya M, Kondoh H, Takada S (2002) Wnt signaling plays an essential role in neuronal specification of the dorsal spinal cord. *Genes Dev* 16, 548-553.

[44] Wang X, Kopinke D, Lin J, McPherson AD, Duncan RN, Otsuna H, Moro E, Hoshijima K, Grunwald DJ, Argenton F, Chien CB, Murtaugh LC, Dorsky RI (2012) Wnt sig-

naling regulates postembryonic hypothalamic progenitor differentiation. *Dev Cell* 23, 624-636.

[45] Slawny NA, O'Shea KS (2011) Dynamic changes in Wnt signaling are required for neuronal differentiation of mouse embryonic stem cells. *Mol Cell Neurosci* 48, 205-216.

[46] Lie DC, Colamarino SA, Song HJ, Desire L, Mira H, Consiglio A, Lein ES, Jessberger S, Lansford H, Dearie AR, Gage FH (2005) Wnt signalling regulates adult hippocampal neurogenesis. *Nature* 437, 1370-1375.

[47] Song H, Stevens CF, Gage FH (2002) Astroglia induce neurogenesis from adult neural stem cells. *Nature* 417, 39-44.

[48] Kuwabara T, Hsieh J, Muotri A, Yeo G, Warashina M, Lie DC, Moore L, Nakashima K, Asashima M, Gage FH (2009) Wnt-mediated activation of NeuroD1 and retro-elements during adult neurogenesis. *Nat Neurosci* 12, 1097-1105.

[49] He TC, Sparks AB, Rago C, Hermeking H, Zawel L, da Costa LT, Morin PJ, Vogelstein B, Kinzler KW (1998) Identification of c-MYC as a target of the APC pathway. *Science* 281, 1509-1512.

[50] Boutin C, Hardt O, de Chevigny A, Core N, Goebbels S, Seidenfaden R, Bosio A, Cremer H (2010) NeuroD1 induces terminal neuronal differentiation in olfactory neurogenesis. *Proc Natl Acad Sci U S A* 107, 1201-1206.

[51] Gao Z, Ure K, Ables JL, Lagace DC, Nave KA, Goebbels S, Eisch AJ, Hsieh J (2009) Neurod1 is essential for the survival and maturation of adult-born neurons. *Nat Neurosci* 12, 1090-1092.

[52] Karalay O, Doberauer K, Vadodaria KC, Knobloch M, Berti L, Miquelajauregui A, Schwark M, Jagasia R, Taketo MM, Tarabykin V, Lie DC, Jessberger S (2011) Prospero-related homeobox 1 gene (Prox1) is regulated by canonical Wnt signaling and has a stage-specific role in adult hippocampal neurogenesis. *Proc Natl Acad Sci U S A* 108, 5807-5812.

[53] Haegele L, Ingold B, Naumann H, Tabatabai G, Ledermann B, Brandner S (2003) Wnt signalling inhibits neural differentiation of embryonic stem cells by controlling bone morphogenetic protein expression. *Mol Cell Neurosci* 24, 696-708.

[54] Kielman MF, Rindapaa M, Gaspar C, van Poppel N, Breukel C, van Leeuwen S, Taketo MM, Roberts S, Smits R, Fodde R (2002) Apc modulates embryonic stem-cell differentiation by controlling the dosage of beta-catenin signaling. *Nat Genet* 32, 594-605.

[55] Aubert J, Dunstan H, Chambers I, Smith A (2002) Functional gene screening in embryonic stem cells implicates Wnt antagonism in neural differentiation. *Nat Biotechnol* 20, 1240-1245.

[56] Cajanek L, Ribeiro D, Liste I, Parish CL, Bryja V, Arenas E (2009) Wnt/beta-catenin signaling blockade promotes neuronal induction and dopaminergic differentiation in embryonic stem cells. *Stem Cells* 27, 2917-2927.

[57] Doble BW, Patel S, Wood GA, Kockeritz LK, Woodgett JR (2007) Functional redundancy of GSK-3alpha and GSK-3beta in Wnt/beta-catenin signaling shown by using an allelic series of embryonic stem cell lines. *Dev Cell* 12, 957-971.

[58] Kelly KF, Ng DY, Jayakumaran G, Wood GA, Koide H, Doble BW (2011) beta-catenin enhances Oct-4 activity and reinforces pluripotency through a TCF-independent mechanism. *Cell Stem Cell* 8, 214-227.

[59] Takao Y, Yokota T, Koide H (2007) Beta-catenin up-regulates Nanog expression through interaction with Oct-3/4 in embryonic stem cells. *Biochem Biophys Res Commun* 353, 699-705.

[60] Pulverer BJ, Fisher C, Vousden K, Littlewood T, Evan G, Woodgett JR (1994) Site-specific modulation of c-Myc cotransformation by residues phosphorylated in vivo. *Oncogene* 9, 59-70.

[61] Welcker M, Orian A, Jin J, Grim JE, Harper JW, Eisenman RN, Clurman BE (2004) The Fbw7 tumor suppressor regulates glycogen synthase kinase 3 phosphorylation-dependent c-Myc protein degradation. *Proc Natl Acad Sci U S A* 101, 9085-9090.

[62] Knoepfler PS, Cheng PF, Eisenman RN (2002) N-myc is essential during neurogenesis for the rapid expansion of progenitor cell populations and the inhibition of neuronal differentiation. *Genes Dev* 16, 2699-2712.

[63] Hatton KS, Mahon K, Chin L, Chiu FC, Lee HW, Peng D, Morgenbesser SD, Horner J, DePinho RA (1996) Expression and activity of L-Myc in normal mouse development. *Mol Cell Biol* 16, 1794-1804.

[64] Knoepfler PS, Kenney AM (2006) Neural precursor cycling at sonic speed: N-Myc pedals, GSK-3 brakes. *Cell Cycle* 5, 47-52.

[65] Sjostrom SK, Finn G, Hahn WC, Rowitch DH, Kenney AM (2005) The Cdk1 complex plays a prime role in regulating N-myc phosphorylation and turnover in neural precursors. *Dev Cell* 9, 327-338.

[66] Zhao Q, Kho A, Kenney AM, Yuk Di DI, Kohane I, Rowitch DH (2002) Identification of genes expressed with temporal-spatial restriction to developing cerebellar neuron precursors by a functional genomic approach. *Proc Natl Acad Sci U S A* 99, 5704-5709.

[67] Kenney AM, Widlund HR, Rowitch DH (2004) Hedgehog and PI-3 kinase signaling converge on Nmyc1 to promote cell cycle progression in cerebellar neuronal precursors. *Development* 131, 217-228.

[68] Oliver TG, Grasfeder LL, Carroll AL, Kaiser C, Gillingham CL, Lin SM, Wickramasinghe R, Scott MP, Wechsler-Reya RJ (2003) Transcriptional profiling of the Sonic

hedgehog response: a critical role for N-myc in proliferation of neuronal precursors. *Proc Natl Acad Sci U S A* 100, 7331-7336.

[69] Mottet D, Dumont V, Deccache Y, Demazy C, Ninane N, Raes M, Michiels C (2003) Regulation of hypoxia-inducible factor-1alpha protein level during hypoxic conditions by the phosphatidylinositol 3-kinase/Akt/glycogen synthase kinase 3beta pathway in HepG2 cells. *J Biol Chem* 278, 31277-31285.

[70] Flugel D, Gorlach A, Michiels C, Kietzmann T (2007) Glycogen synthase kinase 3 phosphorylates hypoxia-inducible factor 1alpha and mediates its destabilization in a VHL-independent manner. *Mol Cell Biol* 27, 3253-3265.

[71] Mazumdar J, O'Brien WT, Johnson RS, LaManna JC, Chavez JC, Klein PS, Simon MC (2010) O2 regulates stem cells through Wnt/beta-catenin signalling. *Nat Cell Biol* 12, 1007-1013.

[72] Roh MS, Eom TY, Zmijewska AA, De Sarno P, Roth KA, Jope RS (2005) Hypoxia activates glycogen synthase kinase-3 in mouse brain in vivo: protection by mood stabilizers and imipramine. *Biol Psychiatry* 57, 278-286.

[73] Singh KK, De Rienzo G, Drane L, Mao Y, Flood Z, Madison J, Ferreira M, Bergen S, King C, Sklar P, Sive H, Tsai LH (2011) Common DISC1 polymorphisms disrupt Wnt/GSK3beta signaling and brain development. *Neuron* 72, 545-558.

[74] Ishizuka K, Kamiya A, Oh EC, Kanki H, Seshadri S, Robinson JF, Murdoch H, Dunlop AJ, Kubo K, Furukori K, Huang B, Zeledon M, Hayashi-Takagi A, Okano H, Nakajima K, Houslay MD, Katsanis N, Sawa A (2011) DISC1-dependent switch from progenitor proliferation to migration in the developing cortex. *Nature* 473, 92-96.

[75] Emamian ES, Hall D, Birnbaum MJ, Karayiorgou M, Gogos JA (2004) Convergent evidence for impaired AKT1-GSK3beta signaling in schizophrenia. *Nat Genet* 36, 131-137.

[76] Hall D, Gogos JA, Karayiorgou M (2004) The contribution of three strong candidate schizophrenia susceptibility genes in demographically distinct populations. *Genes Brain Behav* 3, 240-248.

[77] Beaulieu JM, Sotnikova TD, Yao WD, Kockeritz L, Woodgett JR, Gainetdinov RR, Caron MG (2004) Lithium antagonizes dopamine-dependent behaviors mediated by an AKT/glycogen synthase kinase 3 signaling cascade. *Proc Natl Acad Sci U S A* 101, 5099-5104.

[78] Beaulieu JM, Sotnikova TD, Marion S, Lefkowitz RJ, Gainetdinov RR, Caron MG (2005) An Akt/beta-arrestin 2/PP2A signaling complex mediates dopaminergic neurotransmission and behavior. *Cell* 122, 261-273.

[79] Stambolic V, Ruel L, Woodgett JR (1996) Lithium inhibits glycogen synthase kinase-3 activity and mimics wingless signalling in intact cells. *Curr Biol* 6, 1664-1668.

[80] Beaulieu JM (2007) Not only lithium: regulation of glycogen synthase kinase-3 by antipsychotics and serotonergic drugs. *Int J Neuropsychopharmacol* 10, 3-6.

[81] Benedetti F, Bernasconi A, Lorenzi C, Pontiggia A, Serretti A, Colombo C, Smeraldi E (2004) A single nucleotide polymorphism in glycogen synthase kinase 3-beta promoter gene influences onset of illness in patients affected by bipolar disorder. *Neurosci Lett* 355, 37-40.

[82] Reif A, Fritzen S, Finger M, Strobel A, Lauer M, Schmitt A, Lesch KP (2006) Neural stem cell proliferation is decreased in schizophrenia, but not in depression. *Mol Psychiatry* 11, 514-522.

[83] Maciag D, Hughes J, O'Dwyer G, Pride Y, Stockmeier CA, Sanacora G, Rajkowska G (2010) Reduced density of calbindin immunoreactive GABAergic neurons in the occipital cortex in major depression: relevance to neuroimaging studies. *Biol Psychiatry* 67, 465-470.

[84] Higashi M, Maruta N, Bernstein A, Ikenaka K, Hitoshi S (2008) Mood stabilizing drugs expand the neural stem cell pool in the adult brain through activation of notch signaling. *Stem Cells* 26, 1758-1767.

[85] Wexler EM, Geschwind DH, Palmer TD (2008) Lithium regulates adult hippocampal progenitor development through canonical Wnt pathway activation. *Mol Psychiatry* 13, 285-292.

[86] Morgan TH (1917) The theory of the gene. *American Naturalist* 51.

[87] Poulson DF (1937) Chromosomal deficiencies and the embryonic development of Drosophila melanogaster. *Proc Natl Acad Sci U S A* 23, 133-137.

[88] Furukawa T, Mukherjee S, Bao ZZ, Morrow EM, Cepko CL (2000) rax, Hes1, and notch1 promote the formation of Muller glia by postnatal retinal progenitor cells. *Neuron* 26, 383-394.

[89] Scheer N, Groth A, Hans S, Campos-Ortega JA (2001) An instructive function for Notch in promoting gliogenesis in the zebrafish retina. *Development* 128, 1099-1107.

[90] Redmond L, Oh SR, Hicks C, Weinmaster G, Ghosh A (2000) Nuclear Notch1 signaling and the regulation of dendritic development. *Nat Neurosci* 3, 30-40.

[91] Costa RM, Honjo T, Silva AJ (2003) Learning and memory deficits in Notch mutant mice. *Curr Biol* 13, 1348-1354.

[92] Ruel L, Bourouis M, Heitzler P, Pantesco V, Simpson P (1993) Drosophila shaggy kinase and rat glycogen synthase kinase-3 have conserved activities and act downstream of Notch. *Nature* 362, 557-560.

[93] Foltz DR, Santiago MC, Berechid BE, Nye JS (2002) Glycogen synthase kinase-3beta modulates notch signaling and stability. *Curr Biol* 12, 1006-1011.

[94] Espinosa L, Ingles-Esteve J, Aguilera C, Bigas A (2003) Phosphorylation by glycogen synthase kinase-3 beta down-regulates Notch activity, a link for Notch and Wnt pathways. *J Biol Chem* 278, 32227-32235.

[95] Jin YH, Kim H, Oh M, Ki H, Kim K (2009) Regulation of Notch1/NICD and Hes1 expressions by GSK-3alpha/beta. *Mol Cells* 27, 15-19.

[96] Fryer CJ, White JB, Jones KA (2004) Mastermind recruits CycC:CDK8 to phosphorylate the Notch ICD and coordinate activation with turnover. *Mol Cell* 16, 509-520.

[97] Kwon C, Cheng P, King IN, Andersen P, Shenje L, Nigam V, Srivastava D (2011) Notch post-translationally regulates beta-catenin protein in stem and progenitor cells. *Nat Cell Biol* 13, 1244-1251.

[98] Shimizu T, Kagawa T, Inoue T, Nonaka A, Takada S, Aburatani H, Taga T (2008) Stabilized beta-catenin functions through TCF/LEF proteins and the Notch/RBP-Jkappa complex to promote proliferation and suppress differentiation of neural precursor cells. *Mol Cell Biol* 28, 7427-7441.

[99] Torres MA, Eldar-Finkelman H, Krebs EG, Moon RT (1999) Regulation of ribosomal S6 protein kinase-p90(rsk), glycogen synthase kinase 3, and beta-catenin in early Xenopus development. *Mol Cell Biol* 19, 1427-1437.

[100] Holnthoner W, Pillinger M, Groger M, Wolff K, Ashton AW, Albanese C, Neumeister P, Pestell RG, Petzelbauer P (2002) Fibroblast growth factor-2 induces Lef/Tcf-dependent transcription in human endothelial cells. *J Biol Chem* 277, 45847-45853.

[101] Jia J, Amanai K, Wang G, Tang J, Wang B, Jiang J (2002) Shaggy/GSK3 antagonizes Hedgehog signalling by regulating Cubitus interruptus. *Nature* 416, 548-552.

[102] Price MA, Kalderon D (2002) Proteolysis of the Hedgehog signaling effector Cubitus interruptus requires phosphorylation by Glycogen Synthase Kinase 3 and Casein Kinase 1. *Cell* 108, 823-835.

[103] Wang B, Li Y (2006) Evidence for the direct involvement of {beta}TrCP in Gli3 protein processing. *Proc Natl Acad Sci U S A* 103, 33-38.

[104] Pan Y, Bai CB, Joyner AL, Wang B (2006) Sonic hedgehog signaling regulates Gli2 transcriptional activity by suppressing its processing and degradation. *Mol Cell Biol* 26, 3365-3377.

[105] Tempe D, Casas M, Karaz S, Blanchet-Tournier MF, Concordet JP (2006) Multisite protein kinase A and glycogen synthase kinase 3beta phosphorylation leads to Gli3 ubiquitination by SCFbetaTrCP. *Mol Cell Biol* 26, 4316-4326.

[106] Chen Y, Yue S, Xie L, Pu XH, Jin T, Cheng SY (2011) Dual Phosphorylation of suppressor of fused (Sufu) by PKA and GSK3beta regulates its stability and localization in the primary cilium. *J Biol Chem* 286, 13502-13511.

[107] Tanji C, Yamamoto H, Yorioka N, Kohno N, Kikuchi K, Kikuchi A (2002) A-kinase anchoring protein AKAP220 binds to glycogen synthase kinase-3beta (GSK-3beta)

and mediates protein kinase A-dependent inhibition of GSK-3beta. *J Biol Chem* 277, 36955-36961.

[108] Logue JS, Whiting JL, Tunquist B, Sacks DB, Langeberg LK, Wordeman L, Scott JD (2011) AKAP220 protein organizes signaling elements that impact cell migration. *J Biol Chem* 286, 39269-39281.

[109] Kuhn HG, Winkler J, Kempermann G, Thal LJ, Gage FH (1997) Epidermal growth factor and fibroblast growth factor-2 have different effects on neural progenitors in the adult rat brain. *J Neurosci* 17, 5820-5829.

[110] Craig CG, Tropepe V, Morshead CM, Reynolds BA, Weiss S, van der Kooy D (1996) In vivo growth factor expansion of endogenous subependymal neural precursor cell populations in the adult mouse brain. *J Neurosci* 16, 2649-2658.

[111] Emsley JG, Hagg T (2003) Endogenous and exogenous ciliary neurotrophic factor enhances forebrain neurogenesis in adult mice. *Exp Neurol* 183, 298-310.

[112] Zigova T, Pencea V, Wiegand SJ, Luskin MB (1998) Intraventricular administration of BDNF increases the number of newly generated neurons in the adult olfactory bulb. *Mol Cell Neurosci* 11, 234-245.

[113] Bath KG, Mandairon N, Jing D, Rajagopal R, Kapoor R, Chen ZY, Khan T, Proenca CC, Kraemer R, Cleland TA, Hempstead BL, Chao MV, Lee FS (2008) Variant brain-derived neurotrophic factor (Val66Met) alters adult olfactory bulb neurogenesis and spontaneous olfactory discrimination. *J Neurosci* 28, 2383-2393.

[114] Farinas I, Wilkinson GA, Backus C, Reichardt LF, Patapoutian A (1998) Characterization of neurotrophin and Trk receptor functions in developing sensory ganglia: direct NT-3 activation of TrkB neurons in vivo. *Neuron* 21, 325-334.

[115] Kirschenbaum B, Goldman SA (1995) Brain-derived neurotrophic factor promotes the survival of neurons arising from the adult rat forebrain subependymal zone. *Proc Natl Acad Sci U S A* 92, 210-214.

[116] Mattson MP (2008) Glutamate and neurotrophic factors in neuronal plasticity and disease. *Ann N Y Acad Sci* 1144, 97-112.

[117] Nagahara AH, Tuszynski MH (2011) Potential therapeutic uses of BDNF in neurological and psychiatric disorders. *Nat Rev Drug Discov* 10, 209-219.

[118] Mines MA, Beurel E, Jope RS (2011) Regulation of cell survival mechanisms in Alzheimer's disease by glycogen synthase kinase-3. *Int J Alzheimers Dis* 2011, 861072.

[119] Pap M, Cooper GM (1998) Role of glycogen synthase kinase-3 in the phosphatidylinositol 3-Kinase/Akt cell survival pathway. *J Biol Chem* 273, 19929-19932.

[120] Bijur GN, De Sarno P, Jope RS (2000) Glycogen synthase kinase-3beta facilitates staurosporine- and heat shock-induced apoptosis. Protection by lithium. *J Biol Chem* 275, 7583-7590.

[121] Maurer U, Charvet C, Wagman AS, Dejardin E, Green DR (2006) Glycogen synthase kinase-3 regulates mitochondrial outer membrane permeabilization and apoptosis by destabilization of MCL-1. *Mol Cell* 21, 749-760.

[122] Ding Q, He X, Hsu JM, Xia W, Chen CT, Li LY, Lee DF, Liu JC, Zhong Q, Wang X, Hung MC (2007) Degradation of Mcl-1 by beta-TrCP mediates glycogen synthase kinase 3-induced tumor suppression and chemosensitization. *Mol Cell Biol* 27, 4006-4017.

[123] Oishi K, Kamakura S, Isazawa Y, Yoshimatsu T, Kuida K, Nakafuku M, Masuyama N, Gotoh Y (2004) Notch promotes survival of neural precursor cells via mechanisms distinct from those regulating neurogenesis. *Dev Biol* 276, 172-184.

[124] Arbour N, Vanderluit JL, Le Grand JN, Jahani-Asl A, Ruzhynsky VA, Cheung EC, Kelly MA, MacKenzie AE, Park DS, Opferman JT, Slack RS (2008) Mcl-1 is a key regulator of apoptosis during CNS development and after DNA damage. *J Neurosci* 28, 6068-6078.

[125] Germain M, Nguyen AP, Le Grand JN, Arbour N, Vanderluit JL, Park DS, Opferman JT, Slack RS (2011) MCL-1 is a stress sensor that regulates autophagy in a developmentally regulated manner. *EMBO J* 30, 395-407.

[126] Magiera MM, Mora S, Mojsa B, Robbins I, Lassot I, Desagher S (2012) Trim17-mediated ubiquitination and degradation of Mcl-1 initiate apoptosis in neurons. *Cell Death Differ.*

[127] Somervaille TC, Linch DC, Khwaja A (2001) Growth factor withdrawal from primary human erythroid progenitors induces apoptosis through a pathway involving glycogen synthase kinase-3 and Bax. *Blood* 98, 1374-1381.

[128] Linseman DA, Butts BD, Precht TA, Phelps RA, Le SS, Laessig TA, Bouchard RJ, Florez-McClure ML, Heidenreich KA (2004) Glycogen synthase kinase-3beta phosphorylates Bax and promotes its mitochondrial localization during neuronal apoptosis. *J Neurosci* 24, 9993-10002.

[129] Chu B, Zhong R, Soncin F, Stevenson MA, Calderwood SK (1998) Transcriptional activity of heat shock factor 1 at 37 degrees C is repressed through phosphorylation on two distinct serine residues by glycogen synthase kinase 3 and protein kinases Calpha and Czeta. *J Biol Chem* 273, 18640-18646.

[130] Wang X, She H, Mao Z (2009) Phosphorylation of neuronal survival factor MEF2D by glycogen synthase kinase 3beta in neuronal apoptosis. *J Biol Chem* 284, 32619-32626.

[131] Viatour P, Dejardin E, Warnier M, Lair F, Claudio E, Bureau F, Marine JC, Merville MP, Maurer U, Green D, Piette J, Siebenlist U, Bours V, Chariot A (2004) GSK3-mediated BCL-3 phosphorylation modulates its degradation and its oncogenicity. *Mol Cell* 16, 35-45.

[132] Pazyra-Murphy MF, Hans A, Courchesne SL, Karch C, Cosker KE, Heerssen HM, Watson FL, Kim T, Greenberg ME, Segal RA (2009) A retrograde neuronal survival

response: target-derived neurotrophins regulate MEF2D and bcl-w. *J Neurosci* 29, 6700-6709.

[133] Moberg KH, Mukherjee A, Veraksa A, Artavanis-Tsakonas S, Hariharan IK (2004) The Drosophila F box protein archipelago regulates dMyc protein levels in vivo. *Curr Biol* 14, 965-974.

[134] Yada M, Hatakeyama S, Kamura T, Nishiyama M, Tsunematsu R, Imaki H, Ishida N, Okumura F, Nakayama K, Nakayama KI (2004) Phosphorylation-dependent degradation of c-Myc is mediated by the F-box protein Fbw7. *EMBO J* 23, 2116-2125.

[135] Wei W, Jin J, Schlisio S, Harper JW, Kaelin WG, Jr. (2005) The v-Jun point mutation allows c-Jun to escape GSK3-dependent recognition and destruction by the Fbw7 ubiquitin ligase. *Cancer Cell* 8, 25-33.

[136] Liu N, Li H, Li S, Shen M, Xiao N, Chen Y, Wang Y, Wang W, Wang R, Wang Q, Sun J, Wang P (2010) The Fbw7/human CDC4 tumor suppressor targets proproliferative factor KLF5 for ubiquitination and degradation through multiple phosphodegron motifs. *J Biol Chem* 285, 18858-18867.

[137] Zhao D, Zheng HQ, Zhou Z, Chen C (2010) The Fbw7 tumor suppressor targets KLF5 for ubiquitin-mediated degradation and suppresses breast cell proliferation. *Cancer Res* 70, 4728-4738.

[138] Welcker M, Singer J, Loeb KR, Grim J, Bloecher A, Gurien-West M, Clurman BE, Roberts JM (2003) Multisite phosphorylation by Cdk2 and GSK3 controls cyclin E degradation. *Mol Cell* 12, 381-392.

[139] Zhou BP, Deng J, Xia W, Xu J, Li YM, Gunduz M, Hung MC (2004) Dual regulation of Snail by GSK-3beta-mediated phosphorylation in control of epithelial-mesenchymal transition. *Nat Cell Biol* 6, 931-940.

[140] Cartwright P, McLean C, Sheppard A, Rivett D, Jones K, Dalton S (2005) LIF/STAT3 controls ES cell self-renewal and pluripotency by a Myc-dependent mechanism. *Development* 132, 885-896.

[141] Wang Z, Inuzuka H, Zhong J, Wan L, Fukushima H, Sarkar FH, Wei W (2012) Tumor suppressor functions of FBW7 in cancer development and progression. *FEBS Lett* 586, 1409-1418.

[142] Hoeck JD, Jandke A, Blake SM, Nye E, Spencer-Dene B, Brandner S, Behrens A (2010) Fbw7 controls neural stem cell differentiation and progenitor apoptosis via Notch and c-Jun. *Nat Neurosci* 13, 1365-1372.

[143] Jandke A, Da Costa C, Sancho R, Nye E, Spencer-Dene B, Behrens A (2011) The F-box protein Fbw7 is required for cerebellar development. *Dev Biol* 358, 201-212.

[144] Matsumoto A, Onoyama I, Sunabori T, Kageyama R, Okano H, Nakayama KI (2011) Fbxw7-dependent degradation of Notch is required for control of "stemness" and neuronal-glial differentiation in neural stem cells. *J Biol Chem* 286, 13754-13764.

[145] Sutherland C (2011) What Are the bona fide GSK3 Substrates? *Int J Alzheimers Dis* 2011, 505607.

[146] Cole AR (2012) GSK3 as a Sensor Determining Cell Fate in the Brain. *Front Mol Neurosci* 5, 4.

[147] Asada N, Sanada K (2010) LKB1-mediated spatial control of GSK3beta and adenomatous polyposis coli contributes to centrosomal forward movement and neuronal migration in the developing neocortex. *J Neurosci* 30, 8852-8865.

[148] Eickholt BJ, Walsh FS, Doherty P (2002) An inactive pool of GSK-3 at the leading edge of growth cones is implicated in Semaphorin 3A signaling. *J Cell Biol* 157, 211-217.

[149] Etienne-Manneville S, Hall A (2003) Cdc42 regulates GSK-3beta and adenomatous polyposis coli to control cell polarity. *Nature* 421, 753-756.

[150] Jiang H, Guo W, Liang X, Rao Y (2005) Both the establishment and the maintenance of neuronal polarity require active mechanisms: critical roles of GSK-3beta and its upstream regulators. *Cell* 120, 123-135.

[151] Shi SH, Cheng T, Jan LY, Jan YN (2004) APC and GSK-3beta are involved in mPar3 targeting to the nascent axon and establishment of neuronal polarity. *Curr Biol* 14, 2025-2032.

[152] Yoshimura T, Kawano Y, Arimura N, Kawabata S, Kikuchi A, Kaibuchi K (2005) GSK-3beta regulates phosphorylation of CRMP-2 and neuronal polarity. *Cell* 120, 137-149.

[153] Guo W, Jiang H, Gray V, Dedhar S, Rao Y (2007) Role of the integrin-linked kinase (ILK) in determining neuronal polarity. *Dev Biol* 306, 457-468.

[154] Cole AR, Sutherland C (2008) Measuring GSK3 expression and activity in cells. *Methods Mol Biol* 468, 45-65.

[155] Cole AR, Causeret F, Yadirgi G, Hastie CJ, McLauchlan H, McManus EJ, Hernandez F, Eickholt BJ, Nikolic M, Sutherland C (2006) Distinct priming kinases contribute to differential regulation of collapsin response mediator proteins by glycogen synthase kinase-3 in vivo. *J Biol Chem* 281, 16591-16598.

[156] Seeling JM, Miller JR, Gil R, Moon RT, White R, Virshup DM (1999) Regulation of beta-catenin signaling by the B56 subunit of protein phosphatase 2A. *Science* 283, 2089-2091.

[157] Hernandez F, Langa E, Cuadros R, Avila J, Villanueva N (2010) Regulation of GSK3 isoforms by phosphatases PP1 and PP2A. *Mol Cell Biochem* 344, 211-215.

Chapter 6

Roles of Wnt/β-Catenin Signaling in Controlling the Dopaminergic Neuronal Cell Commitment of Midbrain and Therapeutic Application for Parkinson's Disease

Liang-Wei Chen

Additional information is available at the end of the chapter

1. Introduction

Parkinson's disease (PD) is a severe deliberating neurodegenerative disease resulting from progressive and massive cell death of dopaminergic (DA) neurons in the substantia nigra [1]. While cell therapy strategy is strongly suggested for clinical cure of PD and DA progenitors are identified at different developing stages of midbrain, full understanding of key cell signaling or mechanism in controlling of DA neuronal differentiation from neural stem cells *in vivo* raises a great interest in cell therapeutic application for PD [2, 3]. A growing line of studies has shown that Wnts are lipid-modified factor for stem cell growth and cell differentiation and regulate midbrain DA neuronal development and hippocampal neurogenesis through both canonical and non-canonical Wnt signaling pathways [4-7]. The canonical Wnt/β-catenin signaling appeals a key mechanism in controlling DA neuronal fate decision from neural stem cells or progenitors in the ventral midbrain during embryonic development and adulthood [8]. This chapter has focused on fast growing knowledge on Wnt/β-catenin signaling pathway, intracellular cascade or crosstalk, functional roles in controlling DA neuronal fate decision and neural repair under physiological development and pathological events, and potential manipulation of Wnt/β-catenin signaling pathway as cell therapeutic target for treatment of PD in human beings.

2. The Wnt/β-catenin signaling pathway

The Wnt signaling pathway, conserved from low animals to primates, was originally identified as the morphogenic signaling for organogenesis. Among three branches of Wnt signaling pathways, the best studied one is the canonical Wnt pathway, which is highlighted by β-catenin-dependent regulation of down-streaming genes. The canonical Wnt ligands, e.g. Wnt1, Wnt2 and Wnt3a, can be secreted by surrounding neuronal and glial cells in the nervous system, bind to Frizzled and Lrp5/6 receptors in the target cells. At absence of binding with ligand Wnts, a protein complex in the cytoplasm, namely Axin2/GSK3β/APC complex makes phosphorylation of β-catenin and degradation of phosphorylated β-catenin, and keeps cytoplasmic β-catenin at such a low level that β-catenin can not be translocated into nucleus. Upon Wnt stimulation, the Axin2/GSK3β/APC complex can be deaggregated, the cytoplasmic β-catenin is accumulated and increased β-catenin imported into nucleus. In the nucleus, β-catenin is recruited by transcription factors TCF1-4 to the promoter regions of the target genes for specific biological effects. These TCF-4 downstream targeting genes include c-myc, mmp-7, cyclin D1, CD44 that are actively and mainly involved in cell proliferation, cycling and cell differentiation (Figure 1). On the other hand, the non-canonical Wnt signaling pathways, i.e. PCP pathway and Ca^{2+} pathway, Wnt ligands bind to Frizzled receptors, then activate GTPase or increase intracellular Ca2+, transmitting signals by JNK cascade or without any nucleus events [4-6].

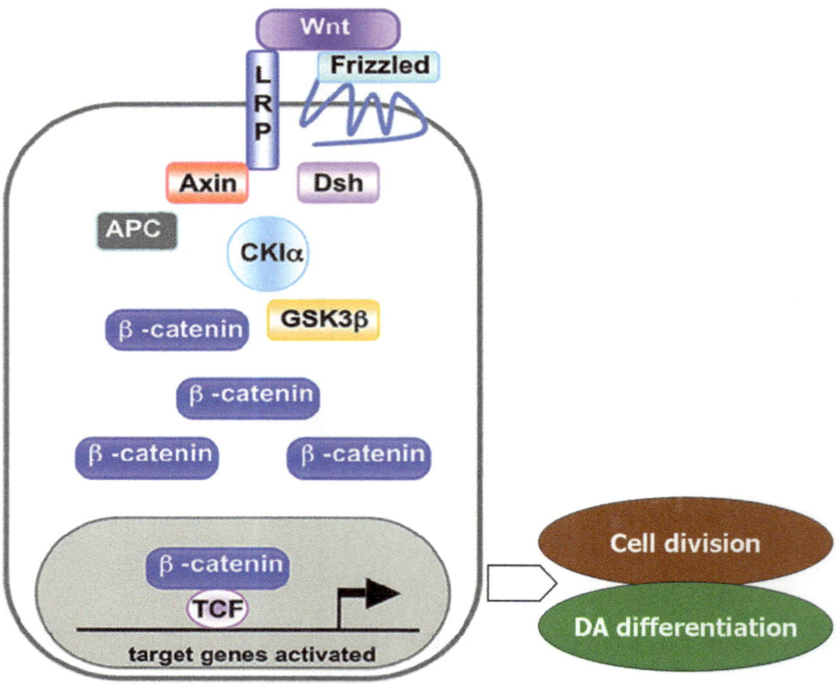

Figure 1. The canonical Wnt/β-catenin signaling pathway in regulation of downstream target genes of DA neurogenesis (*From Ref. 48, Ding, et al., 2011*)

3. Role of Wnt/β-catenin signaling in facilitating DA neuronal development

The canonical Wnt/β-catenin signaling pathways is critical for generation of DA neurons during development. Differential regulation of midbrain DA neurogenesis by Wnt1, Wnt3a, and Wnt5a was well studied [9]. The β-catenin was detected in DA precursor cells and β-catenin signaling took place in the precursor cells by assessment of TOPgal reporter mice. Wnt3a promoted proliferation of precursor cells expressing the orphan nuclear receptor-related factor 1 (Nurr1) but did not increase the number of DA neurons. The Wnt1 and Wnt5a increased the number of midbrain DA neurons in E14.5 possibly by two mechanisms. Wnt1 predominantly increased the proliferation of Nurr1+ precursors that acquired a neuronal DA phenotype, up-regulated cyclins D1 and D3, and down-regulated p27 and p57 expression. In contrast, Wnt5a increased proportion of Nurr1+ precursors and up-regulated expression of Ptx3 and c-ret mRNA. Moreover, the soluble cysteine-rich domain of Frizzled-8 (a Wnt inhibitor) blocked endogenous Wnts and effects of Wnt1 and Wnt5a on proliferation and acquisition of DA phenotype. For the embryonic expression, Wnt1 was throughout of midbrain at E8.5, and then restricted to the roof plate, a subset of floor plate cells and isthemus of midbrain at E9.5. From E10 to E12, Wnt2 was observed in the ventral midbrain, with highest in the intermediate and marginal zone of ventral midbrain. Wnt3a was expressed in dorsal midbrain of rat at E11.5. The Wnt5a appeared at E9.5 and became restricted to the floor plate of midbrain from E11.5 to E13.5. Functionally, mutation of Wnt1 led to reduced DA neurons in late embryos. Mechanistic study showed that Wnt1 and its downstream gene Lmx1 formed a loop to regulate the expression of Octx2, Nurr1 and Pitx3, thereby establishing identity of DA precursors *in vivo* [10]. This Wnt1-lmx1a regulatory loop synergistically controlled DA differentiation in the midbrain by antagonizing Shh signaling pathway [11]. Wnt 2 mutation resulted in a decrease in proliferation of DA progenitors and subsequently loss of DA neurons, partially by phosphorylation of Lrp5/6 and Dishevelled 2/3. Wnt 3a promoted the proliferation of Nurr1-positive DA progenitors. The Wnt5a, derived by the astrocytes and radial glial cells, was demonstrated to promote cell fate commitment of precursors into DA neurons and development of A9-A10 DA neurons *in vivo* [12, 13]. The Wnt5a also regulated DA axon growth and guidance in midbrain development [14]. In mouse embryo at E11.5, Wnt5a was abundantly expressed in the ventral midbrain where it promoted DA neurite and axonal growth. By E14.5, when DA axons were approaching their striatal target, Wnt5a caused DA neurite retraction. Co-culture of ventral midbrain explants with Wnt5a-overexpressing cell aggregates revealed that Wnt5a was capable of repelling DA neurites. Antagonism experiments revealed that the effects of Wnt5a were mediated by the Frizzled receptors and by small GTPase, Rac1. Moreover, this effect was specifically blocked by Wnt5a antibody. Role of Wnt5a in DA neuronal axon morphogenesis was further verified in Wnt5a-/-mice, where fasciculation of the medial forebrain bundle as well as the density of DA neurites and striatal terminals were disrupted. Although Wnts can function via intracellularβ-catenin, Ca2+, and JNK signaling, the canonical Wnt/β-catenin signaling pathway shows a major position in regulation of DA neurogenesis. It appeared that all Wnt1, Wnt3a and Wnt5a act in proliferation and DA differentiation of precursor cells with sequence of proliferation stimulating effect of Wnt1≥Wnt3a≥Wnt5a, or differentiation facilitating effects of Wnt5a≥Wnt1≥Wnt3a. These findings have evidenced that the Wnt/β-catenin signaling is a key regulator of proliferation and differentiation of DA precursors and different Wnts might have specific and unique activity profiles during DA neurogenesis.

Dynamic temporal and cell type-specific expression of Wnt signaling components was found in the developing midbrain [15]. The DA neuronal cluster size was determined during early forebrain patterning [16]. Furthermore, temporally controlling modulation of FGF/ERK signaling directed midbrain DA neural progenitor fate in mouse and human pluripotent stem cells [17]. Dickkopf-1 (Dkk1), a specific Wnt signaling inhibitor, regulated ventral midbrain DA neuronal differentiation and morphogenesis [18]. Blockade of Wnt/β-catenin signaling pathway promoted neuronal induction and DA-phenotype differentiation in embryonic stem cells [19]. Delayed DA neuron differentiation was seen in the Lrp6 mutant mice [20]. Signaling interactions between Wnt/β-catenin and sonic hedgehog (Shh) mechanisms functioned to regulate the production of DA neurons. Specific deletion of intracellular β-catenin in Shh expressing cells resulted in diminished DA progenitors, NgN2, BrdU labeling cells, and subsequently DA neurons. Permanent stabilization of β-catenin in Shh expressing cells led to more DA progenitors and DA neurons accordingly, and inhibition of GSK-3β also increases the differentiation of DA precursors [21]. HPRT deficiency coordinately dysregulated canonical Wnt signaling in neuro-developmental regulatory process [22]. Wnts showed antagonism of Shh signaling pathway and facilitated neurogenesis in the midbrain floor plate [23]. The β-arrestin was also a necessary component of Wnt/beta-catenin signaling linking Dvl and axin *in vitro* and *in vivo* functions [24]. Wnt5a induced the DA differentiation of midbrain neural stem cells *in vitro*, and the effect was mediated by the phosphorylation of Dishevelled protein and activation of GTPase RAC1. Wnt5A stimulated the GDP/GTP exchange at pertussis toxin-sensitive heterotrimeric G proteins [25]. As to Wnt receptors, mutation of Lrp6 might not affect the patterning; proliferation and cell death in the ventral midbrain, but displayed a delay in the onset of DA precursor differentiation. Lrp6(-/-) mice exhibited 50% reduction in DA neurons and expression of DA markers such as Nurrl and Pitx3 as well as a defect in midbrain morphogenesis in the mutant embryos at E11.5. The extracellular domain of Lrp5/6 inhibited the non-canonical Wnt signaling *in vivo* condition [26]. The mitogen-activated protein kinases promoted Wnt/β-catenin signaling via phosphorylation of LRP6 [27]. Ectopic Wnt/β-catenin signaling was also involved in induction of neurogenesis in spinal cord [28]. In addition, Wnt5a was required for the endothelial differentiation of embryonic stem cells and vascularization via both Wnt/β-catenin signaling and protein kinase C pathways [29].

4. Role of Wnt/β-catenin signaling in DA neural plasticity or repair in adulthood

The Wnt/β-catenin signaling pathway also actively functions in neural plasticity and repair of DA neurons in the midbrain of disease conditions Interestingly, the crosstalk between Wnt/β-catenin signaling and inflammatory was observed in plasticity of subventricular zone progenitors in response to 1-methyl-4-phenyl-1,2,3,6-tetrahydropyridine (MPTP) model of PD, suggesting its involvement in consequences for neuroprotection and functional repair

[30]. Accumulating evidence indicated that a population of astrocyte was functionally activated, named reactive astrocytes with active proliferation, morphological expanding of cell bodies and increasing generation of various neurotrophic factors, and with predominate distribution in the nigra and striatum of PD condition. These reactive astrocytes and Wnt/β-catenin signaling showed a link of nigrostriatal injury to repair in MPTP model of PD. The Wnt signaling components Frizzled-1 and β-catenin were dynamically regulated in response to MPTP insult-induced DA neuronal degeneration and reactive glial activation. Activated or reactive astrocytes in the ventral midbrain were identified as candidate source of Wnt1. Blocking Wnt/Fzd signaling with Dkk1 also counteracted astrocyte-induced neuroprotection against MPP (+) toxicity in primary mesencephalic astrocyte-neuron cultures. Moreover, astrocyte-derived Wnt1 promoted DA neurogenesis from adult midbrain stem cells or progenitor cells. Conversely, lack of Wnt1 transcription in response to MPTP in aged animals and failure of DA neurons to recover could be reversed by activation of Wnt/β-catenin signaling *in vivo*, suggesting MPTP-reactive astrocytes and Wnt1 worked as neuroprotective activity in DA neural plasticity [31]. Obviously, Wnt1 regulated Frizzled-1/β-catenin signaling pathway as a candidate regulatory circuit for DA neuron-astrocyte crosstalk in the ventral midbrain, also implying that Wnt signals might act as the critical messages in neuron-glial intercommunication in the adult mammalian nervous system [32].

Moreover, The Wnt/β-catenin signaling also involved in Parkin protection of DA neurons [33]. Differential expression of Wnts was observed after spinal cord contusion injury in adult rodents [34]. Wnt signaling in the activated microglia; cells exhibited proinflammatory effect. Gene-expression profiling revealed that Wnt3A specifically increased expression of proinflammatory immune response genes in microglia and exacerbated release of IL-6, IL-12, and tumor necrosis factor α [35]. Heterotrimeric G protein-dependent Wnt5A signaling to ERK1/2 mediated distinct aspects of proinflammatory transformation in microglial cells [36]. While combining nitric oxide release with anti-inflammatory activity preserved DA innervation and prevented motor impairment in the MPTP model of PD [37], switching the microglial harmful phenotype promoted lifelong restoration of DA neurons from inflammatory degeneration in the substantia nigra of aged mice [38]. In addition, activation or inhibition of Wnt/β-catenin signaling could regulate neuronal and glial differentiation in neurospheres, respectively. Inhibition of Wnt signaling promoted gliogenesis from neural stem cells. Long-term activation of Wnt signaling pathway by Wnt-7a or GSK3 inhibitors promoted a moderate increase of neuronal differentiation and blocked gliogenesis. In contrast, Wnt pathway inhibition by Dkk1overexpression robustly increased gliogenesis [39]. Accumulating evidences suggested that the glial cells including reactive astrocytes and microglial cells might present as crucial turning points for the therapeutic strategy against PD [40, 41]

5. Prospect on manipulation of Wnt/β-catenin signaling for regeneration medicine

The studies have indicated that transplantation of Wnt primed neural stem cells might result in improvements of cellular and functional recovery in PD condition. The midbrain neural stem cells with Wnt5a-treatment showed beneficial effect for DA cell replacement therapy in parkinsonian animal model [42], and purified Wnt5a increased dishevelled phosphorylation and DA neuronal differentiation in the midbrain [43]. Both GSK-3β inhibition and β-catenin stabilization increased commitment into DA neurons of neural precursors in the ventral midbrain [44], and the application of GSK-3β inhibitor lithium also influenced DA differentiation potential of human NT2 cells [45]. Generation of DA phenotype in neural stem cells could be carried out by engineering Nurr1 and Wnt signals [46]. Wnts also showed regulating role on differentiation of noradrenergic neuronal precursors in locus coeruleus [47]. In addition, the functional involvement of Wnt/β-catenin signaling pathway in link of reactive astrocytes and plasticity or repair of nigrostriatal system further suggests Wnt/β-catenin signaling as neuroprotection therapeutic targets [30, 31]. It is hopefully that DA differentiation of the neural stem cells and the nigrostriatal plasticity may be effectively and specifically enhanced or improved by manipulation targeting on Wnt/β-catenin signaling pathway [48].

6. Summary

Although the DA neuronal cell commitment from neural stem cells or progenitor cells is highly complicated and precisely regulated process, the canonical Wnt/β-catenin pathway shows a critical role in controlling differentiation of DA neurons in the ventral midbrain during development and plasticity or neural repair in adulthood. In addition, Wnt singling might also act via Ca2+, JNK signaling and function candidate messages in DA neuron-glial cross-talk as well. Taken together, it is hopefully expected that molecular target manipulation of Wnt/β-catenin signaling cascades will benefit controlling of DA neurogenesis and establishing novel cell therapy for PD in human beings.

Acknowledgements

This work was supported by grants from the Basic Research Program of China (2011CB504103, 2012CB525002) and the National Natural Science Foundation of China (30970862, 81071609, 81272346).

Author details

Liang-Wei Chen

Address all correspondence to: lwchen@fmmu.edu.cn

Institute of Neurosciences, The Fourth Military Medical University, Xi'an, China

References

[1] Fernandez-Espejo E. Pathogenesis of Parkinson's disease: prospects of neuroprotective and restorative therapies. Mol. Neurobiol., 2004; 29:15-30.

[2] Lie DC, Song H, Colamarino SA, Ming GL, Gage FH. Neurogenesis in the adult brain: new strategies for central nervous system diseases. Annu. Rev. Pharmacol. Toxicol., 2004; 44:399-421.

[3] Jönsson ME, Ono Y, Björklund A, Thompson LH. Identification of transplantable dopamine neuron precursors at different stages of midbrain neurogenesis. Exp. Neurol., 2009; 219:341-354.

[4] Willert K, Brown JD, Danenberg E, Duncan AW, Weissman IL, Reya T, Yates JR 3rd, Nusse R. Wnt proteins are lipid-modified and can act as stem cell growth factors. Nature, 2003, 423:448-452.

[5] Prakash N, Wurst W. A Wnt signal regulates stem cell fate and differentiation in vivo. Neurodegener. Dis., 2007; 4:333-338.

[6] Widelitz R. Wnt signaling through canonical and non-canonical pathways: recent progress. Growth Factors, 2005; 23:111-116.

[7] Lie DC, Colamarino SA, Song HJ, Désiré L, Mira H, Consiglio A, Lein ES, Jessberger S, Lansford H, Dearie AR, Gage FH. Wnt signalling regulates adult hippocampal neurogenesis. Nature, 2005; 437:1370-1375.

[8] Castelo-Branco G, Arenas E. Function of Wnts in dopaminergic neuron development. Neurodegener. Dis., 2006; 3:5-11.

[9] Castelo-Branco G, Wagner J, Rodriguez FJ, Kele J, Sousa K, Rawal N, Pasolli HA, Fuchs E, Kitajewski J, Arenas E. Differential regulation of midbrain dopaminergic neuron development by Wnt-1, Wnt-3a, and Wnt-5a. Proc. Natl. Acad. Sci. USA., 2003; 100:12747-12752.

[10] Prakash N, Brodski C, Naserke T, Puelles E, Gogoi R, Hall A, Panhuysen M, Echevarria D, Sussel L, Weisenhorn DM, Martinez S, Arenas E, Simeone A, Wurst W. A Wnt1-regulated genetic network controls the identity and fate of midbrain-dopaminergic progenitors in vivo. Development, 2006; 133:89-98.

[11] Chung S, Leung A, Han BS, Chang MY, Moon JI, Kim CH, Hong S, Pruszak J, Isacson O, Kim KS. Wnt1-lmx1a forms a novel autoregulatory loop and controls midbrain dopaminergic differentiation synergistically with the SHH-FoxA2 pathway. Cell Stem Cell, 2009; 5:646-658.

[12] Andersson ER, Prakash N, Cajanek L, Minina E, Bryja V, Bryjova L, Yamaguchi TP, Hall AC, Wurst W, Arenas E. Wnt5a regulates ventral midbrain morphogenesis and the development of A9-A10 dopaminergic cells in vivo. PLoS One, 2008; 3:e3517.

[13] Castelo-Branco G, Sousa KM, Bryja V, Pinto L, Wagner J, Arenas E. Ventral midbrain glia express region-specific transcription factors and regulate dopaminergic neurogenesis through Wnt-5a secretion. Mol. Cell. Neurosci., 2006; 31:251-262.

[14] Blakely BD, Bye CR, Fernando CV, Horne MK, Macheda ML, Stacker SA, Arenas E, Parish CL. Wnt5a regulates midbrain dopaminergic axon growth and guidance. PLoS One, 2011; 6:e18373.

[15] Rawal N, Castelo-Branco G, Sousa KM, Kele J, Kobayashi K, Okano H, Arenas E. Dynamic temporal and cell type-specific expression of Wnt signaling components in the developing midbrain. Exp. Cell Res., 2006; 312:1626-1636.

[16] Russek-Blum N, Gutnick A, Nabel-Rosen H, Blechman J, Staudt N, Dorsky RI, Houart C, Levkowitz G. Dopaminergic neuronal cluster size is determined during early forebrain patterning. Development, 2008; 135:3401-3413.

[17] Jaeger I, Arber C, Risner-Janiczek JR, Kuechler J, Pritzsche D, Chen IC, Naveenan T, Ungless MA, Li M. Temporally controlled modulation of FGF/ERK signaling directs midbrain dopaminergic neural progenitor fate in mouse and human pluripotent stem cells. Development, 2011; 138:4363-4374.

[18] Ribeiro D, Ellwanger K, Glagow D, Theofilopoulos S, Corsini NS, Martin-Villalba A, Niehrs C, Arenas E. Dkk1 regulates ventral midbrain dopaminergic differentiation and morphogenesis. PLoS One, 2011; 6:e15786.

[19] Cajánek L, Ribeiro D, Liste I, Parish CL, Bryja V, Arenas E. Wnt/beta-catenin signaling blockade promotes neuronal induction and dopaminergic differentiation in embryonic stem cells. Stem Cells, 2009; 27:2917-2927.

[20] Castelo-Branco G, Andersson ER, Minina E, Sousa KM, Ribeiro D, Kokubu C, Imai K, Prakash N, Wurst W, Arenas E. Delayed dopaminergic neuron differentiation in Lrp6 mutant mice. Dev. Dyn., 2010; 239:211-221.

[21] Tang M, Villaescusa JC, Luo SX, Guitarte C, Lei S, Miyamoto Y, Taketo MM, Arenas E, Huang EJ. Interactions of Wnt/beta-catenin signaling and sonic hedgehog regulate the neurogenesis of ventral midbrain dopamine neurons. J. Neurosci., 2010; 30:9280-9291.

[22] Kang TH, Guibinga GH, Jinnah HA, Friedmann T. HPRT deficiency coordinately dysregulates canonical Wnt and presenilin-1 signaling: a neuro-developmental regulatory role for a housekeeping gene? PLoS One, 2011; 6:e16572.

[23] Joksimovic M, Yun BA, Kittappa R, Anderegg AM, Chang WW, Taketo MM, McKay RD, Awatramani RB. Wnt antagonism of Shh facilitates midbrain floor plate neurogenesis. Nat. Neurosci., 2009; 12:125-31.

[24] Bryja V, Gradl D, Schambony A, Arenas E, Schulte G. Beta-arrestin is a necessary component of Wnt/beta-catenin signaling in vitro and in vivo. Proc. Natl. Acad. Sci. USA., 2007; 104:6690-6695.

[25] Kilander MB, Dijksterhuis JP, Ganji RS, Bryja V, Schulte G. WNT-5A stimulates the GDP/GTP exchange at pertussis toxin-sensitive heterotrimeric G proteins. Cell Signal, 2011; 23:550-554.

[26] Bryja V, Andersson ER, Schambony A, Esner M, Bryjová L, Biris KK, Hall AC, Kraft B, Cajanek L, Yamaguchi TP, Buckingham M, Arenas E. The extracellular domain of Lrp5/6 inhibits noncanonical Wnt signaling in vivo. Mol. Biol. Cell., 2009; 20:924-936.

[27] Červenka I, Wolf J, Mašek J, Krejci P, Wilcox WR, Kozubík A, Schulte G, Gutkind JS, Bryja V. Mitogen-activated protein kinases promote WNT/beta-catenin signaling via phosphorylation of LRP6. Mol. Cell. Biol., 2011; 31(1):179-189.

[28] Joksimovic M, Patel M, Taketo MM, Johnson R, Awatramani R. Ectopic Wnt/beta-catenin signaling induces neurogenesis in the spinal cord and hindbrain floor plate. PLoS One, 2012; 7:e30266.

[29] Yang DH, Yoon JY, Lee SH, Bryja V, Andersson ER, Arenas E, Kwon YG, Choi KY. Wnt5a is required for endothelial differentiation of embryonic stem cells and vascularization via pathways involving both Wnt/beta-catenin and protein kinase Calpha. Circ. Res., 2009; 104:372-379.

[30] L'Episcopo F, Tirolo C, Testa N, Caniglia S, Morale MC, Deleidi M, Serapide MF, Pluchino S, Marchetti B. Plasticity of subventricular zone neuroprogenitors in MPTP (1-methyl-4-phenyl- 1,2,3,6-tetrahydropyridine) mouse model of Parkinson's disease involves cross talk between inflammatory and Wnt/β-catenin signaling pathways: functional consequences for neuroprotection and repair. J. Neurosci., 2012; 32:2062-2085.

[31] L'Episcopo F, Tirolo C, Testa N, Caniglia S, Morale MC, Cossetti C, D'Adamo P, Zardini E, Andreoni L, Ihekwaba AE, Serra PA, Franciotta D, Martino G, Pluchino S, Marchetti B. Reactive astrocytes and Wnt/β-catenin signaling link nigrostriatal injury to repair in 1-methyl-4-phenyl- 1,2,3,6-tetrahydropyridine model of Parkinson's disease. Neurobiol. Dis., 2011; 41:508-527.

[32] L'episcopo F, Serapide MF, Tirolo C, Testa N, Caniglia S, Morale MC, Pluchino S, Marchetti B. A Wnt1 regulated Frizzled-1/β-Catenin signaling pathway as a candidate regulatory circuit controlling mesencephalic dopaminergic neuron-astrocyte crosstalk: Therapeutical relevance for neuron survival and neuroprotection. Mol. Neurodegener., 2011; 6:49.

[33] Rawal N, Corti O, Sacchetti P, Ardilla-Osorio H, Sehat B, Brice A, Arenas E. Parkin protects dopaminergic neurons from excessive Wnt/beta-catenin signaling. Biochem. Biophys. Res. Commun., 2009; 388:473-478.

[34] Fernández-Martos CM, González-Fernández C, González P, Maqueda A, Arenas E, Rodríguez FJ. Differential expression of Wnts after spinal cord contusion injury in adult rats. PLoS One, 2011; 6:e27000.

[35] Halleskog C, Mulder J, Dahlström J, Mackie K, Hortobágyi T, Tanila H, Kumar Puli L, Färber K, Harkany T, Schulte G. WNT signaling in activated microglia is proinflammatory. Glia, 2011; 59:119-131.

[36] Halleskog C, Dijksterhuis JP, Kilander MB, Becerril-Ortega J, Villaescusa CJ, Lindgren E, Arenas E, Schulte G. Heterotrimeric G protein-dependent WNT-5A signaling to ERK1/2 mediates distinct aspects of microglia proinflammatory transformation. J. Neuroinflammation., 2012; 9:111.

[37] L'Episcopo F, Tirolo C, Caniglia S, Testa N, Serra PA, Impagnatiello F, Morale MC, Marchetti B. Combining nitric oxide release with anti-inflammatory activity preserves nigrostriatal dopaminergic innervation and prevents motor impairment in a 1-methyl-4-phenyl-1,2,3,6- tetrahydropyridine model of Parkinson's disease. J Neuroinflammation. 2010 Nov 23; 7:83.

[38] L'episcopo F, Tirolo C, Testa N, Caniglia S, Morale MC, Impagnatiello F, Marchetti B. Switching the microglial harmful phenotype promotes lifelong restoration of subtantia nigra dopaminergic neurons from inflammatory neurodegeneration in aged mice. Rejuvenation Res., 2011; 14:411-424.

[39] Kunke D, Bryja V, Mygland L, Arenas E, Krauss S. Inhibition of canonical Wnt signaling promotes gliogenesis in P0-NSCs. Biochem. Biophys. Res. Commun., 2009; 386:628-633.

[40] L' Episcopo F, Tirolo C, Testa N, Caniglia S, Morale MC, Marchetti B. Glia as a turning point in the therapeutic strategy of Parkinson's disease. CNS Neurol. Disord. Drug Targets, 2010; 9:349-372.

[41] Chen LW, Yung KL, Chan YS. Reactive astrocytes as potential manipulation targets in novel cell replacement therapy of Parkinson's disease. Current Drug Targets, 2005; 6:821-833.

[42] Parish CL, Castelo-Branco G, Rawal N, Tonnesen J, Sorensen AT, Salto C, Kokaia M, Lindvall O, Arenas E. Wnt5a-treated midbrain neural stem cells improve dopamine cell replacement therapy in parkinsonian mice. J. Clin. Invest., 2008; 118:149-160.

[43] Schulte G, Bryja V, Rawal N, Castelo-Branco G, Sousa KM, Arenas E. Purified Wnt-5a increases differentiation of midbrain dopaminergic cells and dishevelled phosphorylation. J. Neurochem., 2005; 92:1550-1553.

[44] Castelo-Branco G, Rawal N, Arenas E. GSK-3beta inhibition/beta-catenin stabilization in ventral midbrain precursors increases differentiation into dopamine neurons. J. Cell Sci., 2004; 117:5731-5737.

[45] Misiuta IE, Saporta S, Sanberg PR, Zigova T, Willing AE. Influence of retinoic acid and lithium on proliferation and dopaminergic potential of human NT2 cells. J. Neurosci. Res., 2006; 83:668-679.

[46] Arenas E. Engineering a dopaminergic phenotype in stem/precursor cells: role of Nurr1, glia-derived signals, and Wnts. Ann. N. Y. Acad. Sci., 2005; 1049:51-66.

[47] Holm PC, Rodríguez FJ, Kele J, Castelo-Branco G, Kitajewski J, Arenas E. BMPs, FGF8 and Wnts regulate the differentiation of locus coeruleus noradrenergic neuronal precursors. J. Neurochem., 2006; 99:343-352.

[48] Ding YX, Wei LC, Wang YZ, Cao R, Wang X, Chen LW. Molecular manipulation targeting regulation of dopaminergic differentiation and proliferation of neural stem cells or pluripotent stem cells. CNS Neurol. Disord. Drug Targets, 2011; 10:517-528.

Section 3

Neurotrophin and Neuronal Fate Decision

Chapter 7

Neurotrophin Signaling and Alzheimer's Disease Neurodegeneration – Focus on BDNF/TrkB Signaling

Jenny Wong

Additional information is available at the end of the chapter

1. Introduction

1.1. Neurotrophins

Neurotrophins are small proteins vital for neuronal growth, differentiation, survival, and plasticity [1]. Members of the mammalian neurotrophin family include nerve growth factor (NGF), brain-derived neurotrophic factor (BDNF), neurotrophin-3 (NT-3), and neurotrophin-4/5 (NT-4/5). Their neurotrophic effects are mediated by the tropomyosin receptor kinase (Trk) receptors, membrane-bound receptor tyrosine kinases (NGF for TrkA, BDNF and NT4/5 for TrkB, and NT-3 for TrkC) which activate various cell signaling pathways linked to growth, differentiation, and survival [2]. The importance of neurotrophin signaling in brain development is highlighted by findings showing that knockout mice for any one of the neurotrophins or their receptors are fatal or exhibit severe neural defects [3].

1.2. BDNF and Alzheimer's disease

The neurotrophin, NGF, is reduced in the nucleus basalis, a region concentrated in basal forebrain cholinergic neurons, which show substantial degeneration in Alzheimer's disease (AD) [4, 5]. However, there is conflicting evidence demonstrating that NGF levels are unchanged or even increased in other brain regions including the frontal cortex and hippocampus, two major brain regions affected in AD [6-9]. In contrast, BDNF is more highly expressed and widely distributed in the brain compared to NGF, and its expression and growth promoting actions are critical for survival and plasticity of a variety of neurons throughout the brain, particularly in brain regions heavily affected in AD such as hippocampal, cortical, and cholinergic neurons [10-14]. Moreover, in cell culture and animal models, functioning of the BDNF signaling pathway has been repeatedly demonstrated to be critical for neuronal differentiation, survival, plasticity, and cognition [3, 11, 13, 15-21]. Independent lines of evidence suggest that dysfunction in BDNF signaling may contribute to the neurodegeneration in AD. Brain regions associated with reduced BDNF expression are those displaying the highest levels of neurodegeneration (eg. hippocampus). The role of BDNF in AD has been studied extensively. In AD brains, BDNF mRNA and protein levels have been found to be reduced in the hippocampus and neocortex [8, 22-27]. With findings of reduced BDNF expression in AD, interest emerged in the role of the TrkB receptor, as reductions in BDNF signaling may also occur through alterations in and/or through decreased expression of this BDNF receptor.

1.3. The BDNF receptor – TrkB

The TrkB receptor is the principal component of the BDNF signaling pathway. In the human brain, multiple isoforms of TrkB are expressed. There are three major isoforms of the TrkB receptor characterized to date: the full-length (TrkB-TK+) and two C-terminal truncated TrkB receptors (TrkB-TK- and TrkB-Shc) that are generated by alternative splicing of the TrkB pre-mRNA [28]. The full-length TrkB receptor, TrkB-TK+, is the principal mediator of the neurotrophic effects of BDNF. Upon ligand binding, monomeric TrkB-TK+ homodimerizes and undergoes trans-phosphorylation at key tyrosine residues in the C-terminal domain that couple it to downstream signaling pathways that promote neuronal survival, growth, differentiation, and plasticity including mitogen-activated protein kinase kinase (MEK), phosphatidyl inositol 3 kinase (PI3K), and phospholipase C-gamma (PLCγ) [29-32] (Figure 1). The two truncated TrkB receptor isoforms include TrkB-TK- and TrkB-Shc. Both truncated isoforms are generated from alternatively spliced transcripts and are truncated at the C-terminus, thus lacking the tyrosine kinase domain [28, 33]. However, the TrkB-TK- and TrkB-Shc receptors differ in that each contain unique amino acid sequences at their C-terminus. The TrkB-Shc isoform includes the sarc homology containing (Shc) binding domain that is absent in TrkB-TK- [28].

1.4. TrkB and Alzheimer's disease

Previous reports on TrkB-TK+ and TrkB-TK- expression levels in AD have been variable due to brain cohort differences and the variable techniques used to measure their expression. In general, reductions in TrkB-TK+ in neurons have mostly been found in the hippocampus and the frontal and temporal cortices in AD [27, 34]. Conversely, up-regulation of TrkB-TK- has been found in association with senile plaques in AD, and is suggested to be linked to increases in reactive glial cells [9, 27, 34]. Furthermore, increases in TrkB-TK+ have also been found in glial cells in the hippocampus [27]. Surprisingly, while the existence of TrkB-Shc has been known for some time, its role in AD has not been defined.

1.5. Importance of TrkB

Neuron viability and function is dependent upon BDNF-stimulated TrkB-TK+ signaling. In AD, much evidence suggests that BDNF/TrkB-TK+ signaling is reduced [8, 22-27, 34-36]. In addition to changes in BDNF expression, neuronal BDNF/TrkB-TK+ signaling can also be modulated by alterations in the ratio of full-length (TrkB-TK+) to truncated (TrkB-TK- and

TrkB-Shc) TrkB expressed [31, 37]. Homodimers of TrkB-TK+ receptors bind to BDNF and initiates intracellular second messenger signaling (Figure 1). Changes in TrkB alternative transcript expression or protein stability, such as increased TrkB-TK- and/or TrkB-Shc, will have a profound negative impact on BDNF/TrkB-TK+ signaling as homodimers of truncated receptors and heterodimers of full-length and truncated receptors can not initiate BDNF-stimulated second messenger signaling (Figure 2). This is important because changes in the ratio of full-length to truncated TrkB expression in neurons may underlie reductions in neurotrophic support in AD, which ultimately lead to neurodegeneration and profound neuron and brain volume loss. Considering that TrkB-Shc is a brain- and neuron-specific TrkB isoform that has been demonstrated to inhibit BDNF/TrkB-TK+ signaling, it is important to establish what role TrkB-Shc plays in AD development and progression.

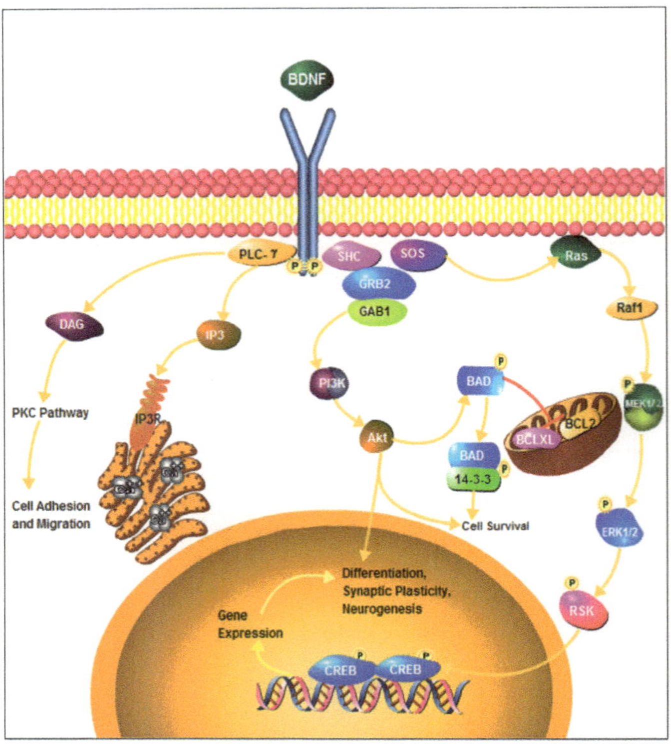

Figure 1. BDNF/TrkB-TK+ signaling pathway. Activation of TrkB-TK+ by BDNF leads to auto-phosphorylation of tyrosine residues in the intracellular C-terminal domain. This leads to the activation of TrkB-TK+-linked second messenger signaling pathways including PLCγ (phospholipase C-gamma), MEK (mitogen-activated protein kinase kinase), and PI3K (phosphatidyl inositol 3 kinase), which are linked to downstream processes involved in cell adhesion/migration, cells survival, synaptic plasticity, neurogenesis, and neuronal differentiation. This figure is modified from the BDNF Pathway Figure (Protein Lounge Pathway Templates) from ProteinLounge using Pathway Builder Tool.

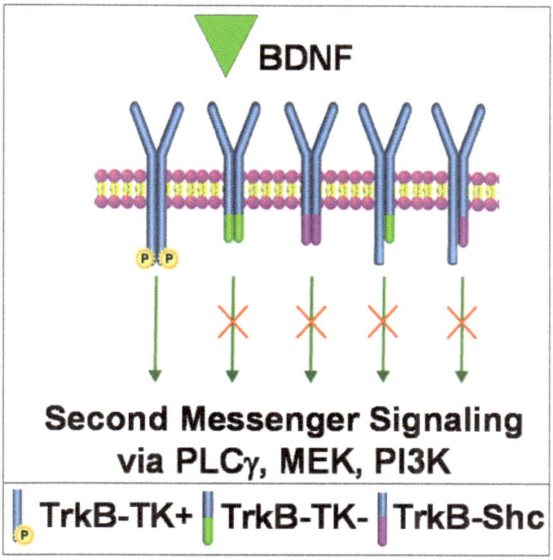

Figure 2. TrkB receptor dimer combinations. All dimer combinations of TrkB receptors can bind to BDNF. However, only a homodimer of TrkB-TK+ can initiate second messenger signaling. This figure utilizes modified ProteinLounge graphics created using the Pathway Builder Tool (www.proteinlounge.com).

2. Evidence that TrkB-Shc alternative transcripts are selectively increased in the hippocampus during severe, late stage AD

In Wong et al. (2012) [38], we measured changes in TrkB alternate transcript levels in control and AD postmortem human brain tissue derived from the hippocampus, temporal cortex, occipital cortex, and cerebellum (Braak stages V and VI) [38]. By quantitative real-time PCR, using primers specific for each TrkB alternative transcript, we found significant increases in TrkB-Shc mRNA expression in the hippocampus but not in any other brain region (Figure 3).

Considering that brain homogenates contain a mixed population of cells, we determined whether the changes found in TrkB transcript expression using the hippocampal tissue homogenates also occur in neurons exposed to an amyloidogenic environment. Here, changes in TrkB transcripts were assessed by incubating differentiated SHSY5Y cells (a human neuroblastoma cell-line which express TrkB) with different species of amyloid beta 1-42 ($A\beta_{42}$) peptides at various stages of aggregation. Oligomers and fibrils were prepared as described in Ryan et al. [39] and characterized by western blotting and atomic force microscopy imaging [38]. A significant increase in TrkB-Shc mRNA levels was found when cells were incubated with preparations of $A\beta_{42}$ containing fibrils compared to controls (Figure 4). The small magnitude of change was expected as the $A\beta_{42}$ fibril preparation contained mixed $A\beta_{42}$ species and the absolute amount of fibrils would be low (fibrils were absent in the monomer and oligomer $A\beta_{42}$ preparations). Further, in comparison to the $A\beta_{42}$ monomer and oligomer preparations, the $A\beta_{42}$ fibril preparations would be most representative of all $A\beta_{42}$ species present in the AD hippocampus as this preparation comprises a mix of all three species [38]. These results were consistent with findings of increased TrkB-Shc mRNA levels in the AD hippocampus (Figures 3 and 4).

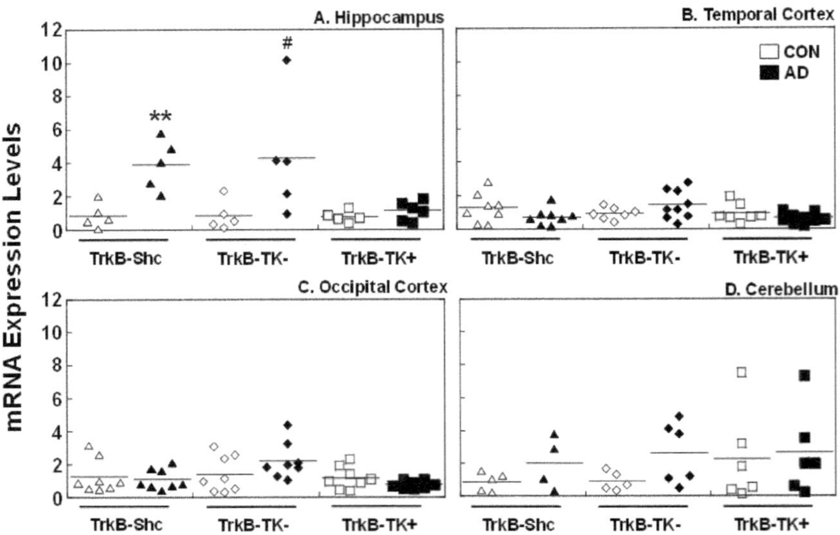

Figure 3. TrkB alternative transcript expression in various control and AD brain regions. Expression of TrkB alternative transcripts in the (A) hippocampus, (B) temporal cortex, (C) occipital cortex, and (D) cerebellum of control (CON) (white) and Alzheimer's disease (AD) (black) postmortem human brain tissue were measured by qPCR. ** P=0.004; # P=0.07. Figure is from Wong J, et al. Amyloid beta selectively modulates neuronal TrkB alternative transcript expression with implications for Alzheimer's disease. Neuroscience 2012;210 363-374.

In regards to the brain regions examined, AD brain pathology from most severe to least affected is: hippocampus>temporal cortex>occipital cortex>cerebellum. The selective increase in TrkB-Shc transcripts observed only in the hippocampus suggested that the elevated TrkB-Shc transcript levels were occurring in brain regions that are most severely affected in the diseased state and that the observed increase may likely be influenced by the neuronal cell population present. This was supported by our *in vitro* AD cell culture model showing that TrkB-Shc mRNA levels in the differentiated SHSY5Y neuronal cells can be increased by exposure to preparations of $A\beta_{42}$ containing fibrils. $A\beta_{42}$ fibril species are increased in the advanced stages of AD [40]. While it is widely accepted that soluble oligomers are the more neurotoxic of the $A\beta_{42}$ species, evidence also suggest that the neurotoxicity of $A\beta_{42}$ requires its aggregation in the fibrillar form, particularly in the form of protofibrils [41, 42]. In our $A\beta_{42}$ preparations, we detected various sizes of fibrils in the $A\beta_{42}$ fibril preparations, includ-

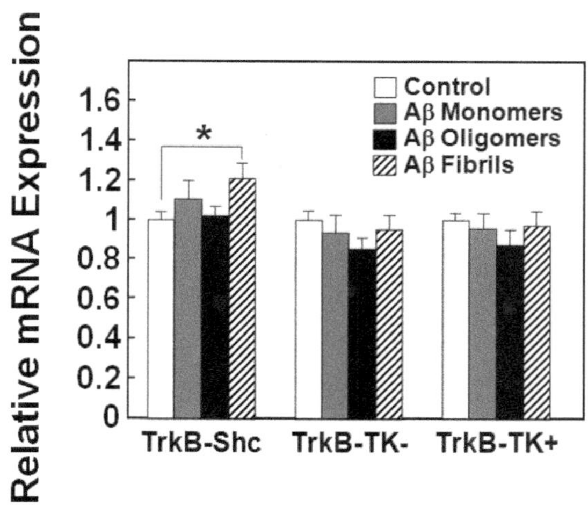

Figure 4. Effect of different structural forms of $A\beta_{42}$ on TrkB alternative transcript expression in differentiated SHSY5Y neuronal cells. SHSY5Y cells were differentiated for 9 d and incubated in the absence (white bars) or presence of 1 μM $A\beta_{42}$ monomers (AβM) (gray bars), oligomers (AβO) (black bars), and fibrils (AβF) (hatched bars) for 6 h and harvested. Expression of TrkB alternative transcripts were then measured by qPCR. Data are expressed as mean + SEM relative to the control (white bars) condition that was set to 1. * P=0.03. Figure is from Wong J, et al. Amyloid beta selectively modulates neuronal TrkB alternative transcript expression with implications for Alzheimer's disease. Neuroscience 2012;210 363-374.

ing protofibrils which can be ~100 nm in length. If we consider that $A\beta_{42}$ fibrils are predominant in the advanced stages of AD [40], that the hippocampus is the most affected brain region, and that the CA1 subregion (the hippocampal region assessed) is the most severely impacted subregion of the hippocampus in AD, altogether, our findings suggest that the selective increase in the TrkB-Shc alternative splice transcript in the AD hippocampus may be specific to severe, late stage pathology.

3. TrkB-Shc inhibits TrkB-TK+ function and BDNF/TrkB-TK+ signaling

The elevated levels of TrkB-Shc in AD suggested that it may have a functional impact on cellular TrkB-TK+ signaling *in vivo*. Previous studies have demonstrated that TrkB-Shc can function as a dominant negative receptor by inhibiting TrkB-TK+ phosphorylation [28]. In Wong et al. (2012) [38], we confirmed this finding and extended it by showing that TrkB-Shc can decrease downstream second messenger signaling linked to TrkB-TK+, supporting a dominant negative function of TrkB-Shc on BDNF/TrkB-TK+ signaling. In particular, we found that when TrkB-Shc was overexpressed in SHSY5Y cells (which express endogenous TrkB-TK+), BDNF/TrkB-TK+ stimulated MEK pathway signaling was selectively attenuated. The ratio of phosphorylated ERK1/2:total ERK1/2 (a measure of ERK1/2 activity) was reduced but little change was observed for phosphorylated TrkB:total TrkB-TK+ and phosphorylated AKT:total AKT ratios (Figure 5).

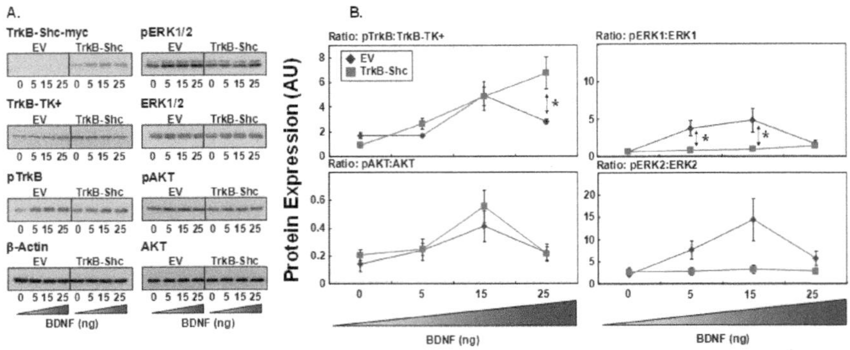

Figure 5. Effect of TrkB-Shc overexpression on BDNF-stimulated TrkB-TK+ second messenger signaling in differentiated SHSY5Y neuronal cells. Differentiated SHSY5Y cells were transfected with either empty vector (EV; blue) or myc-tagged TrkB-Shc (pink) for 24 h and treated with increasing concentrations of BDNF for 15 min and harvested. Proteins were separated by Western blotting and immunoprobed. (A) Representative Western blot images. (B) Bands were quantitated by densitometry and presented as protein expression ratios of phosphorylated protein to non-phosphorylated protein (pTrkB-TK+:TrkB-TK+; pAKT:AKT; pERK1:ERK1; pERK2:ERK2) -/+ SEM. * P=0.02 for pTrkB:TrkB-TK+ at 25 ng, P=0.03 for pERK1:ERK1 at 5 ng BDNF and P=0.049 for pERK1:ERK1 at 15 ng BDNF. Figure is from Wong J, et al. Amyloid beta selectively modulates neuronal TrkB alternative transcript expression with implications for Alzheimer's disease. Neuroscience 2012;210 363-374.

In a parallel study [43], we determined how TrkB-Shc exerts its dominant negative effect on BDNF-stimulated TrkB-TK+ signaling. Using a non-neuronal cell-line, Chinese Hamster Ovary K1 (CHOK1) cells (which do not express endogenous TrkB receptors), we transiently overexpressed TrkB-Shc protein and examined its effect on TrkB-TK+ protein stability. We used cycloheximide to block protein synthesis as this would prevent newly synthesized protein from replacing protein that has been degraded. From this, we found that TrkB-Shc protein levels were rapidly decreased when cells were exposed to exogenous BDNF. Moreover, in co-expression experiments where TrkB-Shc and TrkB-TK+ were co-expressed, cycloheximide treatment revealed increased protein degradation of phosphorylated TrkB-TK+ protein, a process that is accelerated by BDNF exposure (Figure 6A and B) [43]. Interestingly, while the reduction of phosphorylated TrkB-TK+ protein was more pronounced in the presence of TrkB-Shc following BDNF exposure, the stability of TrkB-Shc protein itself was increased (Figure 6C).

4. Discussion

Our recent findings have important implications in regards to the role of TrkB-Shc and its impact on BDNF-mediated TrkB-TK+ signaling in neurons in AD. MEK signaling through

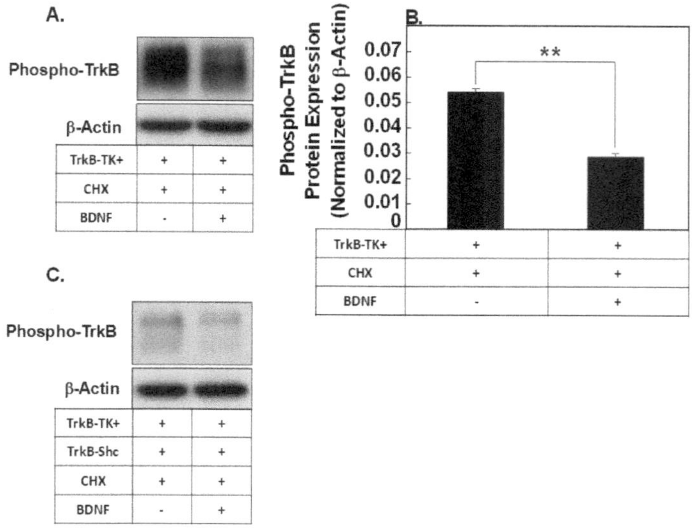

Figure 6. Effect of TrkB-Shc on the stability of phosphorylated TrkB-TK+. CHOK1 cells co-transfected with either empty vector + TrkB-TK+ or TrkB-TK+ + TrkB-Shc for 24 h were treated with 15 ng BDNF for 15 min and then incubated with cycloheximide for 3 h before harvest. Proteins were separated by Western blotting and immunoprobed. (A and C) Representative Western blot images. (A) and (C) are from the same blot and have the same exposure. (B) Bands in (A) were quantitated by densitometry and presented as protein expression normalized to β-actin + SEM. **P = 0.007. Figure is from Wong, J and Garner, B. Biochemical and Biophysical Research Communications 2012; 420 331–335.

ERK1/2 phosphorylation is increased in vulnerable neurons in AD and is implicated in the abnormal phosphorylation of tau and neurofilament proteins [44]. Our finding of a selective attenuation in MEK signaling activity in neurons with elevated levels of cellular TrkB-Shc implicates that elevated levels of this neuron-specific truncated TrkB receptor in AD may occur as a response to the disease. However, our finding that cells may increase TrkB-Shc protein levels in response to BDNF stimulation to regulate TrkB-TK+ activity by increasing degradation of activated receptor complexes also has ramifications for BDNF/TrkB-TK+ signaling in AD. In the non-diseased or control state, this process is akin to feedback regulatory loops observed in metabolic pathways (Figure 7). While BDNF/TrkB-TK+ signaling is important in multiple aspects related to neuronal viability and differentiation, overactivation or inappropriate temporal and spatial activation of BDNF/TrkB-TK+ signaling during brain development or "leakage" of BDNF to adjacent neurons or brain regions can negatively impact brain function. However, in AD, elevated levels of TrkB-Shc in association with reduced BDNF protein levels (which is well documented) and no change in TrkB-TK+ expression may also result in an overall increase in the degradation of phosphorylated TrkB-TK+ receptors, and thus, reduce overall BDNF/TrkB-TK+ activity in neurons in AD.

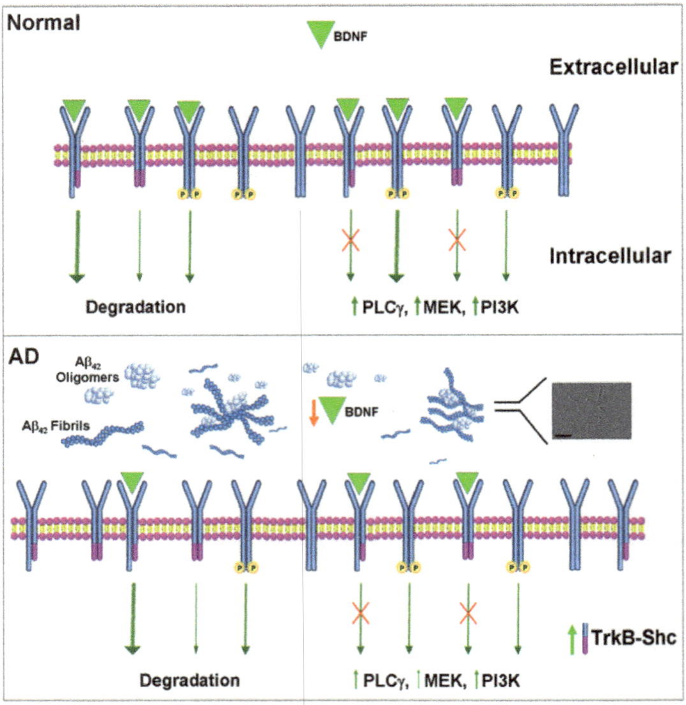

Figure 7. Summary diagram. Upper panel: In the normal, non-diseased state, binding of BDNF to TrkB leads to autophosphorylation of TrkB-TK+ homodimers (but not other TrkB dimer combinations). This leads to activation of downstream second messenger signaling pathways including PLCγ (phospholipase C-gamma), MEK (mitogen-activated protein kinase kinase), and PI3K (phosphatidyl inositol 3 kinase), which are critical for neuronal viability and function. TrkB-TK+ homodimers can also be auto-phosphorylated in the absence of BDNF, although activation of downstream signaling pathways are less intense. BDNF-stimulation of TrkB receptors also leads to their degradation. The arrow thickness indicates the magnitude of effect. The magnitude of decrease in protein levels are greatest for the following receptor combinations when stimulated with exogenous BDNF: TrkB-TK+/TrkB-Shc>TrkB-TK+/TrkB-TK+>TrkB-Shc/TrkB-Shc. Lower panel: In AD, there is Aβ plaque accumulation. Neurons are exposed to mixed species of Aβ, including $A\beta_{42}$ fibrils and oligomers at various stages of aggregation. BDNF protein expression has been reported to be reduced in AD (indicated by red arrow) and TrkB-Shc levels have been reported by us to be increased in AD (hippocampus, CA1) (indicated by green arrow) and in response to $A\beta_{42}$ fibril exposure. The increase in TrkB-Shc is predicted to increase heterodimer combinations of TrkB-TK+/TrkB-Shc and homodimer combinations of TrkB-Shc, which would lead to an overall reduction in downstream signaling. Moreover, the increase in TrkB-Shc dimer combinations also increases TrkB receptor degradation. Thus, the combination of reduced BDNF expression and increased TrkB-Shc expression in the AD hippocampus would likely result in an overall decrease in BDNF/TrkB-TK+ signaling. Figure utilizes modified ProteinLounge graphics created using the Pathway Builder Tool (www.proteinlounge.com). Insert panel: Atomic force microscopy image of the $A\beta_{42}$ fibril preparation used in Wong J, et al. Amyloid beta selectively modulates neuronal TrkB alternative transcript expression with implications for Alzheimer's disease. Neuroscience 2012;210 363-374. This contains mixed species of $A\beta_{42}$ monomers, oligomers, and fibrils of various sizes. Scale represents 1 μm.

5. Conclusion

Neurotrophin signaling via BDNF/TrkB-TK+ is critical for neuronal viability and function. Further research into this topic area is required to determine when changes in BDNF/TrkB-TK+ signaling begin to occur and whether changes in TrkB-Shc expression, function, and interaction with TrkB-TK+ at different stages of the disease process, in response to Aβ, or in response to other amyloidogenic factors may be protective or deleterious.

Nomenclature

Aβ (amyloid beta), AD (Alzheimer's disease), Akt (protein kinase B), BDNF (brain-derived neurotrophic factor), CA1 (Cornu Ammonis area 1), CHO (Chinese hamster ovary), ERK (extracellular signal-regulated kinase), MEK (mitogen-activated protein kinase kinase), NGF (nerve growth factor), NT (neurotrophin), PI3K (phosphatidyl inositol 3 kinase), PLCγ (phospholipase C-gamma), Shc (sarc homology containing), Trk (tropomyosin receptor kinase).

Acknowledgements

Many thanks to Dr John BJ Kwok from Neuroscience Research Australia for providing feedback on the chapter drafts.

Author details

Jenny Wong[1,2]

Address all correspondence to: jwong@uow.edu.au

1 Illawarra Health and Medical Research Institute, University of Wollongong, Wollongong, NSW, 2522, Australia

2 School of Biological Sciences, University of Wollongong, Wollongong, NSW, 2522, Australia

References

[1] Schindowski K, Belarbi K, and Buee L. Neurotrophic factors in Alzheimer's disease: role of axonal transport. Genes, Brain, and Behavior 2008;7 Suppl 143-56.

[2] Patapoutian A and Reichardt LF. Trk receptors: mediators of neurotrophin action. Current Opinion in Neurobiology 2001;11(3) 272-280.

[3] Bartkowska K, Turlejski K, and Djavadian RL. Neurotrophins and their receptors in early development of the mammalian nervous system. Acta Neurobiologiae Experimentalis 2010;70(4) 454-467.

[4] Scott SA, et al. Nerve growth factor in Alzheimer's disease: increased levels throughout the brain coupled with declines in nucleus basalis. Journal of Neuroscience 1995;15(9) 6213-6221.

[5] Teipel SJ, et al. Measurement of basal forebrain atrophy in Alzheimer's disease using MRI. Brain 2005;128(Pt 11) 2626-2644.

[6] Goedert M, et al. Nerve growth factor mRNA in peripheral and central rat tissues and in the human central nervous system: lesion effects in the rat brain and levels in Alzheimer's disease. Brain Research 1986;387(1) 85-92.

[7] Jette N, Cole MS, and Fahnestock M. NGF mRNA is not decreased in frontal cortex from Alzheimer's disease patients. Brain Research Molecular Brain Research 1994;25(3-4) 242-250.

[8] Hock C, et al. Region-specific neurotrophin imbalances in Alzheimer disease: decreased levels of brain-derived neurotrophic factor and increased levels of nerve growth factor in hippocampus and cortical areas. Archives of Neurology 2000;57(6) 846-851.

[9] Connor B, et al. Trk receptor alterations in Alzheimer's disease. Brain Research Molecular Brain Research 1996;42(1) 1-17.

[10] Ghosh A, Carnahan J, and Greenberg ME. Requirement for BDNF in activity-dependent survival of cortical neurons. Science 1994;263(5153) 1618-1623.

[11] Lowenstein DH and Arsenault L. The effects of growth factors on the survival and differentiation of cultured dentate gyrus neurons. Journal of Neuroscience 1996;16(5) 1759-1769.

[12] Lindholm D, et al. Autocrine-paracrine regulation of hippocampal neuron survival by IGF-1 and the neurotrophins BDNF, NT-3 and NT-4. European Journal of Neuroscience 1996;8(7) 1452-1460.

[13] Alderson RF, et al. Brain-derived neurotrophic factor increases survival and differentiated functions of rat septal cholinergic neurons in culture. Neuron 1990;5(3) 297-306.

[14] Knusel B, et al. Promotion of central cholinergic and dopaminergic neuron differentiation by brain-derived neurotrophic factor but not neurotrophin 3. Proceedings of the National Academy of Sciences of the United States of America 1991;88(3) 961-965.

[15] McAllister AK, Katz LC, and Lo DC. Neurotrophin regulation of cortical dendritic growth requires activity. Neuron 1996;17(6) 1057-1064.

[16] Medina DL, et al. TrkB regulates neocortex formation through the Shc/PLCgamma-mediated control of neuronal migration. The Embo Journal 2004;23(19) 3803-3814.

[17] Korte M, et al. Hippocampal long-term potentiation is impaired in mice lacking brain-derived neurotrophic factor. Proceedings of the National Academy of Sciences of the United States of America 1995;92(19) 8856-8860.

[18] Minichiello L, et al. Essential role for TrkB receptors in hippocampus-mediated learning. Neuron 1999;24(2) 401-414.

[19] Yamada MK, et al. Brain-derived neurotrophic factor promotes the maturation of GABAergic mechanisms in cultured hippocampal neurons. Journal of Neuroscience 2002;22(17) 7580-7585.

[20] Massa SM, et al. Small molecule BDNF mimetics activate TrkB signaling and prevent neuronal degeneration in rodents. Journal of Clinical Investigation 2010;120(5) 1774-1785.

[21] Marty S, et al. Brain-derived neurotrophic factor promotes the differentiation of various hippocampal nonpyramidal neurons, including Cajal-Retzius cells, in organotypic slice cultures. Journal of Neuroscience 1996;16(2) 675-687.

[22] Connor B, et al. Brain-derived neurotrophic factor is reduced in Alzheimer's disease. Brain Research Molecular Brain Research 1997;49(1-2) 71-81.

[23] Garzon D, Yu G, and Fahnestock M. A new brain-derived neurotrophic factor transcript and decrease in brain-derived neurotrophic factor transcripts 1, 2 and 3 in Alzheimer's disease parietal cortex. Journal of Neurochemistry 2002;82(5) 1058-1064.

[24] Fahnestock M, et al. Neurotrophic factors and Alzheimer's disease: are we focusing on the wrong molecule? Journal of Neural Transmission. Supplementa 2002(62) 241-252.

[25] Holsinger RM, et al. Quantitation of BDNF mRNA in human parietal cortex by competitive reverse transcription-polymerase chain reaction: decreased levels in Alzheimer's disease. Brain Research Molecular Brain Research 2000;76(2) 347-354.

[26] Phillips HS, et al. BDNF mRNA is decreased in the hippocampus of individuals with Alzheimer's disease. Neuron 1991;7(5) 695-702.

[27] Ferrer I, et al. BDNF and full-length and truncated TrkB expression in Alzheimer disease. Implications in therapeutic strategies. Journal of Neuropathology and Experimental Neurology 1999;58(7) 729-739.

[28] Stoilov P, Castren E, and Stamm S. Analysis of the human TrkB gene genomic organization reveals novel TrkB isoforms, unusual gene length, and splicing mechanism. Biochemical and Biophysical Research Communications 2002;290(3) 1054-1065.

[29] Biffo S, et al. Selective binding and internalisation by truncated receptors restrict the availability of BDNF during development. Development 1995;121(8) 2461-2470.

[30] Snapyan M, et al. Vasculature guides migrating neuronal precursors in the adult mammalian forebrain via brain-derived neurotrophic factor signaling. Journal of Neuroscience 2009;29(13) 4172-4188.

[31] Eide FF, et al. Naturally occurring truncated trkB receptors have dominant inhibitory effects on brain-derived neurotrophic factor signaling. Journal of Neuroscience 1996;16(10) 3123-3129.

[32] Ninkina N, et al. Expression and function of TrkB variants in developing sensory neurons. The Embo Journal 1996;15(23) 6385-6393.

[33] Klein R, et al. The trkB tyrosine protein kinase gene codes for a second neurogenic receptor that lacks the catalytic kinase domain. Cell 1990;61(4) 647-656.

[34] Allen SJ, Wilcock GK, and Dawbarn D. Profound and selective loss of catalytic TrkB immunoreactivity in Alzheimer's disease. Biochemical and Biophysical Research Communications 1999;264(3) 648-651.

[35] Michalski B and Fahnestock M. Pro-brain-derived neurotrophic factor is decreased in parietal cortex in Alzheimer's disease. Brain Research Molecular Brain Research 2003;111(1-2) 148-154.

[36] Peng S, et al. Precursor form of brain-derived neurotrophic factor and mature brain-derived neurotrophic factor are decreased in the pre-clinical stages of Alzheimer's disease. Journal of Neurochemistry 2005;93(6) 1412-1421.

[37] Arevalo JC and Wu SH. Neurotrophin signaling: many exciting surprises! Cellular and Molecular Life Sciences 2006;63(13) 1523-1537.

[38] Wong J, et al. Amyloid beta selectively modulates neuronal TrkB alternative transcript expression with implications for Alzheimer's disease. Neuroscience 2012;210363-374.

[39] Ryan DA, et al. An improved method for generating consistent soluble amyloid-beta oligomer preparations for in vitro neurotoxicity studies. Journal of Neuroscience Methods 2010;190(2) 171-179.

[40] Hoozemans JJ, et al. Always around, never the same: pathways of amyloid beta induced neurodegeneration throughout the pathogenic cascade of Alzheimer's disease. Current Medicinal Chemistry 2006;13(22) 2599-2605.

[41] Serpell LC. Alzheimer's amyloid fibrils: structure and assembly. Biochimica et Biophysica Acta 2000;1502(1) 16-30.

[42] Walsh DM, et al. Amyloid beta-protein fibrillogenesis. Structure and biological activity of protofibrillar intermediates. Journal of Biological Chemistry 1999;274(36) 25945-25952.

[43] Wong J and Garner B. Evidence that truncated TrkB isoform, TrkB-Shc can regulate phosphorylated TrkB protein levels. Biochemical and Biophysical Research Communications 2012;420331–335.

[44] Perry G, et al. Activation of neuronal extracellular receptor kinase (ERK) in Alzheimer disease links oxidative stress to abnormal phosphorylation. Neuroreport 1999;10(11) 2411-2415.

Section 4

NF-K-b and Neuronal Fate Decision

Chapter 8

NFκB Signaling Directs Neuronal Fate Decision

Yonggang Zhang and Wenhui Hu

Additional information is available at the end of the chapter

1. Introduction

During neural induction, the ectoderm stem cells overlying the notochord of the mesoderm convert into neuroepithelial cells (NECs) that proliferate/differentiate rapidly to form neural plate in response to diffusible inhibitory signals (neural inducer) produced from the notochord. Neural plate folds to form neural groove, which fuses to form neural tube. Within the neural tube, NECs undergo asymmetric dividing to generate neural stem cells (NSCs, or called radial glia cells) due to the expression of B-cell translocation gene 2 (BTG2) [1, 2, 3, 4]. NSCs differentiate sequentially into neural progenitor cells (NPCs) and various lineage-restricted neural blast cells, which include neuroblast and glioblast. These neural blast cells migrate to the target region where they mature and integrate into the existing neural network [5]. The generation of different lineage occurs in a temporally distinct yet overlapping pattern. In rodents, neuronogenesis peaks at embryonic day (E) 14, astrocytogenesis at postnatal day (P) 2, and oligodendrocytogenesis at P14 [6, 7]. It remains largely unclear at which step the fate of neuronal lineage has been decided, from embryonic stem (ES) cells to NECs, to NSCs and to terminally-differentiated neurons. The transcriptional factor NFκB plays a pivotal role in inflammation, immunity, cancer and neural plasticity [8, 9]. Constitutive and inducible activation of NFκB has been reported in many types of human tumors and chronic diseases including neurodegenerative diseases [10, 11, 12, 13, 14]. However, moderate activation of NFκB signaling on many physiological conditions may benefit the whole process of neuronal fate decision, including neurodevelopment and adult neurogenesis [15].

2. NFκB initiates and maintains neuronal fate decision from neural stem cells

NFκB is activated through a series of signaling cascades (Figure 1). The NFκB family contains 5 members including RelA(p65), RelB, c-Rel, p50/p105 (NFκB1) and p52/p100 (NFκB2), which form various combination of homodimers or heterodimers [8, 16]. In non-stimulated cells, the NFκB dimer is sequestered in the cytoplasm by the Inhibitor of NFκB (IκB), which include at least 8 members. Upon stimulation, IκB is degraded via a phosphorylation-dependent proteasome-mediated mechanism and the released NFκB is translocated to the nucleus where it binds to the κB-sites and regulates the transcription of target genes. The phosphorylation of IκB is regulated by the IκB kinase (IKK) that is activated by its upstream IKK kinases. The classical IKK complex contains 2 catalytic subunits IKK1/2 or IKKα/β and 1 regulatory subunit IKKγ [8, 16]. Three distinct signaling pathways for NFκB activation have been identified: classical (canonical), non-classical (non-canonical, alternative) and atypical pathways, all of them rely on sequentially activated kinases (Figure 1) [17]. The classical pathway involves the activation of classical IKK complex [9]. This pathway generally regulates the activation of classical NFκB complexes (e.g. p65/p50), in response to a wide range of stimuli such as pro-inflammatory cytokines tumor necrosis factor α (TNFα) and interleukin (IL) 1β, Toll-like receptor agonists (LPS), antigens, etc. The activated IKK complex phosphorylates IκB members (IκBα, IκBβ, IκBε and p105) on a consensus motif DSGFxS (e.g. Ser-32/Ser-36 for IκBα and Ser-19/Ser-23 for IκBβ) and the phosphorylated serines act as binding site for β-TrCP, the substrate recognition subunit of a Skp1-Cullin-F-box (SCF)–type E3 ubiquitin-protein ligase complex, named $SCF^{\beta\text{-TrCP}}$. This process, then, leads to the ubiquitination on specific lysine and the ubiquitinated IκBs are directed to 26S proteasome for full degradation, leaving free NFκB complexes to enter into the nucleus. The kinetics of phosphorylation and degradation of IκBβ or IκBε are much slower than that of IκBα and may reflect different substrate specificities of the IKK complex. The non-classical pathway involves TNF receptor associated factor 3 (TRAF3)-mediated activation of the NFκB-inducing kinase (NIK) and IKKα [18, 19]. Activated IKKα phosphorylates p100 on specific serine residues. After phosphorylation, p100 is ubiquitinated by $SCF^{\beta\text{-TrCP}}$ E3 ligase and cleaved by 19S proteasome, instead of completely degraded by 26S proteasome, to generate the NFκB subunit p52. This process is generally slower than the activation of the classical pathway and leads to a delayed activation of nuclear p52-containing complexes, such as RelB/p52. The mechanisms of p52 generation are either constitutive (by cotranslational processing) or inducible (by post-translational cleavage). The non-classical pathway is triggered by some particular members of TNF family, such as Lymphotoxin (LT) β, B-cell activation factor (BAFF), CD40 ligand (CD40L). The function of classical pathway has been well investigated but non-classical pathway remains in its infancy. In the following discussion, the role of NFκB signaling in the nervous system relates primarily to classical pathway.

In adult nervous system, NFκB signaling plays a sword-edge role after injuries or diseases [15, 20, 21, 22, 23]. The final outcome is attributable to the cell types, disease stages, and target genes. In most cases, NFκB signaling in immune cells, microglia/macrophage and astrocytes is neurodestructive due to overwhelming production of inflammatory mediators and neurotoxic molecules [22, 23]. However, neuronal NFκB signaling is neuroprotective via its crucial role in maintaining neuronal survival, synaptogenesis, neural plasticity, learning and memory [22, 23, 24, 25]. Recent studies demonstrate a striking enrichment of phosphorylated IκBα and IKK in the axon initial segment [26, 27] and the nodes of Ranvier [28], suggesting a novel role of NFκB signaling in regulating axonal polarity and initial axonal formation.

In a mouse inducible IκBα transgenic model, NFκB in NSCs/NPCs is necessary for axogenesis and maturation [21].

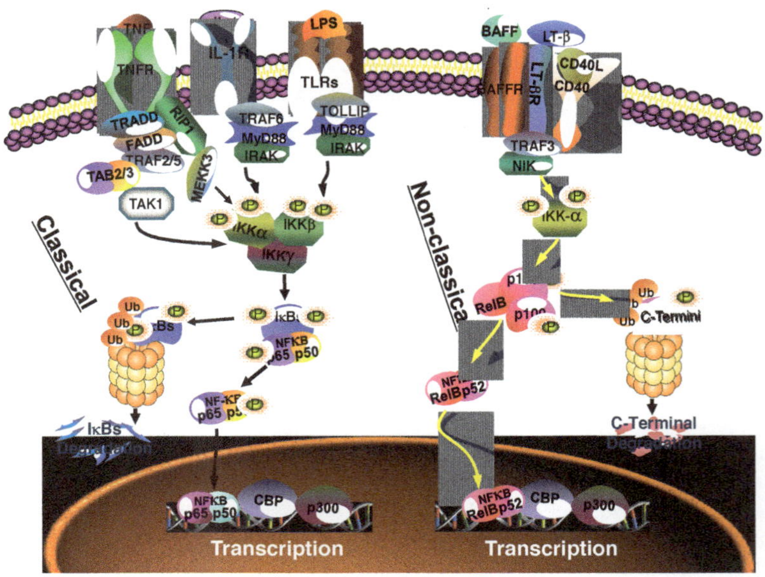

Figure 1. Classical and non-classical signaling pathways of NFκB activation.

In the zones of active neurogenesis in both postnatal and adult mouse brain, various members of the NFκB family are highly expressed [29], indicating for the first time that NFκB is actively involved in the proliferation, migration and differentiation of adult NSCs/NPCs [30, 31]. The presence of NFκB in adult neurogenic zone is further validated by the studies using immunofluorescent microscopy [32, 33]. Direct evidence for the *in vivo* effect of NFκB signaling on the proliferation of NSCs/NPCs derives from p65 and p50 double knockout mice [34] as well as overexpression of super inhibitor IκBα mutant in NSCs/NPCs [35, 36, 37, 38]. Little is known about the role of NFκB signaling in regulating neural differentiation of NSCs/NPCs. A recent study demonstrates that toll-like receptor 2 (TLR2) induces neuronal differentiation via protein kinase C (PKC)-dependent activation of NFκB whereas TLR4 inhibites proliferation and neuronal differentiation of NPCs [30]. In p50-deficient mice, the neuronal differentiation of adult hippocampal NSCs is reduced by 50% while the proliferation does not change [39]. In our recent study, we demonstrate that NFκB signaling regulates the early differentiation of NSCs [32]. During early differentiation of NSCs, NFκB signaling becomes activated [32]. Addition of TNFα to activate NFκB signaling under proliferation conditions induces neural differentiation of NSCs/NPCs [32, 40, 41]. TNF-like weak inducer of apoptosis (TWEAK) induces neuronal differentiation of NSCs/NPCs, under proliferation condition, through NFκB-dependent down-regulation of Hes1 that prevents neuronal differentiation

[42]. Selective inhibition of classical NFκB signaling by various pharmacologic inhibitors, small interfering RNA and NSC-specific transgene dominant-negative IκBα retain the tripotential ability of differentiation and restore or enhance self-renewal capability of NSCs, suggesting that NFκB signaling is essential for early neural differentiation [32]. The critical role of NFκB in the initial differentiation step of NSCs highlights a novel molecular mechanism for neurogenesis. We hypothesize that moderate activation of NFκB signaling promotes NSC differentiation into NPCs and maintains a continuous source for adult neurogenesis under physiological conditions. However, persistent and repeated overactivation of NFκB signaling in NSCs may exhaust NSC pool and thus lead to reduced neurogenesis as seen in aging patients [43, 44] and chronic stress [45].

To further test this hypothesis, we generated double transgenic mice expressing constitutively active form of IKKβ ($IKK\beta^{CA}$) [46, 47] driven by the promoter of glial fibrillary acid protein (GFAP) by crossbreeding GFAP-Cre mice (Jackson Lab, 004600) with Rosa26-$Stop^{Floxed}$-$IKK\beta^{CA}$ mice (Jackson Lab, 008242). *In vitro* studies using the NSCs/NPCs cultured from the brain of GFAP-$IKK\beta^{CA}$ mice validated the over-activation of NFκB signaling (Figure 2), the loss of NSCs during passage as determined by the reduced number of $GFAP^{+}$/$Nestin^{+}$ NSCs (Figure 3) as well as the inhibition of NSC selfrenewing and tripotential capacity (Figure 4) [32]. The *in vivo* effect of persistent over-activation of NFκB on $GFAP^{+}$ NSCs and their progeny in brain neurogenic zones of adult animals and their correlations with aging are currently under investigation.

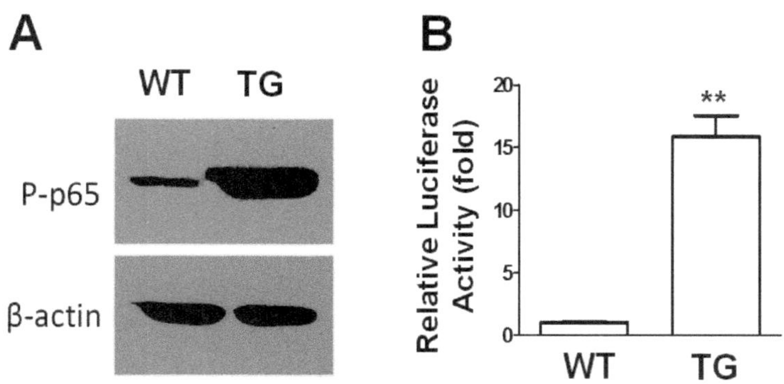

Figure 2. Over-activation of NFκB signaling in brain neural stem/progenitor cells from GFAP-Cre-$IKK\beta^{CA}$ mice determined by Western blot analysis (A) and adenovirus-mediated NFκB-luciferase reporter assay (B). *A.* Whole cell lysates of primary neurospheres cultured from brain subventricular zones (SVZ) of littermate wild-type (WT) or transgenic (TG) adult mouse were immunoblotted with antibodies against phosphorylated p65 (Ser-536) or β-actin (as loading control). *B.* Dissociated neural stem/progenitor cells were plated on 96-well plate and infected with adenovirus carrying NFκB *firefly*-luciferase at 50 multiplicity of infection (MOI) for 24 h. Luciferase activity was measured with *OneGlo*™ luciferase assay and cell viability was determined with *CellTiter-Glo*™ luminescent assay. Data are expressed as relative fold change after cell number normalization. ** $p<0.01$ indicates statistical significance from WT control.

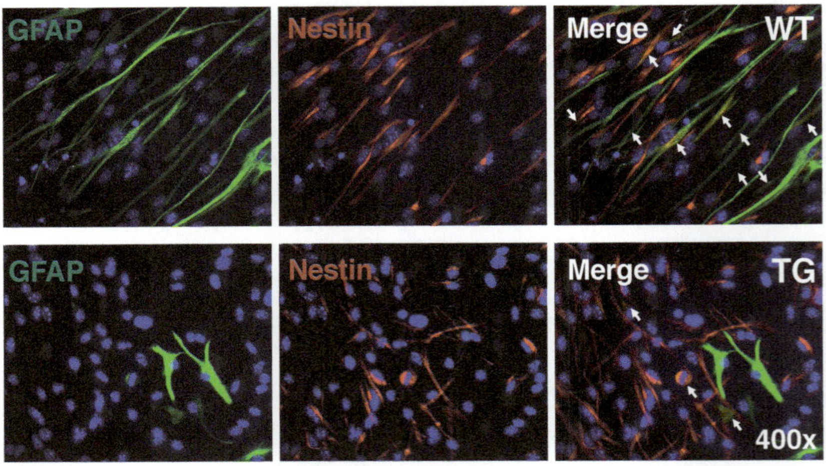

Figure 3. Over-activation of NFκB signaling in cultured brain neural stem/progenitor cells from GFAP-Cre-IKKβ^{CA} mice reduced the number of GFAP$^+$/Nestin$^+$ neural stem cells (Arrow). Passage 2 neurospheres cultured from brain subventricular zones (SVZ) of littermate wild-type (WT) or transgenic (TG) 5-week-old mouse were dissociated into single cells. Cells were plated in matrigel-coated 8-well chamber slide and cultured under proliferation media containing 20 ng/mL of epidermal growth factor (EGF) and basic fibroblast growth factor (bFGF) for 3 d. After fixation for 10 min at room temperature with 4% paraformaldehyde, the cells were immunostained simultaneously with goat anti-GFAP polyclonal antibody and mouse anti-Nestin monoclonal antibody followed by donkey anti-goat *Alexa Fluor*® 488 and donkey anti-mouse *Alexa Fluor*® 594 secondary antibodies. The nuclei were counterstained with Hoechst 33258.

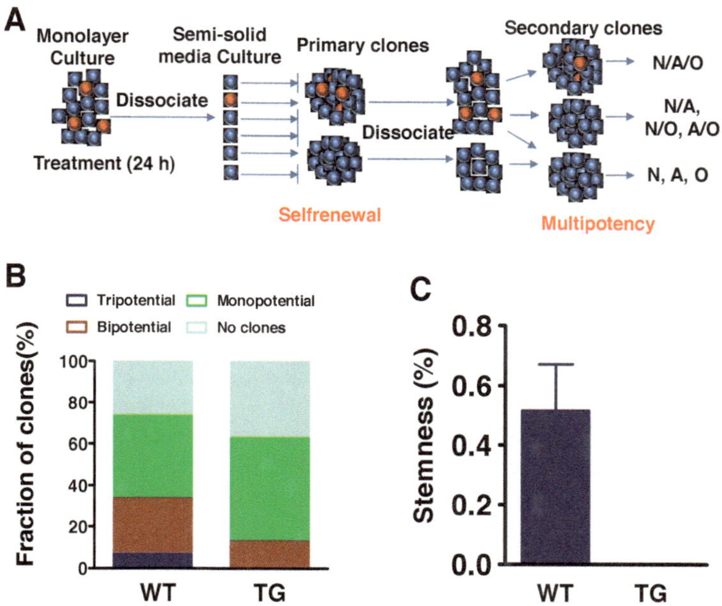

Figure 4. Over-activation of NFκB signaling in cultured brain neural stem/progenitor cells from GFAP-Cre-IKKβ^{CA} mice led to loss of stemness (selfrenewal and tripotency). *A.* Diagram of modified stemness assay. Passage 2 neurospheres cultured from brain subventricular zones (SVZ) of littermate wild-type (WT) or transgenic (TG) 5-week-old mouse were dissociated into single cells for monolayer culture under differentiation media for 24 h. Then dissociated single cells (500 per well) were cultured in semisolid medium containing 20 ng/mL of epidermal growth factor (EGF) and basic fibroblast growth factor (bFGF) for 12 d. The clones with more than 300 μm in diameter were picked, dissociated and cultured as neurosphere. The biggest secondary clones were dissociated into single cells plated on matrigel-coated 96-well plate. After 5 days' differentiation, the cells were fixed in 4% paraformaldehyde and cell lineage differentiations were examined with multi-labeled fluorescent immunocytochemistry using cell type-specific antibodies against neuron (N, Tuji1), astrocytes (A, GFAP) and oligodendrocytes (O, myelin basic protein). *B.* Fraction of primary clones that show different multipotency. Tripotential clone: differentiating into three types of neural cells; bipotential clone: differentiating into either two cell types; monopotential clone: differentiating into one cell type. *C.* The percentage of primary clones with selfrenewal and tripotency over the plated single cells.

3. Regulation of proneuronal genes by NFκB signaling

At each step of neurogenesis, cells undergo symmetric and asymmetric dividing to maintain stemness and generate daughter progeny. The self-renewal and neuronal fate decision of NECs/NSCs during embryonic neurogenesis are regulated by various transcription factors and their signaling pathways including the nuclear hormone receptor TLX (tailless), the high-mobility-group transcription factor Sox2, the basic helix-loop-helix transcriptional factor Hes (hairy and enhancer of split), the tumor suppressor phosphatase Pten (phosphatase and tensin homolog deleted on chromosome 10), and the Drosophila membrane-associated protein Numb homologs, Numb and Numblike [48]. Neuronal fate decision also relies on the intrinsic proneuronal genes in NECs/NSCs/NPCs [49]. The proneuronal factors specify distinct neuronal identities in different regions of the nervous system [49, 50]. Transcriptional activation and epigenic modification of the proneuronal genes are essential for neuronal lineage progression [51]. Little is known about the effect of NFκB signaling on the expression or function of proneuronal factors during neurogenesis. The Hes family plays key but opposing role in regulating neurodevelopment. Hes1 and Hes5 are activated by Notch signaling and repress the expression of proneuronal factors such as Mash1, Neurogenin, Math and NeuroD [52, 53, 54]. In contrast, Hes6 promotes neuronal differentiation but inhibits astrocyte differentiation [55, 56]. Notch signaling is regulated by NFκB signaling, and thus it is speculated that NFκB signaling may regulate the expression of proneuronal genes during neural induction and neurogenesis [57, 58, 59]. The tripartite motif-containing protein 32 (Trim32) promotes asymmetric dividing and neuronal differentiation of NSCs/NPCs by regulating protein degradation and microRNA activity [60, 61], and enhancing retinoic acid receptor-mediated transcription [62]. Our studies demonstrated that NFκB inhibition blocks the asymmetric distribution of Trim32 and maintain NSC selfrenewal [32], implying that NFκB signaling may initiate neuronal differentiation through suppressing Trim32 function.

4. Regulation of neural induction and neural plate patterning by NFκB signaling

NFκB signaling is essential for embryonic development (http://www.bu.edu/nf-kb/gene-resources/gene-knockouts/) because p65 knockout mice died on E15 and p65/p50 or p65/c-rel double knockout mice died on E13 due to liver degeneration [63, 64]. Such embryonic lethality precluded further investigation on the role of NFκB in late embryonic brain development. Additional knockout of TNF receptor 1 (TNFR1) in these p65-null mice rescued embryonic lethality [65], providing an opportunity to investigate the role of NFκB signaling in regulating embryonic neurogenesis [34]. However, the distribution pattern of NSCs/NPCs and cell lineage analysis in neurogenic zones of these mutants have not yet been examined. IKKα/IKKβ double knockout mice died on E12 due to apoptosis of NECs leading to impairments in neurogenesis [66].

Several lines of clinical studies identified the correlation of NFκB signaling defects to various neurodevelopmental disorders. Among 6 genes associated with nonsyndromic autosomal-recessive mental retardation [67, 68, 69], two, NIK- and IKKβ-binding protein (NIBP) [67, 68, 69] and coiled-coil and C2 domain-containing protein 2A (CC2D1A) [70, 71], have been shown to regulate NFκB signaling through the classical IKKβ pathway, implying the important role of NFκB signaling in mental retardation and possibly other neurodevelopmental diseases. In autism spectrum disorders, activation of NFκB signaling is significantly increased [72, 73, 74], although the role and mechanism of the activated NFκB signaling remain to be determined.

During neural induction, the ectodermal epithelial cells transit into NECs due to the inhibition of bone morphogenetic protein (BMP) signaling by the neural inducer (Chordin, Noggin and Follistatin). In this original "default model", high activity of BMP signaling defines epidermis, while absence of BMP specifies neural plate [75, 76, 77]. However, this model can no longer explain the complicate process of neural induction, which involves additional signaling pathways such as Wnt/β-catenin, FGF, Sox2, and Notch signaling [77, 78, 79, 80, 81, 82]. NFκB signaling is shown to inhibit BMP signaling in oesteoblastogenesis [83, 84]. We speculate that NFκB may regulate neural induction. Previous studies showed that the graded activation of NFκB/c-rel protein in the dorsal region determine the dorsal-ventral patterning in Drosophila [85, 86, 87, 88] and Xenopus laevis [89]. During mouse embryogenesis, virtually all members of the NFκB pathway are expressed in embryonic, trophoblast, and uterine cells [90]. It is proposed that NFκB may protect the embryos exposed to embryopathic stresses, possibly through its anti-apoptotic effect [90]. However, there is no direct evidence for the role of NFκB signaling in the *in vivo* neural induction (Figure 5).

5. Importance of NFκB signaling in mediating early differentiation of ES/iPS

In vitro neural induction from cultured ES cells or induced pluripotent stem (iPS) cells has been established [80, 82, 91, 92], but the signaling mechanisms remain largely unknown. Such induction is an excellent *in vitro* model to recapture the *in vivo* neural induction and embryonic neurogenesis [80]. The signaling pathways identified during endogenous embryonic morphogenesis can be applied to the neural induction and patterning, such as BMP, FGF, Wnt, Shh and Notch signaling [77, 78, 79, 80, 81, 82]. We speculate that NFκB signaling, through crosstalk with these signaling pathways, play an important role in the neuronal induction from ES or iPS cells (Figure 5) [80].

During murine spermatogenesis, NFκB is activated in a stage-specific manner [93]. During oocyte maturation and early embryonic development, NFκB is activated [94, 95]. In Drosophila melanogaster, the mRNA of the p65 homologue, named Dorsal, is maternally expressed and is concentrated in the egg cortex [85]. In Xenopus, NFκB activation is observed during oocyte maturation [96] and in late blastulae and gastrulae [97]. In zebrafish, NFκB signaling regulates notochord differentiation via activating the expression of no tail (ntl) gene [98]. In mouse embryos, NFκB activation is crucial to engage development beyond the 2-cell stage [94]. NFκB mediates the neurogenic effect of erythropoietin in neurosphere cultures from E14 mouse ganglionic eminence [99]. Recently, it has been shown that murine and human ES cells possess a low level of NFκB activity that increases significantly during the differentiation process [100, 101, 102]. In human ES cells, the classical NFκB pathway regulates differentiation while the non-classical pathway maintains pluripotency [103]. The transcription factor Nanog is essential in maintaining pluripotency of ES cells [104]. During ES cell differentiation, endogenous NFκB activity and target-gene expression are increased (Figure 5) [101, 102, 105]. NFκB inhibition increases expression of pluripotency markers [106, 107]. Nanog binds to NFκB proteins, inhibits NFκB activity and cooperates with Stat3 to maintain pluripotency [100]. ES cell-specific miR-290 maintains the pluripotency and self-renewal of ES cells through repressing classical NFκB signaling [107]. Forced expression of p65 causes loss of pluripotency, promotes differentiation of ES cells, and leads to an epithelial to mesenchymal transition [107]. These data define p65 as a novel target gene of miR-290 cluster and provide new insight into the function of ES cell-specific miRNAs [107]. Taken altogether, NFκB signaling is activated and required during the early differentiation of various stem cells and embryogenesis (Figure 5).

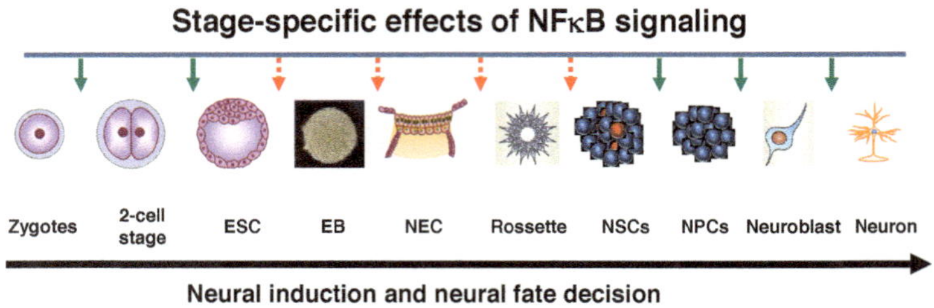

Figure 5. Potential regulatory sites of NFκB signaling during neuronal cell fate decision. Solid green arrows indicate the sites supported by limited reports, while the dotted red arrows indicate the stages that need experimental supports. ESC, embryonic stem cells; EB, embryoid body; NEC, neural epithelial cells; NSCs, neural stem cells; NPCs, neural progenitor cells.

6. Promotion of iPS reprograming by pharmacological or genetic inhibition of NFκB signaling.

Various somatic cells have been successfully reprogramed into the ES-like pluripotent stem cells by a combination of factors or a single factor [108, 109]. During the reprogramming process, the classical NFκB signaling is inhibited [103, 106, 107]. Therefore, we speculate that NFκB inhibition might directly induce or promote the reprograming of iPS. Many specific inhibitors for NFκB signaling have been developed and some of them are applied to clinical trial [110]. In addition, fibroblasts or other somatic cells from transgenic mice deficient in NFκB signaling or clinical patients with mutation of NFκB signaling components can be easily accessible. It will be imperative to use NFκB inhibitors or genetic sources for easy and fast generation of iPS for drug discovery and cell transplantation studies.

7. Concluding remark and future direction

NFκB signaling is a key mediator for numerous niche factors that regulate various stages or phases of neural induction and neurogenesis. The classical pathway of NFκB activation plays important role in regulating selfrenewal/multipotency and early differentiation of

NSCs and ES/iPS cells. During neural induction both *in vitro* and *in vivo*, NFκB signaling is required. However, further studies are needed to determine the expression and function of NFκB signaling during the formation of embryoid body and neural rosette (Figure 5). The upstream regulation and downstream mechanism will be important targets to better understand the essential role of NFκB signaling in initiating early differentiation of both neural induction and neurogenesis. These studies will open a potential avenue for the development of therapeutics for the treatment of neurodevelopmental disorders and neurodegenerative diseases. Emerging evidence suggests that non-classical and atypical NFκB pathways are implicated in ES cell differentiation [101, 102, 111]. It will be important to evaluate the different role of three NFκB pathways during neuronal fate decision.

Author details

Yonggang Zhang and Wenhui Hu*

*Address all correspondence to: whu@temple.edu

Department of Neuroscience, Temple University School of Medicine, Philadelphia, USA

References

[1] Kowalczyk T, Pontious A, Englund C, et al. Intermediate neuronal progenitors (basal progenitors) produce pyramidal-projection neurons for all layers of cerebral cortex. Cereb Cortex 2009;19:2439-2450

[2] Farioli-Vecchioli S, Saraulli D, Costanzi M, et al. The timing of differentiation of adult hippocampal neurons is crucial for spatial memory. PLoS Biol 2008;6:e246

[3] Kosodo Y, Roper K, Haubensak W, et al. Asymmetric distribution of the apical plasma membrane during neurogenic divisions of mammalian neuroepithelial cells. EMBO J 2004;23:2314-2324

[4] Haubensak W, Attardo A, Denk W, et al. Neurons arise in the basal neuroepithelium of the early mammalian telencephalon: a major site of neurogenesis. Proc Natl Acad Sci U S A 2004;101:3196-3201

[5] Farkas LM, Huttner WB. The cell biology of neural stem and progenitor cells and its significance for their proliferation versus differentiation during mammalian brain development. Curr Opin Cell Biol 2008;20:707-715

[6] Sauvageot CM, Stiles CD. Molecular mechanisms controlling cortical gliogenesis. Curr Opin Neurobiol 2002;12:244-249

[7] Wang DD, Bordey A. The astrocyte odyssey. Prog Neurobiol 2008;86:342-367

[8] Perkins ND. Integrating cell-signalling pathways with NF-kappaB and IKK function. Nat Rev Mol Cell Biol 2007;8:49-62

[9] Hacker H, Karin M. Regulation and function of IKK and IKK-related kinases. Sci STKE 2006;2006:re13

[10] Boyce BF, Yao Z, Xing L. Functions of nuclear factor kappaB in bone. Ann N Y Acad Sci 2010;1192:367-375

[11] Mancino A, Lawrence T. Nuclear factor-kappaB and tumor-associated macrophages. Clin Cancer Res 2010;16:784-789

[12] Lin Y, Bai L, Chen W, et al. The NF-kappaB activation pathways, emerging molecular targets for cancer prevention and therapy. Expert Opin Ther Targets 2010;14:45-55

[13] Wong ET, Tergaonkar V. Roles of NF-kappaB in health and disease: mechanisms and therapeutic potential. Clin Sci (Lond) 2009;116:451-465

[14] Teng FY, Tang BL. NF-kappaB signaling in neurite growth and neuronal survival. Rev Neurosci 2010;21:299-313

[15] Gutierrez H, Davies AM. Regulation of neural process growth, elaboration and structural plasticity by NF-kappaB. Trends Neurosci 2011;34:316-325

[16] Chen LF, Greene WC. Shaping the nuclear action of NF-kappaB. Nat Rev Mol Cell Biol 2004;5:392-401

[17] Viatour P, Merville MP, Bours V, et al. Phosphorylation of NF-kappaB and IkappaB proteins: implications in cancer and inflammation. Trends Biochem Sci 2005;30:43-52

[18] Sun SC. The noncanonical NF-kappaB pathway. Immunol Rev 2012;246:125-140

[19] Razani B, Reichardt AD, Cheng G. Non-canonical NF-kappaB signaling activation and regulation: principles and perspectives. Immunol Rev 2011;244:44-54

[20] Kaltschmidt B, Kaltschmidt C. NF-kappaB in the nervous system. Cold Spring Harb Perspect Biol 2009;1:a001271

[21] Imielski Y, Schwamborn JC, Luningschror P, et al. Regrowing the adult brain: NF-kappaB controls functional circuit formation and tissue homeostasis in the dentate gyrus. PLoS One 2012;7:e30838

[22] Mattson MP, Meffert MK. Roles for NF-kappaB in nerve cell survival, plasticity, and disease. Cell Death Differ 2006;13:852-860

[23] Camandola S, Mattson MP. NF-kappa B as a therapeutic target in neurodegenerative diseases. Expert Opin Ther Targets 2007;11:123-132

[24] Fridmacher V, Kaltschmidt B, Goudeau B, et al. Forebrain-specific neuronal inhibition of nuclear factor-kappaB activity leads to loss of neuroprotection. J Neurosci 2003;23:9403-9408

[25] Boersma MC, Dresselhaus EC, De Biase LM, et al. A requirement for nuclear factor-kappaB in developmental and plasticity-associated synaptogenesis. J Neurosci 2011;31:5414-5425

[26] Sanchez-Ponce D, Tapia M, Munoz A, et al. New role of IKK alpha/beta phosphorylated I kappa B alpha in axon outgrowth and axon initial segment development. Mol Cell Neurosci 2008;37:832-844

[27] Schultz C, Konig HG, Del Turco D, et al. Coincident enrichment of phosphorylated IkappaBalpha, activated IKK, and phosphorylated p65 in the axon initial segment of neurons. Mol Cell Neurosci 2006;33:68-80

[28] Politi C, Del Turco D, Sie JM, et al. Accumulation of phosphorylated I kappaB alpha and activated IKK in nodes of Ranvier. Neuropathol Appl Neurobiol 2008;34:357-365

[29] Denis-Donini S, Caprini A, Frassoni C, et al. Members of the NF-kappaB family expressed in zones of active neurogenesis in the postnatal and adult mouse brain. Brain Res Dev Brain Res 2005;154:81-89

[30] Rolls A, Shechter R, London A, et al. Toll-like receptors modulate adult hippocampal neurogenesis. Nat Cell Biol 2007;9:1081-1088

[31] Widera D, Kaus A, Kaltschmidt C, et al. Neural stem cells, inflammation and NF-kappaB: basic principle of maintenance and repair or origin of brain tumours? J Cell Mol Med 2008;12:459-470

[32] Zhang Y, Liu J, Yao S, et al. Nuclear factor kappa B signaling initiates early differentiation of neural stem cells. Stem Cells 2012;30:510-524

[33] Meneghini V, Francese MT, Carraro L, et al. A novel role for the Receptor for Advanced Glycation End-products in neural progenitor cells derived from adult Sub-Ventricular Zone. Mol Cell Neurosci 2010;45:139-150

[34] Young KM, Bartlett PF, Coulson EJ. Neural progenitor number is regulated by nuclear factor-kappaB p65 and p50 subunit-dependent proliferation rather than cell survival. J Neurosci Res 2006;83:39-49

[35] Zhu C, Liu Z, Gui L, et al. Mutated IkappaBalpha represses proliferation of immortalized neural progenitor cells and prevents their apoptosis after oxygen-glucose deprivation. Brain Res 2008;1244:24-31

[36] Wu JP, Kuo JS, Liu YL, et al. Tumor necrosis factor-alpha modulates the proliferation of neural progenitors in the subventricular/ventricular zone of adult rat brain. Neurosci Lett 2000;292:203-206

[37] Widera D, Mikenberg I, Elvers M, et al. Tumor necrosis factor alpha triggers proliferation of adult neural stem cells via IKK/NF-kappaB signaling. BMC Neurosci 2006;7:64

[38] Rubio-Araiz A, Arevalo-Martin A, Gomez-Torres O, et al. The endocannabinoid system modulates a transient TNF pathway that induces neural stem cell proliferation. Mol Cell Neurosci 2008;38:374-380

[39] Denis-Donini S, Dellarole A, Crociara P, et al. Impaired adult neurogenesis associated with short-term memory defects in NF-kappaB p50-deficient mice. J Neurosci 2008;28:3911-3919

[40] Bernardino L, Agasse F, Silva B, et al. Tumor necrosis factor-alpha modulates survival, proliferation, and neuronal differentiation in neonatal subventricular zone cell cultures. Stem Cells 2008;26:2361-2371

[41] Lou SJ, Gu P, Xu H, et al. [Effect of tumor necrosis factor-alpha on differentiation of mesencephalic neural stem cells and proliferation of oligodendrocytes in the rat]. Sheng Li Xue Bao 2003;55:183-186

[42] Scholzke MN, Rottinger A, Murikinati S, et al. TWEAK regulates proliferation and differentiation of adult neural progenitor cells. Mol Cell Neurosci 2011;46:325-332

[43] Encinas JM, Sierra A. Neural stem cell deforestation as the main force driving the age-related decline in adult hippocampal neurogenesis. Behav Brain Res 2012;227:433-439

[44] Villeda SA, Luo J, Mosher KI, et al. The ageing systemic milieu negatively regulates neurogenesis and cognitive function. Nature 2011;477:90-94

[45] Koo JW, Russo SJ, Ferguson D, et al. Nuclear factor-kappaB is a critical mediator of stress-impaired neurogenesis and depressive behavior. Proc Natl Acad Sci U S A 2010;107:2669-2674

[46] Calado DP, Zhang B, Srinivasan L, et al. Constitutive canonical NF-kappaB activation cooperates with disruption of BLIMP1 in the pathogenesis of activated B cell-like diffuse large cell lymphoma. Cancer Cell 2010;18:580-589

[47] Vlantis K, Wullaert A, Sasaki Y, et al. Constitutive IKK2 activation in intestinal epithelial cells induces intestinal tumors in mice. J Clin Invest 2011;121:2781-2793

[48] Shi Y, Sun G, Zhao C, et al. Neural stem cell self-renewal. Crit Rev Oncol Hematol 2008;65:43-53

[49] Bertrand N, Castro DS, Guillemot F. Proneural genes and the specification of neural cell types. Nat Rev Neurosci 2002;3:517-530

[50] Shaker T, Dennis D, Kurrasch DM, et al. Neurog1 and Neurog2 coordinately regulate development of the olfactory system. Neural Dev 2012;7:28

[51] Castro DS, Guillemot F. Old and new functions of proneural factors revealed by the genome-wide characterization of their transcriptional targets. Cell Cycle 2011;10:4026-4031

[52] Cau E, Gradwohl G, Casarosa S, et al. Hes genes regulate sequential stages of neurogenesis in the olfactory epithelium. Development 2000;127:2323-2332

[53] Kageyama R, Ohtsuka T, Kobayashi T. Roles of Hes genes in neural development. Dev Growth Differ 2008;50 Suppl 1:S97-103

[54] Wang R, Liu K, Chen L, et al. Neural fate decisions mediated by trans-activation and cis-inhibition in Notch signaling. Bioinformatics 2011;27:3158-3165

[55] Vilas-Boas F, Henrique D. HES6-1 and HES6-2 function through different mechanisms during neuronal differentiation. PLoS One 2010;5:e15459

[56] Fior R, Henrique D. A novel hes5/hes6 circuitry of negative regulation controls Notch activity during neurogenesis. Dev Biol 2005;281:318-333

[57] Bonini SA, Ferrari-Toninelli G, Uberti D, et al. Nuclear factor kappaB-dependent neurite remodeling is mediated by Notch pathway. J Neurosci 2011;31:11697-11705

[58] Ang HL, Tergaonkar V. Notch and NFkappaB signaling pathways: Do they collaborate in normal vertebrate brain development and function? Bioessays 2007;29:1039-1047

[59] Fujita K, Yasui S, Shinohara T, et al. Interaction between NF-kappaB signaling and Notch signaling in gliogenesis of mouse mesencephalic neural crest cells. Mech Dev 2011;128:496-509

[60] Schwamborn JC, Berezikov E, Knoblich JA. The TRIM-NHL protein TRIM32 activates microRNAs and prevents self-renewal in mouse neural progenitors. Cell 2009;136:913-925

[61] Hillje AL, Worlitzer MM, Palm T, et al. Neural stem cells maintain their stemness through protein kinase C zeta-mediated inhibition of TRIM32. Stem Cells 2011;29:1437-1447

[62] Sato T, Okumura F, Kano S, et al. TRIM32 promotes neural differentiation through retinoic acid receptor-mediated transcription. J Cell Sci 2011;124:3492-3502

[63] Beg AA, Sha WC, Bronson RT, et al. Embryonic lethality and liver degeneration in mice lacking the RelA component of NF-kappa B. Nature 1995;376:167-170

[64] Grossmann M, Metcalf D, Merryfull J, et al. The combined absence of the transcription factors Rel and RelA leads to multiple hemopoietic cell defects. Proc Natl Acad Sci U S A 1999;96:11848-11853

[65] Alcamo E, Mizgerd JP, Horwitz BH, et al. Targeted mutation of TNF receptor I rescues the RelA-deficient mouse and reveals a critical role for NF-kappa B in leukocyte recruitment. J Immunol 2001;167:1592-1600

[66] Li Q, Estepa G, Memet S, et al. Complete lack of NF-kappaB activity in IKK1 and IKK2 double-deficient mice: additional defect in neurulation. Genes Dev 2000;14:1729-1733

[67] Mir A, Kaufman L, Noor A, et al. Identification of mutations in TRAPPC9, which encodes the NIK- and IKK-beta-binding protein, in nonsyndromic autosomal-recessive mental retardation. Am J Hum Genet 2009;85:909-915

[68] Mochida GH, Mahajnah M, Hill AD, et al. A truncating mutation of TRAPPC9 is associated with autosomal-recessive intellectual disability and postnatal microcephaly. Am J Hum Genet 2009;85:897-902

[69] Philippe O, Rio M, Carioux A, et al. Combination of linkage mapping and microarray-expression analysis identifies NF-kappaB signaling defect as a cause of autosomal-recessive mental retardation. Am J Hum Genet 2009;85:903-908

[70] Zhao M, Raingo J, Chen ZJ, et al. Cc2d1a, a C2 domain containing protein linked to nonsyndromic mental retardation, controls functional maturation of central synapses. J Neurophysiol 2011;105:1506-1515

[71] Noor A, Windpassinger C, Patel M, et al. CC2D2A, encoding a coiled-coil and C2 domain protein, causes autosomal-recessive mental retardation with retinitis pigmentosa. Am J Hum Genet 2008;82:1011-1018

[72] Ziats MN, Rennert OM. Expression profiling of autism candidate genes during human brain development implicates central immune signaling pathways. PLoS One 2011;6:e24691

[73] Naik US, Gangadharan C, Abbagani K, et al. A study of nuclear transcription factor-kappa B in childhood autism. PLoS One 2011;6:e19488

[74] Go HS, Seo JE, Kim KC, et al. Valproic acid inhibits neural progenitor cell death by activation of NF-kappaB signaling pathway and up-regulation of Bcl-XL. J Biomed Sci 2011;18:48

[75] Levine AJ, Brivanlou AH. Proposal of a model of mammalian neural induction. Dev Biol 2007;308:247-256

[76] Lenka N, Ramasamy SK. Neural induction from ES cells portrays default commitment but instructive maturation. PLoS One 2007;2:e1349

[77] Stern CD. Neural induction: 10 years on since the 'default model'. Curr Opin Cell Biol 2006;18:692-697

[78] Mason I. Initiation to end point: the multiple roles of fibroblast growth factors in neural development. Nat Rev Neurosci 2007;8:583-596

[79] Stuhlmiller TJ, Garcia-Castro MI. Current perspectives of the signaling pathways directing neural crest induction. Cell Mol Life Sci 2012

[80] Osakada F, Takahashi M. Neural induction and patterning in Mammalian pluripotent stem cells. CNS Neurol Disord Drug Targets 2011;10:419-432

[81] de Almeida I, Rolo A, Batut J, et al. Unexpected activities of Smad7 in Xenopus mesodermal and neural induction. Mech Dev 2008;125:421-431

[82] Salewski RP, Buttigieg J, Mitchell RA, et al. The generation of definitive neural stem cells from piggyBac transposon induced pluripotent stem cells can be enhanced by induction of the NOTCH signalling pathway. Stem Cells Dev 2012

[83] Tang Y, Xie H, Chen J, et al. Activated NF-kB in bone marrow mesenchymal stem cells from SLE patients inhibits osteogenic differentiation through down-regulating Smad signaling. Stem Cells Dev 2012

[84] Yamaguchi M, Weitzmann MN, Murata T. Exogenous regucalcin stimulates osteoclastogenesis and suppresses osteoblastogenesis through NF-kappaB activation. Mol Cell Biochem 2012;359:193-203

[85] Chen G, Handel K, Roth S. The maternal NF-kappaB/dorsal gradient of Tribolium castaneum: dynamics of early dorsoventral patterning in a short-germ beetle. Development 2000;127:5145-5156

[86] DeLotto R, DeLotto Y, Steward R, et al. Nucleocytoplasmic shuttling mediates the dynamic maintenance of nuclear Dorsal levels during Drosophila embryogenesis. Development 2007;134:4233-4241

[87] Reeves GT, Stathopoulos A. Graded dorsal and differential gene regulation in the Drosophila embryo. Cold Spring Harb Perspect Biol 2009;1:a000836

[88] Ayyar S, Pistillo D, Calleja M, et al. NF-kappaB/Rel-mediated regulation of the neural fate in Drosophila. PLoS One 2007;2:e1178

[89] Lake BB, Ford R, Kao KR. Xrel3 is required for head development in Xenopus laevis. Development 2001;128:263-273

[90] Torchinsky A, Toder V. To die or not to die: the function of the transcription factor NF-kappaB in embryos exposed to stress. Am J Reprod Immunol 2004;51:138-143

[91] Chambers SM, Fasano CA, Papapetrou EP, et al. Highly efficient neural conversion of human ES and iPS cells by dual inhibition of SMAD signaling. Nat Biotechnol 2009;27:275-280

[92] Tsuji O, Miura K, Fujiyoshi K, et al. Cell therapy for spinal cord injury by neural stem/progenitor cells derived from iPS/ES cells. Neurotherapeutics 2011;8:668-676

[93] Lilienbaum A, Sage J, Memet S, et al. NF-kappa B is developmentally regulated during spermatogenesis in mice. Dev Dyn 2000;219:333-340

[94] Nishikimi A, Mukai J, Yamada M. Nuclear translocation of nuclear factor kappa B in early 1-cell mouse embryos. Biol Reprod 1999;60:1536-1541

[95] Paciolla M, Boni R, Fusco F, et al. Nuclear factor-kappa-B-inhibitor alpha (NFKBIA) is a developmental marker of NF-kappaB/p65 activation during in vitro oocyte maturation and early embryogenesis. Hum Reprod 2011;26:1191-1201

[96] Dominguez I, Sanz L, Arenzana-Seisdedos F, et al. Inhibition of protein kinase C zeta subspecies blocks the activation of an NF-kappa B-like activity in Xenopus laevis oocytes. Mol Cell Biol 1993;13:1290-1295

[97] Richardson JC, Garcia Estrabot AM, Woodland HR. XrelA, a Xenopus maternal and zygotic homologue of the p65 subunit of NF-kappa B. Characterisation of transcriptional properties in the developing embryo and identification of a negative interference mutant. Mech Dev 1994;45:173-189

[98] Correa RG, Tergaonkar V, Ng JK, et al. Characterization of NF-kappa B/I kappa B proteins in zebra fish and their involvement in notochord development. Mol Cell Biol 2004;24:5257-5268

[99] Shingo T, Sorokan ST, Shimazaki T, et al. Erythropoietin regulates the in vitro and in vivo production of neuronal progenitors by mammalian forebrain neural stem cells. J Neurosci 2001;21:9733-9743

[100] Torres J, Watt FM. Nanog maintains pluripotency of mouse embryonic stem cells by inhibiting NFkappaB and cooperating with Stat3. Nat Cell Biol 2008;10:194-201

[101] Kim YE, Kang HB, Park JA, et al. Upregulation of NF-kappaB upon differentiation of mouse embryonic stem cells. BMB Rep 2008;41:705-709

[102] Kang HB, Kim YE, Kwon HJ, et al. Enhancement of NF-kappaB expression and activity upon differentiation of human embryonic stem cell line SNUhES3. Stem Cells Dev 2007;16:615-623

[103] Yang C, Atkinson SP, Vilella F, et al. Opposing putative roles for canonical and non-canonical NFkappaB signaling on the survival, proliferation, and differentiation potential of human embryonic stem cells. Stem Cells 2010;28:1970-1980

[104] Mitsui K, Tokuzawa Y, Itoh H, et al. The homeoprotein Nanog is required for maintenance of pluripotency in mouse epiblast and ES cells. Cell 2003;113:631-642

[105] Guan X, Yabuuchi A, Huo H, et al. Derivation of human embryonic stem cells with NEMO deficiency. Stem Cell Res 2012;8:410-415

[106] Dutta D, Ray S, Home P, et al. Self-renewal versus lineage commitment of embryonic stem cells: protein kinase C signaling shifts the balance. Stem Cells 2011;29:618-628

[107] Luningschror P, Stocker B, Kaltschmidt B, et al. miR-290 Cluster Modulates Pluripotency by Repressing Canonical NF-kappaB Signaling. Stem Cells 2012;30:655-664

[108] Saporta MA, Grskovic M, Dimos JT. Induced pluripotent stem cells in the study of neurological diseases. Stem Cell Res Ther 2011;2:37

[109] Rajasingh J. Reprogramming of somatic cells. Prog Mol Biol Transl Sci 2012;111:51-82

[110] Kwak JH, Jung JK, Lee H. Nuclear factor-kappa B inhibitors; a patent review (2006-2010). Expert Opin Ther Pat 2011;21:1897-1910

[111] Saldanha-Araujo F, Haddad R, Malmegrim de Farias KC, et al. Mesenchymal stem cells promote the sustained expression of CD69 on activated T-lymphocytes: roles of canonical and non-canonical NF-kappaB signaling. J Cell Mol Med 2011

Section 5

Stem Cells and Signaling Pathways

Regulation of Basal and Injury-Induced Fate Decisions of Adult Neural Precursor Cells: Focus on SOCS2 and Related Signalling Pathways

Harleen S. Basrai, Kimberly J. Christie and
Ann M. Turnley

Additional information is available at the end of the chapter

1. Introduction

Two decades ago it was discovered that the adult mammalian brain contains neural stem cells (NSCs) and neural precursor cells (NPCs) capable of producing new neurons and glial cells [1-3]. This has led to a great deal of research to understand the biology of these cells and to determine signalling pathways that can be targeted to promote repair of the damaged nervous system. There are two primary regions in the adult mammalian brain that contain adult NSCs/NPCs. These are the subventricular zone (SVZ) lining the lateral walls of the lateral ventricles and the subgranular zone (SGZ) of the hippocampal dentate gyrus. NPC fate is regulated by intrinsic (e.g. transcription factors and signalling mediators) and extrinsic (e.g growth factors and extracellular matrix) factors which involve effects on proliferation, migration and differentiation of new neurons and glial cells.

This review will highlight the major signalling cascades involved in neuronal fate from birth to integration. It will begin with a discussion of pathways involved under normal physiological conditions, which will be followed by discussion of changes to these signalling cascades following neural damage due to injury or disease. Finally, there will be a more focused examination of the roles of suppressor of cytokine signalling (SOCS) molecules and related pathways in the context of signalling in adult neurogenesis under basal conditions and following neural damage.

2. Adult neurogenesis

2.1. Hippocampal neurogenesis

NPCs in the SGZ become neurons of the granular cell layer of the dentate gyrus in the hippocampus. In the SGZ, the most immature NPCs (Type 1) are radial and horizontal NPCs that transition to intermediate progenitors (type-2a, 2b and 3) and then to immature granule neurons which become dentate granular neurons. These then make large mossy fibre projections with CA3 pyramidal neurons [4].

2.2. SVZ neurogenesis

The SVZ produces NPCs that form neuroblasts which migrate along the rostral migratory stream and become neurons in the olfactory bulb. These new neurons primarily become GABAergic granule neurons that provide lateral inhibition between mitral and tufted cells. A minority of the new neurons become periglomerular neurons that are involved in lateral inhibition between glomeruli, and a small number of these cells are dopaminergic. Similar to the SGZ, there is a progression of NPC development in the SVZ. Slowly proliferating astrocytes in the SVZ (Type B cells) are the NSCs and these generate the highly proliferative transit-amplifying Type C cells. These then generate post-mitotic neuroblasts (the Type A cells) destined for the olfactory bulb via migration along the rostral migratory stream (RMS) [5-7].

3. Signalling cascades regulating NPC fate under basal conditions

NPCs from the dentate gyrus and SVZ have the potential to differentiate into neurons and glial cells. Multiple signalling pathways are activated to produce a neuron from NSCs. These cascades can involve both intrinsic and extrinsic factors as the NSC is created, migrates, and finally integrates into its final location.

3.1. Proliferation and neuronal fate

Many pathways important for embryonic neural development are conserved in adult neurogenesis. The Wnt pathway, for example, is a key regulator of proliferation and differentiation in development and a key regulator of adult hippocampal neurogenesis [8]. Wnt signalling results in the activation of the GSK3β/β-catenin that leads to the increased expression of NeuroD1 and promotes neuronal differentiation in NSCs [9]. Activation of Wnt, Sonic Hedgehog (Shh), Notch, and the Sox family of genes, in particular *Sox2*, are also important for the formation and proliferation of NSCs [10-12]. At early stages of differentiation, *Sox2* is required for neuronal fate; while downregulation of *Sox9* by miR-124 is required for neuronal differentiation [13, 14]. Other Sox members are important for neuronal specification, including *Sox3, Sox 4* and *Sox 11* [15-19]. Notch signalling is important for maintaining NSCs/NPCs, however this is dependent on the mitotic state of NSCs/NPCs [20]. Bone morphogenic protein (BMP) signalling inhibits neuronal differentiation; however expression of noggin and neurogenin-1 (Ngn1) in the SVZ and SGZ can obstruct this cascade [21-23]. Inhibition of the BMP pathway increases neurogenesis initially, however it results in depletion of the NSC pool leading to decreased neurogenesis [24]. In the dentate gyrus, the RNA-binding protein FXR2 regulates neurogenesis by reducing the stability of noggin mRNA leading to an increased activation of the BMP pathway [25]. Proliferation in the SVZ is under epigenetic control via histone HZAX phosophorylation which can limit proliferation and overall neurogenesis [26].

Proneural proteins, basic-helix-loop-helix (bHLH) transcription factors also control neuronal fate commitment of NPCs. Type C cells of the SVZ fated to become GABAergic interneurons in the olfactory bulb express *Ascl1* [27]. *Ngn2* and *Tbr2* are expressed in dorsal SVZ progenitors that become glutamatergic juxtaglomerular neurons [28], while *Sp8* is required for parvalbumin-expressing interneurons in the olfactory bulb [29]. In the SGZ, *Neurog2* and *Tbr2* are expressed in NPCs destined to become glutamatergic neurons in the hippocampus [27, 30, 31], while over-expression of *Ascl1* produces oligodendrocytes [32].

Neurotrophic growth factors have been studied extensively in the SVZ. Many, including, epidermal growth factor (EGF), transforming growth factor (TGF), and vascular endothelial growth factor (VEGF) can augment SVZ progenitor proliferation and migration of newly derived cells into structures beside the lateral ventricles; however these cells primarily differentiate into oligodendrocytes [33-36]. Fibroblast growth factor-2 (FGF-2) signalling promotes proliferation in both the SVZ and SGZ [37-39]. FGF-2 and TGF synthesis and secretion can be augmented by ATP, which can increase proliferation, and provide a potential explanation for the reduced neurogenesis in purinergic receptor knockout mice (P2Y1) [40, 41]. Other factors also play a role in neurogenesis, including neuregulin-1, which has been implicated in dentate gyrus neurogenesis in addition to having antidepressant effects [42] and Growth Hormone (GH) which augments EGF and FGF2-induced proliferation [43]. Growth factor signalling often leads to activation of Akt through phosphoinositide-3 kinase (PI-3K); one negative regulator of this pathway is the phosphatase and tumour suppressor PTEN, which has a role in regulating neurogenesis as demonstrated by increased proliferation and differentiation in mutant mice [44]. Furthermore, IGF-2 also regulates proliferation in the dentate gyrus in an Akt-dependent manner [45].

The gp130-associated cytokines, ciliary neurotrophic factor (CNTF) and leukemia inhibitory factor (LIF), activate Janus kinase (JAK/signal transducer of transcription 3 (STAT3)), mitogen activated protein (MAP) kinase and PI-3K/Akt pathways following ligand binding. These cytokines have been shown to regulate NSC proliferation and differentiation [46-49]. Specifically in the dentate gyrus, the activation of STAT3 from CNTF appears to be essential for the formation and maintenance of the NSCs [50]. The role of the JAK/STAT pathway will be discussed in more detail later. The MAPK pathway is important for neurogenesis as demonstrated by conditional knockdown of extracellular signal-related kinase 5 (ERK5) which limits neuronal differentiation and neurogenesis resulting in impaired contextual fear extinction and remote fear memory [51, 52].

Other molecules shown to have a role in controlling neuronal differentiation include Presenilin-1 (PS1), which is the catalytic core of the aspartyl protease gamma-secretase. Reduction of PS1 enhances differentiation, primarily through its transducers the EGF receptor and β-catenin [53]. Interferon-γ, which signals via STAT1, and interferon-β which does not, both inhibit cultured adult NPC proliferation, but only interferon-γ promotes neuronal differentiation [54, 55].

3.2. Migration and integration

Migration from the SVZ along the RMS involves long distances and multiple pathways [56] For example, it is dependent on Shh signalling, as evident by a decrease of neuroblasts in the olfactory bulb following Hedgehog signalling interruption [11]. Shh is a chemoattractant cue extrinsic to the neuroblast that guides migration to the olfactory bulb. Neurotrophic growth factor signalling is also important for migration, in particular insulin-like growth factor (IGF-1) null mice show an abundance of neuroblasts in the SVZ that have failed to migrate to the olfactory bulb [57]. Guidance cues from EphB2/ephrin-B2 pathways also enable formation of the chain migration from the SVZ to the olfactory bulb [58]. Recently, endocannabinoid signalling has been shown to regulate migration and neurogenesis in both the SVZ and dentate gyrus [59, 60]. Other molecules involved in this migration include polysialated neural cell adhesion molecule (PSA-NCAM) [61-63], Slit-Robo [64] and integrins [65, 66]. Many of these factors signal via the Rho kinase pathway, which is a downstream regulator of NPC migration [67]. In addition adult NPCs express a range of chemokine receptors and chemokines are expressed in different brain regions, with the highest levels in the olfactory bulb, suggesting an as yet largely unexplored role for chemokines in regulating basal adult NPC migration [68].

The migration distance for new neurons from the SGZ is relatively short as they travel into the granular layer above the SGZ, where guidance molecules may control this movement. NMDA receptor signalling is required for the proper migration of newborn granular cells in the dentate gyrus [69]. This is achieved through the activation of Disrupted-in-schizophrenia (DISC1), as neurons without DISC1 migrate further into granular layer and into the molecular layer [69, 70]. DISC1 also controls the dendritic maturation of newborn granule cells through GABA depolarization of NKCC1 and activation of the Akt-mTOR pathway [70, 71].

New neurons must integrate into existing circuitry or they will not survive. The vast majority of new neurons do not survive past 4 weeks. Interestingly, NMDA receptors expressed in neuroblasts along the RMS are crucial to the integration of these neurons in existing olfactory bulb circuitry [72]. Glutamate is released from astrocyte-like cells that surround the neuroblasts. NMDA receptor activation in newly-born dentate gyrus granule cells also increases survival. Initial GABA depolarization plays a role in the maturation of neurons in the dentate gyrus and olfactory bulb [73, 74]. This depolarization and subsequent Ca^{2+} influx are required for dendrite initiation and elongation [75]. This process involves coordinated expression of the GABA receptor subunit alpha2 that controls the maturation of the new neurons [76]. In addition, agrin signalling is necessary for integration and survival of newborn neurons in the olfactory bulb, as demonstrated by a loss of agrin leading to improper synapse formation while an overexpression of agrin results in an increase in dendritic spines [77].

Neurotrophin signalling has important role in the survival and integration of new neurons. Brain-derived growth factor (BDNF) binding to the TrkB receptor tyrosine kinases increases the number and survival of NSCs in the SVZ and olfactory bulb [78-80]. Similarly, knock-down of TrkB receptors and disruption of BDNF signalling in dentate gyrus progenitors leads to shorter dendrites and reduced spine formation, culminating in a lack of survival [81]. Fibroblast growth factor (FGF-2) has a role in neurogenesis and memory consolidation in this context [39].

Intrinsic factors are also necessary for the maturation and survival of newly born neurons. In the dentate gyrus, *Prox1* [18], *NeuroD* [82, 83] and Kruppel-like factor 9 [84] play important roles in survival. In the SVZ, *Pax6* and *Dlx-2* influence neuronal fate, leading to the production of dopaminergic periglomerular cells in the olfactory bulb [85-87]. New neurons in the dentate gyrus rely on cyclic response element binding protein (CREB) signalling for maturation and integration into the network. Interestingly, CREB activates miR-132 which regulates dendrite maturation in newborn dentate gyrus granular neurons [88]. The collapsin response mediator protein-5 (CRMP5) is expressed in both the SVZ and dentate gyrus and CRMP5$^{-/-}$ mice show an increase in proliferation and neurogenesis in addition to displaying an increase in apoptosis of granular cells in both the olfactory bulb and dentate gyrus [89].

4. Signalling cascades regulating NPC fate following neural damage

Neurogenesis and gliogenesis are known to be initiated following brain damage, such as ischemia, seizures, traumatic injury and neurodegenerative diseases [90-92]. However, these new neurons and glia usually do not effectively replenish those that were lost. Many of the normal signalling cascades are altered following injury. Below is a discussion of the major changes in these cascades that influence neuronal fate of the NSCs generated in the SVZ and SGZ following injury or disease.

4.1. Brain injury

A traumatic lesion to the brain cortex results in an increase in proliferation of NSCs in the SVZ, although varied locations and degrees of injury have resulted in an incongruity of results across the literature [93-98]. Nonetheless, it is generally agreed that the increase in proliferation results in an increase in neurogenesis at the SVZ [99]. Expression of growth factors such as BDNF, FGF2, GDNF, IGF-1 and VEGF are increased following ischemia and exogenous application further augments NSC proliferation and survival [100-105]. Shh expression is also upregulated in the SVZ following ischemia, potentially playing a role in the increase of proliferation, while Wnt expression does not change [106, 107]. Phosphorylated CREB is upregulated following ischemia and induces hippocampal neurogenesis [108].

Following proliferation these cells must migrate and integrate to damaged cortical tissue. The majority of research on ectopic migration from the SVZ has been performed following an ischemic insult and has demonstrated that cells do reach the injured striatum [90, 109-114]. It appears that the cells no longer migrate in a chain formation and carry on individually, interestingly, at the expense of the RMS population [109, 115]. This change in migration is the direct result of chemoattractive cues expressed from the injury site.

Chemokines and their receptors can attract neuroblasts from the RMS, for example it has been shown that Stromal cell-derived factor-1 (CXCL12) and its receptor CXCR4 are upregulated at the injury site [116, 117]. Expression of several chemokines and their receptors is upregulated on adult NPCs by inflammatory cytokines, such as interferon-γ and TNF-α [68].

Migration is also altered following an epileptic seizure: the NSCs migrate along the RMS more quickly, while in the dentate gyrus there is faster integration and maturation [118, 119]. There are morphological changes to the hippocampal region including mossy fibre sprouting, dispersion of the granular cell layer, and ectopically migrated dentate granule cells in the hilus (reviewed in [120]).

When cells do migrate to the correct location they must differentiate into neurons to recover function of neurons lost. Unfortunately, this does not appear to be consistent. Recent work on ischemia has demonstrated that new neurons from the SVZ are found in the cortex near the lesioned area, while injury of the somatosensory cortex showed the generation of astrocytes and microglia/macrophages without any new neurons [98, 121]. Other work has found the production of astrocytes and oligodendrocytes near the injury site as a result of expression of repressors of neuronal fate [122, 123]. For example, the BMP antagonist, chordin, and the transcription factor Olig2 both induce glial expression in neuroblasts at the injury site [124, 125]. However, following ischemia, pro-neuronal transcription factors are expressed in primate progenitors in the SGZ, including *Emx2*, *Pax6* and *Ngn2* [126]. Recently it has been shown that following thirty and sixty days after stroke, *Ascl1/Mash1* expressing cells in the ischemic striatum gave rise to GABAergic neurons and mature oligodendrocytes [127]. Even when a NSC differentiates into a neuron, the survival of these neurons is very low. Recent work has demonstrated that the Ras-related GTPase, Rit, is an important component in the survival of young granular cells in the dentate gyrus following a brain injury. $Rit^{-/-}$ mice show a marked increase in new neuron death following injury [128]. Recently, the small non-coding RNA molecule, miR-124a, was shown to be altered following stroke. Interestingly, it can mediate stroke induced neurogenesis via the Notch signalling pathway [129]. Inhibition of the Notch pathway increases neurogenesis after spinal cord injury in zebrafish resulting in higher proliferation and more motor neurons [130]. Lentiviral expression of Wnt3 increased neurogenesis following focal ischemia and improved functional recovery [131].

4.2. Neurodegenerative diseases

Reports on neurogenesis in neurodegenerative diseases are highly dependent on the disease model used. Variations in transgenic mice and other drug induced models are the most probable cause for the conflicting results. In many models of Alzheimer's disease, Parkinson's disease and Huntington's disease there is impaired neurogenesis (reviewed in [132]). Alzheimer's disease (AD) is characterized by degeneration of basal forebrain cholinergic neurons in the cortex and hippocampus from the deposition of neurofibrillary tangles and amyloid-β plaques [133]. The neuropathologic hallmark of AD is the amyloid-β plaques; however small oligomeric amyloid-β appears to be the noxious component. Neurogenesis can be both increased and decreased in AD, depending on the transgenic model used (reviewed in [132]). Early in the disease, oligomeric amyloid-β may transiently promote the generation of immature neurons from NPCs. However, reduced concentrations of multiple neurotrophic factors and higher levels of FGF2 seem to induce a developmental arrest of newly generated neurons. Further, there is a down-regulation of *Olig2* and over-expression of *Ascl1* caused by amyloid-β that switches the cell fate to death [134, 135]. Generally, there is a decrease in proliferation and survival of NSCs in the dentate gyrus and SVZ with AD. A better understanding on the effects of amyloid-β on NSC proliferation and maturation is needed to improve this decrease in neurogenesis.

Parkinson's disease (PD) is the outcome of the loss of dopaminergic neurons in the substantia nigra of the midbrain (reviewed in [136]). In transgenic mouse models, there is a decrease in newly generated neurons in both the dentate gyrus and olfactory bulb [137, 138]. Alterations in neurogenesis have been linked to a decrease in *Notch1* and *Hes5* expression [138]. Lack of proliferation could be the explanation for a lack of migration of NSCs to the damaged regions in PD and AD [139]. Along these lines, manipulations that increase proliferation also demonstrate migration, for example intraventricular injection of clustering ephrin-A1-Fc increased proliferation in the SVZ, followed by migration to the striatum and differentiation into dopaminergic neurons in a rodent model of Parkinson's disease [140]. Furthermore, exogenous application of EGF and FGF2 showed similar results [141]. Exciting research in salamanders has shown regeneration of dopamine neurons following ablation involving neurogenesis in quiescent cells. This activation is due to the loss of dopamine, demonstrating a control of dopamine signalling maintaining homeostasis [142]. Replacement of dopaminergic neurons relies on NSC differentiation into the proper neuronal fate. Recent studies have elucidated the transcription factors necessary to produce dopaminergic neurons. The combination of *Ascl1/Mash1*, *Nurr1* and *Lmx1a* result in the generation of functional dopaminergic neurons from mouse and human fibroblasts [143]. Other studies have shown that *Foxa2* in combination with *Nurr1* can also induce the production of nigral (A9)-type midbrain neurons from NPCs [144].

Other neurodegenerative diseases such as Huntington's disease have shown a decrease in neurogenesis. NPC proliferation is decreased in Huntington's disease in both the SGZ and SVZ, with some reports of reduced numbers of newly born neurons (reviewed in [132]). In a rat model of Huntington's disease, SGZ progenitor cell proliferation is decreased due to an increase in *Sox2*-positive quiescent stem cells and a decrease in CREB signalling [145].

Overall, further investigation is needed to clarify the changes in signalling pathways following neurodegenerative disease. One pathway that has been extensively studied both in basal neurogenesis and after injury is the suppressor of cytokine signalling (SOCS) family of proteins. The following section will discuss research involving the SOCS proteins and related pathways.

5. SOCS molecules and cytokine signalling pathways

As discussed in the previous section, a diversity of signalling cascades are involved in regulating neuronal cell proliferation, differentiation and survival. However, JAK-STAT signalling seems to be one of the central pathways in the regulation of adult neurogenesis. Since its discovery twenty years ago, this pathway has been studied extensively due to its key roles in modulating many different physiological processes through responses to various regulatory molecules [146].

5.1. JAK/STAT signalling

The JAK-STAT pathway can be activated by a range of cytokines, growth factors and hormones. In the regulation of adult neurogenesis, activation of this pathway is carried out by a group of neuroregulatory cytokines. Members of this cytokine group include CNTF, LIF and cardiotrophin 1 (CT-1), all of which belong to the interleukin 6 family of cytokines. These cytokines initiate JAK-STAT activation by binding and signalling through the LIF receptor-β (LIFRβ)/ glycoprotein 130 (gp130) receptor complex. The receptor complex bound by CNTF differs slightly in that it has a third extracellular receptor component, the CNTF receptor-α (structurally related to gp130), that is held to the membrane via a glycosylphosphoinositol [147].

Cytokine binding results in the dimerization of LIFRβ and gp130 receptors to form a complex [148]. This initiates autophosphorylation and activation of JAK proteins which are associated with the intracellular domains of the LIFRβ and gp130 receptors [149]. Members of the JAK protein family include JAK1, JAK2, JAK3 and TYK2. Cytokines signalling through the LIFRβ/gp130 pathway have been found to activate at least JAK1, JAK2 and TYK2 [150]. In terms of the CNS, only JAK1 and JAK2 expression has been found at significant levels [151]. JAK2 is highly expressed in the developing brain compared to JAK1, thus, a role for it in the regulation of neurogenesis in the developing brain has been suggested [151].

After activation, JAKs phosphorylate tyrosine residues in the intracellular domains of LIFRβ and gp130. These phosphorylated residues become binding sites for SH2 domain containing proteins such as STAT. STAT proteins are a family of transcription factors comprised of STAT1, STAT2, STAT3, STAT4, STAT5a, STAT5b and STAT6 [152]. Upon binding to the activated receptor complex, STAT proteins are phosphorylated by JAKs resulting in their dimerization. Dimerized STAT proteins are now able to translocate into the nucleus and induce gene expression of target neural genes such as glial fibrillary acidic protein (GFAP), peripherin and vasoactive intestinal peptide [46]. Other SH2 domain containing proteins can also bind the activated LIFRβ/gp130 receptor complex to activate the Ras/MAPK and PI-3K/Akt signalling pathways [49].

The LIFRβ/gp130 pathway is essential for the regulation of astrogliogenesis in the developing and adult brain. In cultured cortical precursors, CNTF, LIF and CT-1 all promote astrocyte formation through LIFRβ/gp130 activation [153-155]. Integral to this pathway is signalling via STAT3, as highlighted by the observation that STAT3 activation in neural stem cells induces glial differentiation, while its inhibition promotes a neuronal fate [156, 157]. Also, in neuroepithelial cells, STAT3 activation promotes astrogliogenisis via LIF induced bone morphogenetic protein 2 expression [158]. In addition to regulating astrogliogenesis, STAT3 induction by CNTF was found to be essential in the maintenance of the SGZ neurogenic niche [50]. Further, it has an important role in the positive regulation of reactive astrocytes in the injured CNS [159].

An important aspect to cytokine signalling via a pathway such as JAK-STAT is the need for its downregulation following activation. Thus far, JAK-STAT signalling is known to be negatively regulated by protein inhibitors of activated STATs (PIAS), the SH2-containing protein tyrosine phosphatases (SHPs) and suppressors of cytokine signalling (SOCS) proteins [160]. In this section, SOCS proteins will be the focus of discussion as the negative regulation of the JAK-STAT signalling pathway by SOCS has several effects on the regulation of neurogenesis and NPC fate.

5.2. The suppressors of cytokine signalling

The SOCS family consists of eight members, namely, SOCS1-7 and cytokine-inducible Src homology 2 (SH2) protein (CIS). They are characterised by a central SH2 domain, a C-terminal SOCS box and a variable N-terminal domain. In addition to these, SOCS1 and SOCS3 also contain a small kinase inhibitory domain. CIS was the first member of this protein family to be cloned. It is also unique to the rest of the SOCS family as a result of its SH2 domain which differs in a few amino acids from most all other known SH2 domains [161].

SOCS expression is induced following activation of the JAK-STAT pathway. This initiates a classic negative feedback loop whereby the SOCS proteins activated by JAK-STAT signalling now go on to inhibit it. SOCS proteins achieve downregulation of signalling by binding to tyrosine phosphorylated proteins via their SH2 domain. The exact mechanism by which signalling inhibition is achieved varies depending on the SOCS protein in question. For example, SOCS1 and SOCS3 both work to block the kinase activity of activated JAK proteins. In the case of SOCS1, this is achieved by directly binding and blocking access to the activated JAK. In the case of SOCS3, this is achieved by its binding to the activated gp130 receptor such that STAT proteins can no longer dock onto the phosphorylated tyrosine residues and be activated by JAK. One mechanism of action for SOCS2 is by blocking STAT access to the activated receptor [162].

SOCS proteins are also able to regulate activity of target proteins, including other SOCS proteins, through interaction with their SOCS box [163, 164]. Interestingly, SOCS2, SOCS6 and SOCS7 have the potential to interact with all members of the SOCS protein family including themselves [164]. In terms of SOCS2, when expressed at high levels, it is able to inhibit the action of SOCS1 and SOCS3 by targeting them for proteasomal degradation [164]. This has also been proposed as a mechanism for the dual action of SOCS2 on GH signalling as observed in the overgrowth phenotypes of SOCS2 knockout and overexpressing mice described below [165].

Signalling via the JAK-STAT pathway has an important role in neural precursor proliferation and differentiation [153, 166-168]. Following the discovery that SOCS proteins regulate the JAK-STAT pathway, the next obvious step was to examine them for possible roles in the nervous system. In doing so, analysis of the SOCS family gene expression in the developing mouse forebrain brought SOCS2 into the spotlight [168]. The genes SOCS1 – SOCS3 and CIS were found to be expressed at all ages (E10 to P25) with a common peak in expression between E14 and P8. However, the level of SOCS2 expression was much higher in comparison. The spatial pattern of SOCS2 expression also distinguished it from the other SOCS genes, with moderate to high levels of expression in neurogenic regions and in newborn neurons. In the adult, SOCS2 was maintained in the CA3 region of the hippocampus and at a moderate level in the dentate gyrus, compared to other SOCS genes whose expression was not localized, if expressed at all under basal conditions. SOCS2 expression was also present in the cerebral cortex and other regions such as the olfactory bulb, forebrain and cerebellum. Interestingly, SOCS2 was first upregulated at the time of neuronal differentiation, which is between the developmental stages E10 and E12, suggesting a role for SOCS2 in neural precursor differentiation [168].

6. SOCS2 in the brain

This interesting spatiotemporal expression of SOCS2 instigated further research into its possible role in neuronal development. The generation of the SOCS2 knockout ($SOCS2^{-/-}$) and SOCS2 overexpressing transgenic (SOCS2Tg) mice has been instrumental in the functional characterisation of SOCS2 [169, 170]. $SOCS2^{-/-}$ mice display an overgrowth phenotype where adult mice are up to 40% heavier than their wild-type counterparts, mainly attributed to an increase in organ size and bone length [170]. This phenotype suggested an involvement of SOCS2 in the negative regulation of GH, a regulator of postnatal growth. To address this hypothesis, SOCS2Tg mice were generated [169]. Interestingly, SOCS2Tg mice also display an enhanced growth phenotype, indicating a potential dual action of SOCS2 where at high levels it may enhance rather than inhibit growth hormone signalling [169].

In-vitro, neural stem cells from $SOCS2^{-/-}$ mice show a marked reduction in the number of neurons generated [171], as opposed to SOCS2Tg mice which show an increase in neuron number [172-174]. Additionally, PC12 cells and neural cells from SOCS2Tg mice demonstrate increased neurite outgrowth in tissue culture [171, 174-176]. GH is an inhibitor of neural differentiation and its negative regulation by SOCS2 is evident by the reduction in neuronal differentiation in neural stem cell cultures of $SOCS2^{-/-}$ mice [171, 174]. The importance of GH/SOCS2 signalling in neuronal differentiation can be illustrated by their involvement in the regulation of the Ngn1 basic helix-loop-helix transcription factor [171]. Ngn1 has an important role in promotion of neurogenesis by at the same time inhibiting glial differentiation [177]. Importantly, Ngn1 is subject to inhibition by GH and this inhibition is overcome by SOCS2 overexpression [171]. Thus, a model has been proposed where GH and SOCS2 regulate neural stem cell differentiation through the modulation of Ngn1 expression [178].

GH binds and signals through the GH receptor (GHR) which belongs to the class I superfamily of cytokine receptors. Like the LIFRβ/gp130 complex, signal transduction is carried out through the JAK-STAT pathway. GH binding activates GHR resulting in JAK activation. JAK2 is the major contributor to GH signalling and it phosphorylates tyrosine residues on the GHR that become binding sites primarily for STAT5a or STAT5b. Activated STAT5 then induces SOCS gene expression [179]. JAK2 may also activate STAT1 and STAT3, however this can be cell type specific [180, 181]. One mechanism by which SOCS2 may block STAT5 activation is via its binding to phosphorylated tyrosine residues at the STAT5 binding site on the GHR [182].

SOCS2 can also regulate signalling via the EGF receptor (EGFR) [175, 176]. The main physiological target for EGFR is EGF. EGFR primarily activates and signals through the Ras/MAPK pathway [183]. In terms of the neuronal effects of EGF, it has been shown to enhance neurite outgrowth and survival of different populations of cultured neurons [175, 183]. Relevant to this review, it also has an important role in neurogenesis. As described above, in the adult SVZ and dentate gyrus, EGF regulates neural precursor cell proliferation [37]. The importance of this role is evident when, in response to brain injury, there is an expansion of neural stem cell numbers in the SVZ as a result of an increased responsiveness to EGF due to EGFR upregulation [184]. Important for SOCS2 interaction, EGF also activates STAT5, a process involving the Src tyrosine kinase [185-187]. Overexpression of SOCS2 in PC12 cells inhibited this EGF induced STAT5 phosphorylation [176]. The EGFR was also constitutively phosphorylated at the Src binding site, Tyr^{845}, in SOCS2 overexpressing PC12 cells. It was therefore proposed that SOCS2 competitively bound to Tyr^{845} and blocked its dephosphorylation by the phosphatase SHP2 to allow prolonged Src activation and enhancement of neurite outgrowth [176].

However, while SOCS2 regulated SVZ-derived neurogenesis in a GH dependent manner during development, in the adult SVZ it appears to regulate neurogenesis via regulation of erythropoietin signalling [188]. Further, the mechanism by which SOCS2 regulates adult hippocampal neurogenesis is different and does not appear to involve GH or erythropoietin, although Epo transiently enhanced SGZ NPC proliferation [189, 190]. Hippocampal neurogenesis was studied under control and voluntary exercise conditions (to enhance basal hippocampal neurogenesis) in wildtype, SOCS2Tg and $GHR^{-/-}$ mice. Mice of all 3 genotypes had similar basal levels of neurogenesis and equivalently increased neurogenesis in response to exercise at early timepoints (8 days) aimed at measuring extent of NPC proliferation. However, at later timepoints (35 days) aimed at examining newborn neuron survival, there was a 50% increase in the survival of adult hippocampal neurons in SOCS2Tg mice, under basal conditions and following voluntary exercise. Additionally, SOCS2Tg mice performed better than wildtype animals in the Morris Water Maze which probes hippocampal-dependent cognition [190]. This was an exciting result, as it identified SOCS2 as a potential therapeutic target that could enhance the survival of newly born neurons following brain injury. However, given that GHR-/- mice showed no differences in adult hippocampal neurogenesis compared to wildtype, the mechanism by which SOCS2 promotes survival in this case remains to be determined. One possible explanation for this increase in neuronal survival in SOCS2Tg mice may be that the enhanced neurite outgrowth observed in SOCS2Tg neurons may aid functional integration into existing circuitry and the consequent maturation and survival of neurons.

7. Roles of other SOCS proteins in the CNS

Other SOCS proteins also have roles in the modulation of signalling in the adult CNS. Other than SOCS2, SOCS3 is the best functionally characterised SOCS protein thus far. SOCS3 plays a role in the regulation of neural stem cell fate. Its overexpression in neural stem cells has been shown to inhibit astrogliogenesis and promote neurogenesis through the inhibition of STAT3 transcriptional activity [156]. More recently, SOCS6 involvement in neuronal differentiation was also established. Exogenous IGF1 was found to enhance neurite outgrowth and dendritic branching of neural stem cells through the induction of SOCS6 expression. The same phenotype was produced independently of IGF-1 by SOCS6 overexpression alone. Similar to SOCS2, SOCS6 is activated through the JAK2/STAT5 pathway, however, in this case it is activated through signalling via the IGF receptor. Activated STAT5 induces SOCS6 expression, which goes on to inhibit STAT5 mediated signalling following the classic negative feedback loop [191]. SOCS7 also plays a major role in the brain with SOCS7 null mice exhibiting severe hydrocephalus in early adulthood [192]. While the mechanism by which this occurs has not been elucidated, given the close relationship of ependymal cells and the ventricular space to NPCs in the SVZ, it is tempting to speculate that SOCS7 may also regulate adult NPC biology.

8. SOCS proteins and CNS injury

SOCS2, SOCS3 and SOCS6 all seem to have potential for use as therapeutic targets involving regulation of NPCs following CNS injury. As described earlier, SOCS2 overexpression increases the survival of newly born neurons in the adult brain under basal, physiological conditions. It would therefore be very interesting to look at the effects of SOCS2 overexpression under injury conditions in order to determine whether this phenotype would aid in functional recovery. Similarly, neurogenesis in an SOCS6 overexpressing system under basal and injury conditions should be examined. SOCS3 does not appear to affect neurogenesis *per se* but instead negatively regulates the proliferative and self-renewal effects of LIF on neural precursor cells [193].

SOCS3 has been studied the most extensively under various neural injury conditions, usually in concert with effects on neuroinflammation and astrocytes [194-196]. SOCS3 expression is induced or upregulated in various brain regions including hippocampus and lateral ventricles in response to CNTF administration [197], ischemic stroke [198, 199] and seizure, which also showed transient downregulation of hippocampal SOCS2 expression but no upregulation of SOCS1 [200]. Conversely, after transient forebrain ischemia, SOCS2 expression was upregulated in the hippocampus, not only in astrocytes but also a subset of nestin positive NPCs [201].

Expression of SOCS molecules following CNS damage has functional consequences. It was proposed that a major contributor to the poor axonal regeneration after injury was a compromised responsiveness to injury-induced growth factors and cytokines [202]. For example, it was suggested that the transient neuroprotective effect of CNTF on injured neurons was due to CNTF induced negative regulation of cytokine signalling by upregulation of SOCS proteins. Use of a cyclic AMP analogue as an inhibitor of SOCS expression enhanced CNTF induced signalling [203], identifying a new route through which the outcome of neurotrauma treatments may be improved. Whether such an approach will also regulate and potentiate effects of cytokines on NPCs remains to be determined. Further, SOCS3 deletion resulted in an enhancement of axonal regeneration in retinal ganglion cells post optic nerve injury in a mouse model, by lifting its inhibitory effects on JAK-STAT signalling [202]. Similarly, PTEN deletion enhanced axon regrowth post injury [204]. PTEN is a negative regulator of signalling via the mammalian target of rapamycin (mTOR) which can be activated through a number of means, one of which being the PI-3K/Akt pathway [205]. Interestingly, much more robust axonal regrowth is achieved upon a simultaneous deletion of PTEN and SOCS3 through a synergistic activation of mTOR and STAT3 signalling pathways [206]. SOCS3 also inhibits the beneficial effects of LIF-mediated oligodendrocyte survival following demyelination, with enhanced STAT3 activation and survival of oligodendrocytes from SOCS3 null mice [207].

Thus, it is apparent that there are many aspects to signalling in the processes of adult neurogenesis. The JAK-STAT signalling pathway is one important player, although it is apparent that SOCS proteins can regulate pathways other than JAK/STAT in a cell type dependent manner. The regulation of JAK-STAT signalling by SOCS proteins has enhanced our understanding of the mechanisms of adult neuro- and astrogliogenesis under basal and injury conditions and has opened avenues into the search for potential therapeutic targets for CNS repair.

Acknowledgments

We acknowledge support from Stem Cells Australia and A.M.T. is supported by an NH&MRC Research Fellowship (#628344).

Author details

Harleen S. Basrai, Kimberly J. Christie and Ann M. Turnley*

*Address all correspondence to: turnley@unimelb.edu.au

Centre for Neuroscience Research, Department of Anatomy and Neuroscience, The University of Melbourne, Victoria, Australia

References

[1] Reynolds BA, Tetzlaff W, Weiss S. A multipotent EGF-responsive striatal embryonic progenitor cell produces neurons and astrocytes. J Neurosci. 1992;12(11) 4565-74.

[2] Reynolds BA, Weiss S. Generation of neurons and astrocytes from isolated cells of the adult mammalian central nervous system. Science. 1992;255(5052) 1707-10.

[3] Richards LJ, Kilpatrick TJ, Bartlett PF. De novo generation of neuronal cells from the adult mouse brain. Proc Natl Acad Sci U S A. 1992;89(18) 8591-5.

[4] Freund TF, Buzsaki G. Interneurons of the hippocampus. Hippocampus. 1996;6(4) 347-470.

[5] Doetsch F, Caille I, Lim DA, Garcia-Verdugo JM, Alvarez-Buylla A. Subventricular zone astrocytes are neural stem cells in the adult mammalian brain. Cell. 1999;97(6) 703-16.

[6] Lois C, Alvarez-Buylla A. Long-distance neuronal migration in the adult mammalian brain. Science. 1994;264(5162) 1145-8.

[7] Luskin MB. Restricted proliferation and migration of postnatally generated neurons derived from the forebrain subventricular zone. Neuron. 1993;11(1) 173-89.

[8] Lie DC, Colamarino SA, Song HJ, Desire L, Mira H, Consiglio A, et al. Wnt signalling regulates adult hippocampal neurogenesis. Nature. 2005;437(7063) 1370-5.

[9] Wexler EM, Paucer A, Kornblum HI, Palmer TD, Geschwind DH. Endogenous Wnt signaling maintains neural progenitor cell potency. Stem Cells. 2009;27(5) 1130-41.

[10] Han YG, Spassky N, Romaguera-Ros M, Garcia-Verdugo JM, Aguilar A, Schneider-Maunoury S, et al. Hedgehog signaling and primary cilia are required for the formation of adult neural stem cells. Nat Neurosci. 2008;11(3) 277-84.

[11] Balordi F, Fishell G. Hedgehog signaling in the subventricular zone is required for both the maintenance of stem cells and the migration of newborn neurons. J Neurosci. 2007;27(22) 5936-47.

[12] Imayoshi I, Sakamoto M, Yamaguchi M, Mori K, Kageyama R. Essential roles of Notch signaling in maintenance of neural stem cells in developing and adult brains. J Neurosci. 2010;30(9) 3489-98.

[13] Cavallaro M, Mariani J, Lancini C, Latorre E, Caccia R, Gullo F, et al. Impaired generation of mature neurons by neural stem cells from hypomorphic Sox2 mutants. Development. 2008;135(3) 541-57.

[14] Cheng LC, Pastrana E, Tavazoie M, Doetsch F. miR-124 regulates adult neurogenesis in the subventricular zone stem cell niche. Nat Neurosci. 2009;12(4) 399-408.

[15] Karalay O, Doberauer K, Vadodaria KC, Knobloch M, Berti L, Miquelajauregui A, et al. Prospero-related homeobox 1 gene (Prox1) is regulated by canonical Wnt signal-

ing and has a stage-specific role in adult hippocampal neurogenesis. Proc Natl Acad Sci U S A. 2011;108(14) 5807-12.

[16] Haslinger A, Schwarz TJ, Covic M, Chichung Lie D. Expression of Sox11 in adult neurogenic niches suggests a stage-specific role in adult neurogenesis. Eur J Neurosci. 2009;29(11) 2103-14.

[17] Hevner RF, Hodge RD, Daza RA, Englund C. Transcription factors in glutamatergic neurogenesis: conserved programs in neocortex, cerebellum, and adult hippocampus. Neurosci Res. 2006;55(3) 223-33.

[18] Lavado A, Lagutin OV, Chow LM, Baker SJ, Oliver G. Prox1 is required for granule cell maturation and intermediate progenitor maintenance during brain neurogenesis. PLoS Biol. 2010;8(8).

[19] Wang TW, Stromberg GP, Whitney JT, Brower NW, Klymkowsky MW, Parent JM. Sox3 expression identifies neural progenitors in persistent neonatal and adult mouse forebrain germinative zones. J Comp Neurol. 2006;497(1) 88-100.

[20] Basak O, Giachino C, Fiorini E, Macdonald HR, Taylor V. Neurogenic subventricular zone stem/progenitor cells are Notch1-dependent in their active but not quiescent state. J Neurosci. 2012;32(16) 5654-66.

[21] Bonaguidi MA, McGuire T, Hu M, Kan L, Samanta J, Kessler JA. LIF and BMP signaling generate separate and discrete types of GFAP-expressing cells. Development. 2005;132(24) 5503-14.

[22] Lim DA, Tramontin AD, Trevejo JM, Herrera DG, Garcia-Verdugo JM, Alvarez-Buylla A. Noggin antagonizes BMP signaling to create a niche for adult neurogenesis. Neuron. 2000;28(3) 713-26.

[23] Ueki T, Tanaka M, Yamashita K, Mikawa S, Qiu Z, Maragakis NJ, et al. A novel secretory factor, Neurogenesin-1, provides neurogenic environmental cues for neural stem cells in the adult hippocampus. J Neurosci. 2003;23(37) 11732-40.

[24] Mira H, Andreu Z, Suh H, Lie DC, Jessberger S, Consiglio A, et al. Signaling through BMPR-IA regulates quiescence and long-term activity of neural stem cells in the adult hippocampus. Cell Stem Cell. 2010;7(1) 78-89.

[25] Guo W, Zhang L, Christopher DM, Teng ZQ, Fausett SR, Liu C, et al. RNA-binding protein FXR2 regulates adult hippocampal neurogenesis by reducing Noggin expression. Neuron. 2011;70(5) 924-38.

[26] Fernando RN, Eleuteri B, Abdelhady S, Nussenzweig A, Andang M, Ernfors P. Cell cycle restriction by histone H2AX limits proliferation of adult neural stem cells. Proc Natl Acad Sci U S A. 2011;108(14) 5837-42.

[27] Kim EJ, Leung CT, Reed RR, Johnson JE. In vivo analysis of Ascl1 defined progenitors reveals distinct developmental dynamics during adult neurogenesis and gliogenesis. J Neurosci. 2007;27(47) 12764-74.

[28] Brill MS, Ninkovic J, Winpenny E, Hodge RD, Ozen I, Yang R, et al. Adult generation of glutamatergic olfactory bulb interneurons. Nat Neurosci. 2009;12(12) 1524-33.

[29] Li X, Sun C, Lin C, Ma T, Madhavan MC, Campbell K, et al. The transcription factor Sp8 is required for the production of parvalbumin-expressing interneurons in the olfactory bulb. J Neurosci. 2011;31(23) 8450-5.

[30] Ozen I, Galichet C, Watts C, Parras C, Guillemot F, Raineteau O. Proliferating neuronal progenitors in the postnatal hippocampus transiently express the proneural gene Ngn2. Eur J Neurosci. 2007;25(9) 2591-603.

[31] Kim EJ, Ables JL, Dickel LK, Eisch AJ, Johnson JE. Ascl1 (Mash1) defines cells with long-term neurogenic potential in subgranular and subventricular zones in adult mouse brain. PLoS One. 2011;6(3) e18472.

[32] Jessberger S, Toni N, Clemenson GD, Jr., Ray J, Gage FH. Directed differentiation of hippocampal stem/progenitor cells in the adult brain. Nat Neurosci. 2008;11(8) 888-93.

[33] Gonzalez-Perez O, Romero-Rodriguez R, Soriano-Navarro M, Garcia-Verdugo JM, Alvarez-Buylla A. Epidermal growth factor induces the progeny of subventricular zone type B cells to migrate and differentiate into oligodendrocytes. Stem Cells. 2009;27(8) 2032-43.

[34] Craig CG, Tropepe V, Morshead CM, Reynolds BA, Weiss S, van der Kooy D. In vivo growth factor expansion of endogenous subependymal neural precursor cell populations in the adult mouse brain. J Neurosci. 1996;16(8) 2649-58.

[35] Wittko IM, Schanzer A, Kuzmichev A, Schneider FT, Shibuya M, Raab S, et al. VEGFR-1 regulates adult olfactory bulb neurogenesis and migration of neural progenitors in the rostral migratory stream in vivo. J Neurosci. 2009;29(27) 8704-14.

[36] Calvo CF, Fontaine RH, Soueid J, Tammela T, Makinen T, Alfaro-Cervello C, et al. Vascular endothelial growth factor receptor 3 directly regulates murine neurogenesis. Genes Dev. 2011;25(8) 831-44.

[37] Kuhn HG, Winkler J, Kempermann G, Thal LJ, Gage FH. Epidermal growth factor and fibroblast growth factor-2 have different effects on neural progenitors in the adult rat brain. J Neurosci. 1997;17(15) 5820-9.

[38] Jin K, Zhu Y, Sun Y, Mao XO, Xie L, Greenberg DA. Vascular endothelial growth factor (VEGF) stimulates neurogenesis in vitro and in vivo. Proc Natl Acad Sci U S A. 2002;99(18) 11946-50.

[39] Zhao M, Li D, Shimazu K, Zhou YX, Lu B, Deng CX. Fibroblast growth factor receptor-1 is required for long-term potentiation, memory consolidation, and neurogenesis. Biol Psychiatry. 2007;62(5) 381-90.

[40] Jia C, Cussen AR, Hegg CC. ATP differentially upregulates fibroblast growth factor 2 and transforming growth factor alpha in neonatal and adult mice: effect on neuroproliferation. Neuroscience. 2011;177 335-46.

[41] Suyama S, Sunabori T, Kanki H, Sawamoto K, Gachet C, Koizumi S, et al. Purinergic Signaling Promotes Proliferation of Adult Mouse Subventricular Zone Cells. J Neurosci. 2012;32(27) 9238-47.

[42] Mahar I, Tan S, Davoli MA, Dominguez-Lopez S, Qiang C, Rachalski A, et al. Subchronic peripheral neuregulin-1 increases ventral hippocampal neurogenesis and induces antidepressant-like effects. PLoS One. 2011;6(10) e26610.

[43] McLenachan S, Lum MG, Waters MJ, Turnley AM. Growth hormone promotes proliferation of adult neurosphere cultures. Growth Horm IGF Res. 2009;19(3) 212-8.

[44] Amiri A, Cho W, Zhou J, Birnbaum SG, Sinton CM, McKay RM, et al. Pten deletion in adult hippocampal neural stem/progenitor cells causes cellular abnormalities and alters neurogenesis. J Neurosci. 2012;32(17) 5880-90.

[45] Bracko O, Singer T, Aigner S, Knobloch M, Winner B, Ray J, et al. Gene expression profiling of neural stem cells and their neuronal progeny reveals IGF2 as a regulator of adult hippocampal neurogenesis. J Neurosci. 2012;32(10) 3376-87.

[46] Turnley AM, Bartlett PF. Cytokines that signal through the leukemia inhibitory factor receptor-beta complex in the nervous system. J Neurochem. 2000;74(3) 889-99.

[47] Heinrich PC, Behrmann I, Haan S, Hermanns HM, Muller-Newen G, Schaper F. Principles of interleukin (IL)-6-type cytokine signalling and its regulation. Biochem J. 2003;374(Pt 1) 1-20.

[48] Kamimura D, Ishihara K, Hirano T. IL-6 signal transduction and its physiological roles: the signal orchestration model. Rev Physiol Biochem Pharmacol. 2003;149 1-38.

[49] Ernst M, Jenkins BJ. Acquiring signalling specificity from the cytokine receptor gp130. Trends Genet. 2004;20(1) 23-32.

[50] Muller S, Chakrapani BP, Schwegler H, Hofmann HD, Kirsch M. Neurogenesis in the dentate gyrus depends on ciliary neurotrophic factor and signal transducer and activator of transcription 3 signaling. Stem Cells. 2009;27(2) 431-41.

[51] Pan YW, Chan GC, Kuo CT, Storm DR, Xia Z. Inhibition of adult neurogenesis by inducible and targeted deletion of ERK5 mitogen-activated protein kinase specifically in adult neurogenic regions impairs contextual fear extinction and remote fear memory. J Neurosci. 2012;32(19) 6444-55.

[52] Pan YW, Zou J, Wang W, Sakagami H, Garelick MG, Abel G, et al. Inducible and Conditional Deletion of Extracellular Signal-regulated Kinase 5 Disrupts Adult Hippocampal Neurogenesis. J Biol Chem. 2012;287(28) 23306-17.

[53] Gadadhar A, Marr R, Lazarov O. Presenilin-1 regulates neural progenitor cell differentiation in the adult brain. J Neurosci. 2011;31(7) 2615-23.

[54] Lum M, Croze E, Wagner C, McLenachan S, Mitrovic B, Turnley AM. Inhibition of neurosphere proliferation by IFNgamma but not IFNbeta is coupled to neuronal differentiation. J Neuroimmunol. 2009;206(1-2) 32-8.

[55] Wong G, Goldshmit Y, Turnley AM. Interferon-gamma but not TNF alpha promotes neuronal differentiation and neurite outgrowth of murine adult neural stem cells. Exp Neurol. 2004;187(1) 171-7.

[56] Leong SY, Turnley AM. Regulation of adult neural precursor cell migration. Neurochem Int. 2011;59(3) 382-93.

[57] Hurtado-Chong A, Yusta-Boyo MJ, Vergano-Vera E, Bulfone A, de Pablo F, Vicario-Abejon C. IGF-I promotes neuronal migration and positioning in the olfactory bulb and the exit of neuroblasts from the subventricular zone. Eur J Neurosci. 2009;30(5) 742-55.

[58] Conover JC, Doetsch F, Garcia-Verdugo JM, Gale NW, Yancopoulos GD, Alvarez-Buylla A. Disruption of Eph/ephrin signaling affects migration and proliferation in the adult subventricular zone. Nat Neurosci. 2000;3(11) 1091-7.

[59] Oudin MJ, Gajendra S, Williams G, Hobbs C, Lalli G, Doherty P. Endocannabinoids regulate the migration of subventricular zone-derived neuroblasts in the postnatal brain. J Neurosci. 2011;31(11) 4000-11.

[60] Oudin MJ, Hobbs C, Doherty P. DAGL-dependent endocannabinoid signalling: roles in axonal pathfinding, synaptic plasticity and adult neurogenesis. Eur J Neurosci. 2011;34(10) 1634-46.

[61] Cremer H, Lange R, Christoph A, Plomann M, Vopper G, Roes J, et al. Inactivation of the N-CAM gene in mice results in size reduction of the olfactory bulb and deficits in spatial learning. Nature. 1994;367(6462) 455-9.

[62] Hu H, Tomasiewicz H, Magnuson T, Rutishauser U. The role of polysialic acid in migration of olfactory bulb interneuron precursors in the subventricular zone. Neuron. 1996;16(4) 735-43.

[63] Chazal G, Durbec P, Jankovski A, Rougon G, Cremer H. Consequences of neural cell adhesion molecule deficiency on cell migration in the rostral migratory stream of the mouse. J Neurosci. 2000;20(4) 1446-57.

[64] Wu W, Wong K, Chen J, Jiang Z, Dupuis S, Wu JY, et al. Directional guidance of neuronal migration in the olfactory system by the protein Slit. Nature. 1999;400(6742) 331-6.

[65] Jacques TS, Relvas JB, Nishimura S, Pytela R, Edwards GM, Streuli CH, et al. Neural precursor cell chain migration and division are regulated through different beta1 integrins. Development. 1998;125(16) 3167-77.

[66] Murase S, Horwitz AF. Deleted in colorectal carcinoma and differentially expressed integrins mediate the directional migration of neural precursors in the rostral migratory stream. J Neurosci. 2002;22(9) 3568-79.

[67] Leong SY, Faux CH, Turbic A, Dixon KJ, Turnley AM. The Rho kinase pathway regulates mouse adult neural precursor cell migration. Stem Cells. 2011;29(2) 332-43.

[68] Turbic A, Leong SY, Turnley AM. Chemokines and inflammatory mediators interact to regulate adult murine neural precursor cell proliferation, survival and differentiation. PLoS One. 2011;6(9) e25406.

[69] Namba T, Ming GL, Song H, Waga C, Enomoto A, Kaibuchi K, et al. NMDA receptor regulates migration of newly generated neurons in the adult hippocampus via Disrupted-In-Schizophrenia 1 (DISC1). J Neurochem. 2011;118(1) 34-44.

[70] Duan X, Chang JH, Ge S, Faulkner RL, Kim JY, Kitabatake Y, et al. Disrupted-In-Schizophrenia 1 regulates integration of newly generated neurons in the adult brain. Cell. 2007;130(6) 1146-58.

[71] Kim JY, Liu CY, Zhang F, Duan X, Wen Z, Song J, et al. Interplay between DISC1 and GABA signaling regulates neurogenesis in mice and risk for schizophrenia. Cell. 2012;148(5) 1051-64.

[72] Platel JC, Dave KA, Gordon V, Lacar B, Rubio ME, Bordey A. NMDA receptors activated by subventricular zone astrocytic glutamate are critical for neuroblast survival prior to entering a synaptic network. Neuron. 2010;65(6) 859-72.

[73] Ge S, Goh EL, Sailor KA, Kitabatake Y, Ming GL, Song H. GABA regulates synaptic integration of newly generated neurons in the adult brain. Nature. 2006;439(7076) 589-93.

[74] Saghatelyan A, Roux P, Migliore M, Rochefort C, Desmaisons D, Charneau P, et al. Activity-dependent adjustments of the inhibitory network in the olfactory bulb following early postnatal deprivation. Neuron. 2005;46(1) 103-16.

[75] Gascon E, Dayer AG, Sauvain MO, Potter G, Jenny B, De Roo M, et al. GABA regulates dendritic growth by stabilizing lamellipodia in newly generated interneurons of the olfactory bulb. J Neurosci. 2006;26(50) 12956-66.

[76] Duveau V, Laustela S, Barth L, Gianolini F, Vogt KE, Keist R, et al. Spatiotemporal specificity of GABAA receptor-mediated regulation of adult hippocampal neurogenesis. Eur J Neurosci. 2011;34(3) 362-73.

[77] Burk K, Desoeuvre A, Boutin C, Smith MA, Kroger S, Bosio A, et al. Agrin-signaling is necessary for the integration of newly generated neurons in the adult olfactory bulb. J Neurosci. 2012;32(11) 3759-64.

[78] Kirschenbaum B, Goldman SA. Brain-derived neurotrophic factor promotes the survival of neurons arising from the adult rat forebrain subependymal zone. Proc Natl Acad Sci U S A. 1995;92(1) 210-4.

[79] Zigova T, Pencea V, Wiegand SJ, Luskin MB. Intraventricular administration of BDNF increases the number of newly generated neurons in the adult olfactory bulb. Mol Cell Neurosci. 1998;11(4) 234-45.

[80] Bath KG, Mandairon N, Jing D, Rajagopal R, Kapoor R, Chen ZY, et al. Variant brain-derived neurotrophic factor (Val66Met) alters adult olfactory bulb neurogenesis and spontaneous olfactory discrimination. J Neurosci. 2008;28(10) 2383-93.

[81] Bergami M, Rimondini R, Santi S, Blum R, Gotz M, Canossa M. Deletion of TrkB in adult progenitors alters newborn neuron integration into hippocampal circuits and increases anxiety-like behavior. Proc Natl Acad Sci U S A. 2008;105(40) 15570-5.

[82] Gao Z, Ure K, Ables JL, Lagace DC, Nave KA, Goebbels S, et al. Neurod1 is essential for the survival and maturation of adult-born neurons. Nat Neurosci. 2009;12(9) 1090-2.

[83] Kuwabara T, Hsieh J, Muotri A, Yeo G, Warashina M, Lie DC, et al. Wnt-mediated activation of NeuroD1 and retro-elements during adult neurogenesis. Nat Neurosci. 2009;12(9) 1097-105.

[84] Scobie KN, Hall BJ, Wilke SA, Klemenhagen KC, Fujii-Kuriyama Y, Ghosh A, et al. Kruppel-like factor 9 is necessary for late-phase neuronal maturation in the developing dentate gyrus and during adult hippocampal neurogenesis. J Neurosci. 2009;29(31) 9875-87.

[85] Doetsch F, Petreanu L, Caille I, Garcia-Verdugo JM, Alvarez-Buylla A. EGF converts transit-amplifying neurogenic precursors in the adult brain into multipotent stem cells. Neuron. 2002;36(6) 1021-34.

[86] Brill MS, Snapyan M, Wohlfrom H, Ninkovic J, Jawerka M, Mastick GS, et al. A dlx2- and pax6-dependent transcriptional code for periglomerular neuron specification in the adult olfactory bulb. J Neurosci. 2008;28(25) 6439-52.

[87] Hack MA, Saghatelyan A, de Chevigny A, Pfeifer A, Ashery-Padan R, Lledo PM, et al. Neuronal fate determinants of adult olfactory bulb neurogenesis. Nat Neurosci. 2005;8(7) 865-72.

[88] Magill ST, Cambronne XA, Luikart BW, Lioy DT, Leighton BH, Westbrook GL, et al. microRNA-132 regulates dendritic growth and arborization of newborn neurons in the adult hippocampus. Proc Natl Acad Sci U S A. 2010;107(47) 20382-7.

[89] Veyrac A, Reibel S, Sacquet J, Mutin M, Camdessanche JP, Kolattukudy P, et al. CRMP5 regulates generation and survival of newborn neurons in olfactory and hippocampal neurogenic areas of the adult mouse brain. PLoS One. 2011;6(10) e23721.

[90] Arvidsson A, Collin T, Kirik D, Kokaia Z, Lindvall O. Neuronal replacement from endogenous precursors in the adult brain after stroke. Nat Med. 2002;8(9) 963-70.

[91] Rice AC, Khaldi A, Harvey HB, Salman NJ, White F, Fillmore H, et al. Proliferation and neuronal differentiation of mitotically active cells following traumatic brain injury. Exp Neurol. 2003;183(2) 406-17.

[92] Parent JM. Adult neurogenesis in the intact and epileptic dentate gyrus. Prog Brain Res. 2007;163 529-40.

[93] Ramaswamy S, Goings GE, Soderstrom KE, Szele FG, Kozlowski DA. Cellular proliferation and migration following a controlled cortical impact in the mouse. Brain Res. 2005;1053(1-2) 38-53.

[94] Carbonell WS, Maris DO, McCall T, Grady MS. Adaptation of the fluid percussion injury model to the mouse. J Neurotrauma. 1998;15(3) 217-29.

[95] Chirumamilla S, Sun D, Bullock MR, Colello RJ. Traumatic brain injury induced cell proliferation in the adult mammalian central nervous system. J Neurotrauma. 2002;19(6) 693-703.

[96] Chen XH, Iwata A, Nonaka M, Browne KD, Smith DH. Neurogenesis and glial proliferation persist for at least one year in the subventricular zone following brain trauma in rats. J Neurotrauma. 2003;20(7) 623-31.

[97] Szele FG, Chesselet MF. Cortical lesions induce an increase in cell number and PSA-NCAM expression in the subventricular zone of adult rats. J Comp Neurol. 1996;368(3) 439-54.

[98] Blizzard CA, Chuckowree JA, King AE, Hosie KA, McCormack GH, Chapman JA, et al. Focal damage to the adult rat neocortex induces wound healing accompanied by axonal sprouting and dendritic structural plasticity. Cereb Cortex. 2011;21(2) 281-91.

[99] Goings GE, Wibisono BL, Szele FG. Cerebral cortex lesions decrease the number of bromodeoxyuridine-positive subventricular zone cells in mice. Neurosci Lett. 2002;329(2) 161-4.

[100] Dempsey RJ, Kalluri HS. Ischemia-induced neurogenesis: role of growth factors. Neurosurg Clin N Am. 2007;18(1) 183-90, xi.

[101] Watanabe T, Okuda Y, Nonoguchi N, Zhao MZ, Kajimoto Y, Furutama D, et al. Postischemic intraventricular administration of FGF-2 expressing adenoviral vectors improves neurologic outcome and reduces infarct volume after transient focal cerebral ischemia in rats. J Cereb Blood Flow Metab. 2004;24(11) 1205-13.

[102] Baldauf K, Reymann KG. Influence of EGF/bFGF treatment on proliferation, early neurogenesis and infarct volume after transient focal ischemia. Brain Res. 2005;1056(2) 158-67.

[103] Tureyen K, Vemuganti R, Bowen KK, Sailor KA, Dempsey RJ. EGF and FGF-2 infusion increases post-ischemic neural progenitor cell proliferation in the adult rat brain. Neurosurgery. 2005;57(6) 1254-63; discussion -63.

[104] Schabitz WR, Steigleder T, Cooper-Kuhn CM, Schwab S, Sommer C, Schneider A, et al. Intravenous brain-derived neurotrophic factor enhances poststroke sensorimotor recovery and stimulates neurogenesis. Stroke. 2007;38(7) 2165-72.

[105] Lu KT, Sun CL, Wo PY, Yen HH, Tang TH, Ng MC, et al. Hippocampal neurogenesis after traumatic brain injury is mediated by vascular endothelial growth factor receptor-2 and the Raf/MEK/ERK cascade. J Neurotrauma. 2011;28(3) 441-50.

[106] Wang X, Mao X, Xie L, Greenberg DA, Jin K. Involvement of Notch1 signaling in neurogenesis in the subventricular zone of normal and ischemic rat brain in vivo. J Cereb Blood Flow Metab. 2009;29(10) 1644-54.

[107] Morris DC, Zhang ZG, Wang Y, Zhang RL, Gregg S, Liu XS, et al. Wnt expression in the adult rat subventricular zone after stroke. Neurosci Lett. 2007;418(2) 170-4.

[108] Boneva NB, Yamashima T. New insights into "GPR40-CREB interaction in adult neurogenesis" specific for primates. Hippocampus. 2012;22(4) 896-905.

[109] Jin K, Sun Y, Xie L, Peel A, Mao XO, Batteur S, et al. Directed migration of neuronal precursors into the ischemic cerebral cortex and striatum. Mol Cell Neurosci. 2003;24(1) 171-89.

[110] Sundholm-Peters NL, Yang HK, Goings GE, Walker AS, Szele FG. Subventricular zone neuroblasts emigrate toward cortical lesions. J Neuropathol Exp Neurol. 2005;64(12) 1089-100.

[111] Ohab JJ, Fleming S, Blesch A, Carmichael ST. A neurovascular niche for neurogenesis after stroke. J Neurosci. 2006;26(50) 13007-16.

[112] Yamashita T, Ninomiya M, Hernandez Acosta P, Garcia-Verdugo JM, Sunabori T, Sakaguchi M, et al. Subventricular zone-derived neuroblasts migrate and differentiate into mature neurons in the post-stroke adult striatum. J Neurosci. 2006;26(24) 6627-36.

[113] Cayre M, Canoll P, Goldman JE. Cell migration in the normal and pathological postnatal mammalian brain. Prog Neurobiol. 2009;88(1) 41-63.

[114] Young CC, Brooks KJ, Buchan AM, Szele FG. Cellular and molecular determinants of stroke-induced changes in subventricular zone cell migration. Antioxid Redox Signal. 2011;14(10) 1877-88.

[115] Goings GE, Sahni V, Szele FG. Migration patterns of subventricular zone cells in adult mice change after cerebral cortex injury. Brain Res. 2004;996(2) 213-26.

[116] Imitola J, Raddassi K, Park KI, Mueller FJ, Nieto M, Teng YD, et al. Directed migration of neural stem cells to sites of CNS injury by the stromal cell-derived factor 1alpha/CXC chemokine receptor 4 pathway. Proc Natl Acad Sci U S A. 2004;101(52) 18117-22.

[117] Robin AM, Zhang ZG, Wang L, Zhang RL, Katakowski M, Zhang L, et al. Stromal cell-derived factor 1alpha mediates neural progenitor cell motility after focal cerebral ischemia. J Cereb Blood Flow Metab. 2006;26(1) 125-34.

[118] Parent JM, Valentin VV, Lowenstein DH. Prolonged seizures increase proliferating neuroblasts in the adult rat subventricular zone-olfactory bulb pathway. J Neurosci. 2002;22(8) 3174-88.

[119] Overstreet-Wadiche LS, Bromberg DA, Bensen AL, Westbrook GL. Seizures accelerate functional integration of adult-generated granule cells. J Neurosci. 2006;26(15) 4095-103.

[120] Parent JM, Kron MM. Neurogenesis and Epilepsy. 2012.

[121] Kreuzberg M, Kanov E, Timofeev O, Schwaninger M, Monyer H, Khodosevich K. Increased subventricular zone-derived cortical neurogenesis after ischemic lesion. Exp Neurol. 2010;226(1) 90-9.

[122] Kernie SG, Erwin TM, Parada LF. Brain remodeling due to neuronal and astrocytic proliferation after controlled cortical injury in mice. J Neurosci Res. 2001;66(3) 317-26.

[123] Shear DA, Tate MC, Archer DR, Hoffman SW, Hulce VD, Laplaca MC, et al. Neural progenitor cell transplants promote long-term functional recovery after traumatic brain injury. Brain Res. 2004;1026(1) 11-22.

[124] Jablonska B, Aguirre A, Raymond M, Szabo G, Kitabatake Y, Sailor KA, et al. Chordin-induced lineage plasticity of adult SVZ neuroblasts after demyelination. Nat Neurosci. 2010;13(5) 541-50.

[125] Buffo A, Vosko MR, Erturk D, Hamann GF, Jucker M, Rowitch D, et al. Expression pattern of the transcription factor Olig2 in response to brain injuries: implications for neuronal repair. Proc Natl Acad Sci U S A. 2005;102(50) 18183-8.

[126] Tonchev AB, Yamashima T. Differential neurogenic potential of progenitor cells in dentate gyrus and CA1 sector of the postischemic adult monkey hippocampus. Exp Neurol. 2006;198(1) 101-13.

[127] Zhang RL, Chopp M, Roberts C, Jia L, Wei M, Lu M, et al. Ascl1 lineage cells contribute to ischemia-induced neurogenesis and oligodendrogenesis. J Cereb Blood Flow Metab. 2011;31(2) 614-25.

[128] Cai W, Carlson SW, Brelsfoard JM, Mannon CE, Moncman CL, Saatman KE, et al. Rit GTPase Signaling Promotes Immature Hippocampal Neuronal Survival. J Neurosci. 2012;32(29) 9887-97.

[129] Liu XS, Chopp M, Zhang RL, Tao T, Wang XL, Kassis H, et al. MicroRNA profiling in subventricular zone after stroke: MiR-124a regulates proliferation of neural progenitor cells through Notch signaling pathway. PLoS One. 2011;6(8) e23461.

[130] Dias TB, Yang YJ, Ogai K, Becker T, Becker CG. Notch signaling controls generation of motor neurons in the lesioned spinal cord of adult zebrafish. J Neurosci. 2012;32(9) 3245-52.

[131] Shruster A, Ben-Zur T, Melamed E, Offen D. Wnt signaling enhances neurogenesis and improves neurological function after focal ischemic injury. PLoS One. 2012;7(7) e40843.

[132] Winner B, Kohl Z, Gage FH. Neurodegenerative disease and adult neurogenesis. Eur J Neurosci. 2011;33(6) 1139-51.

[133] Hardy J, Selkoe DJ. The amyloid hypothesis of Alzheimer's disease: progress and problems on the road to therapeutics. Science. 2002;297(5580) 353-6.

[134] Uchida Y, Nakano S, Gomi F, Takahashi H. Differential regulation of basic helix-loop-helix factors Mash1 and Olig2 by beta-amyloid accelerates both differentiation and death of cultured neural stem/progenitor cells. J Biol Chem. 2007;282(27) 19700-9.

[135] Waldau B, Shetty AK. Behavior of neural stem cells in the Alzheimer brain. Cell Mol Life Sci. 2008;65(15) 2372-84.

[136] Goedert M. Alpha-synuclein and neurodegenerative diseases. Nat Rev Neurosci. 2001;2(7) 492-501.

[137] Winner B, Lie DC, Rockenstein E, Aigner R, Aigner L, Masliah E, et al. Human wild-type alpha-synuclein impairs neurogenesis. J Neuropathol Exp Neurol. 2004;63(11) 1155-66.

[138] Crews L, Mizuno H, Desplats P, Rockenstein E, Adame A, Patrick C, et al. Alpha-synuclein alters Notch-1 expression and neurogenesis in mouse embryonic stem cells and in the hippocampus of transgenic mice. J Neurosci. 2008;28(16) 4250-60.

[139] Saha B, Jaber M, Gaillard A. Potentials of endogenous neural stem cells in cortical repair. Front Cell Neurosci. 2012;6 14.

[140] Jing X, Miwa H, Sawada T, Nakanishi I, Kondo T, Miyajima M, et al. Ephrin-A1-mediated dopaminergic neurogenesis and angiogenesis in a rat model of Parkinson's disease. PLoS One. 2012;7(2) e32019.

[141] Winner B, Couillard-Despres S, Geyer M, Aigner R, Bogdahn U, Aigner L, et al. Dopaminergic lesion enhances growth factor-induced striatal neuroblast migration. J Neuropathol Exp Neurol. 2008;67(2) 105-16.

[142] Berg DA, Kirkham M, Wang H, Frisen J, Simon A. Dopamine controls neurogenesis in the adult salamander midbrain in homeostasis and during regeneration of dopamine neurons. Cell Stem Cell. 2011;8(4) 426-33.

[143] Caiazzo M, Dell'Anno MT, Dvoretskova E, Lazarevic D, Taverna S, Leo D, et al. Direct generation of functional dopaminergic neurons from mouse and human fibroblasts. Nature. 2011;476(7359) 224-7.

[144] Lee HS, Bae EJ, Yi SH, Shim JW, Jo AY, Kang JS, et al. Foxa2 and Nurr1 synergistically yield A9 nigral dopamine neurons exhibiting improved differentiation, function, and cell survival. Stem Cells. 2010;28(3) 501-12.

[145] Kandasamy M, Couillard-Despres S, Raber KA, Stephan M, Lehner B, Winner B, et al. Stem cell quiescence in the hippocampal neurogenic niche is associated with elevated transforming growth factor-beta signaling in an animal model of Huntington disease. J Neuropathol Exp Neurol. 2010;69(7) 717-28.

[146] Stark G, Darnell J. The JAK-STAT Pathway at Twenty. Immunity. 2012;36(4) 503-14.

[147] Davis S, Aldrich TH, Valenzuela DM, Wong V, Furth ME, Squinto SP, et al. The receptor for ciliary neurotrophic factor. Science. 1991;253(5015) 59-63.

[148] Boulanger MJ, Garcia KC. Shared Cytokine Signaling Receptors: Structural Insights from the Gp130 System. In: Garcia KC, editor. Advances in Protein Chemistry: Academic Press; 2004. p. 107-46.

[149] Stahl N, Boulton TG, Farruggella T, Ip NY, Davis S, Witthuhn BA, et al. Association and Activation of Jak-Tyk Kinases by CNTF-LIF-OSM-IL-6 β Receptor Components. Science. 1994;263(5143) 92-5.

[150] Stahl N, Yancopoulos GD. The tripartite CNTF receptor complex: Activation and signaling involves components shared with other cytokines. Journal of Neurobiology. 1994;25(11) 1454-66.

[151] De-Fraja C, Conti L, Magrassi L, Govoni S, Cattaneo E. Members of the JAK/STAT proteins are expressed and regulated during development in the mammalian forebrain. Journal of Neuroscience Research. 1998;54(3) 320-30.

[152] Ihle JN. STATs: Signal Transducers and Activators of Transcription. Cell. 1996;84(3) 331-4.

[153] Bonni A, Sun Y, Nadal-Vicens M, Bhatt A, Frank DA, Rozovsky I, et al. Regulation of gliogenesis in the central nervous system by the JAK-STAT signaling pathway. Science. 1997;278(5337) 477-83.

[154] Ochiai W, Yanagisawa M, Takizawa T, Nakashima K, Taga T. Astrocyte differentiation of fetal neuroepithelial cells involving cardiotrophin-1-induced activation of STAT3. Cytokine. 2001;14(5) 264-71.

[155] Rajan P, McKay RDG. Multiple Routes to Astrocytic Differentiation in the CNS. The Journal of Neuroscience. 1998;18(10) 3620-9.

[156] Cao F, Hata R, Zhu P, Ma YJ, Tanaka J, Hanakawa Y, et al. Overexpression of SOCS3 inhibits astrogliogenesis and promotes maintenance of neural stem cells. J Neurochem. 2006;98(2) 459-70.

[157] Gu F, Hata R, Ma Y-J, Tanaka J, Mitsuda N, Kumon Y, et al. Suppression of Stat3 promotes neurogenesis in cultured neural stem cells. Journal of Neuroscience Research. 2005;81(2) 163-71.

[158] Fukuda S, Abematsu M, Mori H, Yanagisawa M, Kagawa T, Nakashima K, et al. Potentiation of astrogliogenesis by STAT3-mediated activation of bone morphogenetic protein-Smad signaling in neural stem cells. Mol Cell Biol. 2007;27(13) 4931-7.

[159] Okada S, Nakamura M, Katoh H, Miyao T, Shimazaki T, Ishii K, et al. Conditional ablation of Stat3 or Socs3 discloses a dual role for reactive astrocytes after spinal cord injury. Nat Med. 2006;12(7) 829-34.

[160] Kile B, Nicola N, Alexander W. Negative Regulators of Cytokine Signaling. International Journal of Hematology. 2001;73(3) 292-8.

[161] Larsen L, Röpke C. Suppressors of cytokine signalling: SOCS. APMIS. 2002;110(12) 833-44.

[162] Krebs DL, Hilton DJ. SOCS Proteins: Negative Regulators of Cytokine Signaling. STEM CELLS. 2001;19(5) 378-87.

[163] Kile BT, Schulman BA, Alexander WS, Nicola NA, Martin HME, Hilton DJ. The SOCS box: a tale of destruction and degradation. Trends in Biochemical Sciences. 2002;27(5) 235-41.

[164] Piessevaux J, Lavens D, Montoye T, Wauman J, Catteeuw D, Vandekerckhove J, et al. Functional Cross-modulation between SOCS Proteins Can Stimulate Cytokine Signaling. Journal of Biological Chemistry. 2006;281(44) 32953-66.

[165] Piessevaux J, Lavens D, Peelman F, Tavernier J. The many faces of the SOCS box. Cytokine Growth Factor Rev. 2008;19(5-6) 371-81.

[166] Bauer S. Cytokine Control of Adult Neural Stem Cells. Annals of the New York Academy of Sciences. 2009;1153(1) 48-56.

[167] Kahn MA, Huang CJ, Caruso A, Barresi V, Nazarian R, Condorelli DF, et al. Ciliary Neurotrophic Factor Activates JAK/Stat Signal Transduction Cascade and Induces Transcriptional Expression of Glial Fibrillary Acidic Protein in Glial Cells. Journal of Neurochemistry. 1997;68(4) 1413-23.

[168] Polizzotto MN, Bartlett PF, Turnley AM. Expression of "suppressor of cytokine signalling" (SOCS) genes in the developing and adult mouse nervous system. The Journal of Comparative Neurology. 2000;423(2) 348-58.

[169] Greenhalgh CJ, Metcalf D, Thaus AL, Corbin JE, Uren R, Morgan PO, et al. Biological Evidence That SOCS-2 Can Act Either as an Enhancer or Suppressor of Growth Hormone Signaling. Journal of Biological Chemistry. 2002;277(43) 40181-4.

[170] Metcalf D, Greenhalgh CJ, Viney E, Willson TA, Starr R, Nicola NA, et al. Gigantism in mice lacking suppressor of cytokine signalling-2. Nature. [10.1038/35016611]. 2000;405(6790) 1069-73.

[171] Turnley AM, Faux CH, Rietze RL, Coonan JR, Bartlett PF. Suppressor of cytokine signaling 2 regulates neuronal differentiation by inhibiting growth hormone signaling. Nat Neurosci. [10.1038/nn954]. 2002;5(11) 1155-62.

[172] Ransome MI, Goldshmit Y, Bartlett PF, Waters MJ, Turnley AM. Comparative analysis of CNS populations in knockout mice with altered growth hormone responsiveness. Eur J Neurosci. 2004;19(8) 2069-79.

[173] Ransome MI, Turnley AM. Analysis of neuronal subpopulations in mice over-expressing suppressor of cytokine signaling-2. Neuroscience. 2005;132(3) 673-87.

[174] Scott HJ, Stebbing MJ, Walters CE, McLenachan S, Ransome MI, Nichols NR, et al. Differential effects of SOCS2 on neuronal differentiation and morphology. Brain Research. 2006;1067(1) 138-45.

[175] Goldshmit Y, Greenhalgh CJ, Turnley AM. Suppressor of cytokine signalling-2 and epidermal growth factor regulate neurite outgrowth of cortical neurons. European Journal of Neuroscience. 2004;20(9) 2260-6.

[176] Goldshmit Y, Walters CE, Scott HJ, Greenhalgh CJ, Turnley AM. SOCS2 Induces Neurite Outgrowth by Regulation of Epidermal Growth Factor Receptor Activation. Journal of Biological Chemistry. 2004;279(16) 16349-55.

[177] Sun Y, Nadal-Vicens M, Misono S, Lin MZ, Zubiaga A, Hua X, et al. Neurogenin promotes neurogenesis and inhibits glial differentiation by independent mechanisms. Cell. 2001;104(3) 365-76.

[178] Turnley AM. Role of SOCS2 in growth hormone actions. Trends in Endocrinology and Metabolism. 2005;16(2) 53-8.

[179] Jegalian AG, Wu H. Regulation of Socs Gene Expression by the Proto-oncoprotein GFI-1B. Journal of Biological Chemistry. 2002;277(3) 2345-52.

[180] Brooks AJ, Wooh JW, Tunny KA, Waters MJ. Growth hormone receptor; mechanism of action. The International Journal of Biochemistry & Cell Biology. 2008;40(10) 1984-9.

[181] Zhu T, Goh ELK, Graichen R, Ling L, Lobie PE. Signal transduction via the growth hormone receptor. Cellular Signalling. 2001;13(9) 599-616.

[182] Ram PA, Waxman DJ. SOCS/CIS Protein Inhibition of Growth Hormone-stimulated STAT5 Signaling by Multiple Mechanisms. Journal of Biological Chemistry. 1999;274(50) 35553-61.

[183] Wong RWC, Guillaud L. The role of epidermal growth factor and its receptors in mammalian CNS. Cytokine & Growth Factor Reviews. 2004;15(2–3) 147-56.

[184] Alagappan D, Lazzarino DA, Felling RJ, Balan M, Kotenko SV, Levison SW. Brain injury expands the numbers of neural stem cells and progenitors in the SVZ by enhancing their responsiveness to EGF. ASN Neuro. 2009;1(2).

[185] Kloth MT, Laughlin KK, Biscardi JS, Boerner JL, Parsons SJ, Silva CM. STAT5b, a Mediator of Synergism between c-Src and the Epidermal Growth Factor Receptor. Journal of Biological Chemistry. 2003;278(3) 1671-9.

[186] Guren TK, Ødegård J, Abrahamsen H, Thoresen GH, Susa M, Andersson Y, et al. EGF receptor-mediated, c-Src-dependent, activation of Stat5b is downregulated in mitogenically responsive hepatocytes. Journal of Cellular Physiology. 2003;196(1) 113-23.

[187] Olayioye MA, Beuvink I, Horsch K, Daly JM, Hynes NE. ErbB Receptor-induced Activation of Stat Transcription Factors Is Mediated by Src Tyrosine Kinases. J Biol Chem. 1999;274(24) 17209-18.

[188] Wang L, Zhang Z, Zhang R, Hafner MS, Wong HK, Jiao Z, et al. Erythropoietin upregulates SOCS2 in neuronal progenitor cells derived from SVZ of adult rat. Neuroreport. 2004;15(8) 1225-9.

[189] Ransome MI, Turnley AM. Systemically delivered Erythropoietin transiently enhances adult hippocampal neurogenesis. J Neurochem. 2007;102(6) 1953-65.

[190] Ransome MI, Turnley AM. Growth hormone signaling and hippocampal neurogenesis: Insights from genetic models. Hippocampus. 2008;18(10) 1034-50.

[191] Gupta S, Mishra K, Surolia A, Banerjee K. Suppressor of Cytokine Signalling-6 Promotes Neurite Outgrowth via JAK2/STAT5-Mediated Signalling Pathway, Involving Negative Feedback Inhibition. PLoS ONE. 2011;6(11) e26674.

[192] Krebs DL, Metcalf D, Merson TD, Voss AK, Thomas T, Zhang JG, et al. Development of hydrocephalus in mice lacking SOCS7. Proc Natl Acad Sci U S A. 2004;101(43) 15446-51.

[193] Emery B, Merson TD, Snell C, Young KM, Ernst M, Kilpatrick TJ. SOCS3 negatively regulates LIF signaling in neural precursor cells. Mol Cell Neurosci. 2006;31(4) 739-47.

[194] Baker BJ, Akhtar LN, Benveniste EN. SOCS1 and SOCS3 in the control of CNS immunity. Trends Immunol. 2009;30(8) 392-400.

[195] Baker BJ, Qin H, Benveniste EN. Molecular basis of oncostatin M-induced SOCS-3 expression in astrocytes. Glia. 2008;56(11) 1250-62.

[196] Qin H, Niyongere SA, Lee SJ, Baker BJ, Benveniste EN. Expression and functional significance of SOCS-1 and SOCS-3 in astrocytes. J Immunol. 2008;181(5) 3167-76.

[197] Bjorbaek C, Elmquist JK, El-Haschimi K, Kelly J, Ahima RS, Hileman S, et al. Activation of SOCS-3 messenger ribonucleic acid in the hypothalamus by ciliary neurotrophic factor. Endocrinology. 1999;140(5) 2035-43.

[198] Choi JS, Shin YJ, Cha JH, Kim HY, Choi JY, Chun MH, et al. Induction of suppressor of cytokine signaling-3 in astrocytes of the rat hippocampus following transient forebrain ischemia. Neurosci Lett. 2008;441(3) 323-7.

[199] Dinapoli VA, Benkovic SA, Li X, Kelly KA, Miller DB, Rosen CL, et al. Age exaggerates proinflammatory cytokine signaling and truncates signal transducers and activa-

tors of transcription 3 signaling following ischemic stroke in the rat. Neuroscience. 2010;170(2) 633-44.

[200] Rosell DR, Akama KT, Nacher J, McEwen BS. Differential expression of suppressors of cytokine signaling-1, -2, and -3 in the rat hippocampus after seizure: implications for neuromodulation by gp130 cytokines. Neuroscience. 2003;122(2) 349-58.

[201] Choi JS, Shin YJ, Lee JY, Choi JY, Cha JH, Chun MH, et al. Enhanced expression of SOCS-2 in the rat hippocampus after transient forebrain ischemia. J Neurotrauma. 2009;26(11) 2097-106.

[202] Smith PD, Sun F, Park KK, Cai B, Wang C, Kuwako K, et al. SOCS3 deletion promotes optic nerve regeneration in vivo. Neuron. 2009;64(5) 617-23.

[203] Park KK, Hu Y, Muhling J, Pollett MA, Dallimore EJ, Turnley AM, et al. Cytokine-induced SOCS expression is inhibited by cAMP analogue: impact on regeneration in injured retina. Mol Cell Neurosci. 2009;41(3) 313-24.

[204] Park KK, Liu K, Hu Y, Smith PD, Wang C, Cai B, et al. Promoting Axon Regeneration in the Adult CNS by Modulation of the PTEN/mTOR Pathway. Science. 2008;322(5903) 963-6.

[205] Hoeffer CA, Klann E. mTOR signaling: At the crossroads of plasticity, memory and disease. Trends in Neurosciences. 2010;33(2) 67-75.

[206] Sun F, Park KK, Belin S, Wang D, Lu T, Chen G, et al. Sustained axon regeneration induced by co-deletion of PTEN and SOCS3. Nature. 2011;480(7377) 372-5.

[207] Emery B, Cate HS, Marriott M, Merson T, Binder MD, Snell C, et al. Suppressor of cytokine signaling 3 limits protection of leukemia inhibitory factor receptor signaling against central demyelination. Proc Natl Acad Sci U S A. 2006;103(20) 7859-64.

Chapter 10

Telencephalic Neurogenesis Versus Telencephalic Differentiation of Pluripotent Stem Cells

Roxana Nat, Galina Apostolova and Georg Dechant

Additional information is available at the end of the chapter

1. Introduction

The mammalian telencephalon, which comprises the cerebral cortex, olfactory bulb, hippocampus, basal ganglia (striatum and globus pallidum), and amygdala, is a highly complex and evolutionarily advanced brain structure. All higher brain functions including the integration and processing of sensory and motor information, the memory storage and retrieval, and the regulation of emotional and drive states take place at the telencephalic level. In humans, the telencephalon also governs the ability to make rational decisions, to plan for the future and to have the creative impulses [1].

At cellular level, the telencephalon is populated by a large diversity of neurons, including **glutamatergic** projection neurons, **GABA (γ-aminobutyric acid)-ergic** interneurons and projection neurons, as well as **cholinergic** interneurons and projection neurons.

Many neurological pathologies are caused by malfunction of telencephalic neurons, as a result of neurodegenerative processes (e.g. Alzheimer disease), genetic mutations (e.g. Huntington disease), or abnormal development (e.g. autism, schizophrenia and epilepsy), all with devastating consequences for the normal brain function.

During the past ten years much progress has been made in elucidating the mechanisms that orchestrate the generation of different telencephalic neuronal subtypes. A combination of fate-mapping studies with genetic loss-of-function and gain-of-function experiments has been successfully used to uncover important molecular players in the development of the rodent telencephalon.

At early stages of its development, the telencephalon is divided into two main regions: **dorsal** (pallium) and **ventral** (subpallium). The pallium is further subdivided into three longitudinal zones: dorsal, medial, and lateral. The dorsal pallium gives rise to the **neo-**

cortex - the most complex structure of the mammalian brain. The medial pallium develops into the hippocampal formation (archicortex), cortical hem and the choroid field. The lateral pallium matures into the paleocortex (olfactory and some limbic areas). From the **ventral** telencephalon medial, lateral and caudal ganglionic eminences (**MGE, LGE** and **CGE**) emerge giving rise to the **basal ganglia** and parts of the **amygdala**, but also to neurons that migrate into the cortex and olfactory bulbs. The progenitor domains in the embryonic telencephalon generate specific types of neurons which finally form the complex neural networks of the mature telencephalon.

Understanding the developmental ontogeny of the diverse telencephalic neuronal populations provides an essential framework for the design of rational approaches towards pluripotent stem cell differentiation for *cellular models* and *cell replacement therapies* for telencephalic related diseases.

In the first part, we review the stages of the mouse telencephalic development, the morphogens and the transcription factors (TF) that are intimately involved in the telencephalic patterning and neuronal subtype specification (**Sections 2-5**).

In the second part, we present recently reported protocols for differentiation of mouse and human pluripotent stem cells into telencephalic populations, following the development principles and reflecting the *in vivo* signaling pathways; we point on the relevant morphogens and TF in each stage, where the level of expression of relevant sets of TF can be considered as a milestone between each differentiation step *in vitro* [2] (**Sections 6-8**).

Finally, we describe our model system in which the *in vitro* differentiation of human and mouse embryonic stem (ES) cells are temporally aligned to each other and compared with mouse telencephalic neurogenesis *in vivo* [3]. Since the telencephalic development has been extensively studied in animal models, it is important to strengthen the interspecies comparative approaches in order to gain further insights into the human telencephalic development. We provide evidence for differences in the default differentiation of mouse and human pluripotent stem cells that proves the utility of the comparative system for optimizing the directed telencephalic differentiation of human pluripotent stem cells. We also exemplify how Hedgehog (Hh) signaling pathway is implied in telencephalic neuronal fate decision *in vitro* and *in vivo* (**Section 8**).

2. Telencephalic neuronal cell diversity

The neurons populating the mature telencephalon are generally classified based on their intrinsic properties: neurochemical profile, morphology and electrophysiological responses. The understanding of how the telencephalic neuronal subtypes are specified encompasses not only the signaling pathways that act in spatial-temporal sequences to confer positional and molecular identity but also the location of the progenitors early in development and the migration pathways they undertake to reach their final destination in the mature brain. The main neuronal types and telencephalic domains in the adult and embryonic mouse brain are schematically presented in Figure 1.

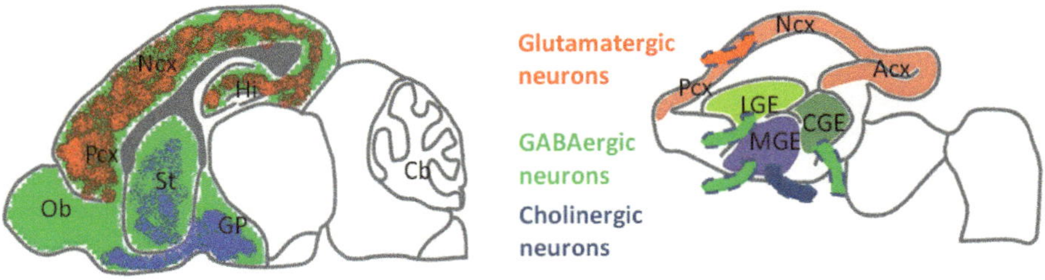

Schematic mouse mature (left side) and embryonic (right) brain; telencephalic subdivision: olfactory bulb (Ob), neocortex (Ncx), palleocortex (Pcx), archicortex (Acx), hippocampus (Hi), striatum (St) and globus pallidum (GP), pallium (pink) medial ganglionic eminence (MGE-violet), lateral ganglion eminence (LGE-light green), caudal ganglionic eminence, (CGE-dark green); domains and origins (as arrows) of telencephalic glutamatergic (red), GABAergic (green) and cholinergic (blue) neurons.

Figure 1. The domains of telencephalic neurons in adult and embryonic mouse brain

Glutamatergic projection (pyramidal) neurons comprise the majority (70-80%) of cortical neurons, they are generated in the dorsal telencephalon; have an excitatory role in the cortical and include many subtypes. Each subtype is characterized by a specific combination of laminar position, morphology, marker expression and connectivity pattern [4;5].

Cajal-Retzius neurons are a transient population expressing reelin and playing a key role in the formation of the cerebral cortex. They die during the first postnatal week [6].

GABAergic neurons are generated in the ventral telencephalon and also include many subtypes of *interneurons* and *projection neurons.*

GABAergic cortical interneurons, comprising 20-30% of the cortical neurons, have an inhibitory role in the cortical circuits; they originate in the ventral telencephalon and subsequently migrate dorsally into the developing cortex.

Other types of GABAergic neurons include the interneurons and projection neurons that populate the striatum, pallidum, olfactory bulb and other forebrain ventral regions.

Different subclasses of GABAergic interneurons arise from different progenitor domains in the subpallium: *somatostatin (Sst)* subclasses of GABAergic interneurons that ultimately reside in the cortex and the basal ganglia are generated in dorsal MGE (dMGE) [7;8]. *Parvalbumin (Pv)* subclasses of GABAergic interneurons, constituting the majority of the cortical interneurons, are generated in ventral MGE (vMGE) [9;10]. *Calretinin (Carl), NPY and reelin*-expressing GABAergic cortical interneurons are produced primarily in CGE [11;12]. Calr expressing GABAergic interneurons, which ultimately reside in the olfactory bulbs and amygdala, arise from the dorsal LGE (dLGE) [13].

GABAergic projection neurons, such as the medium spiny neurons (MSN) which constitute the majority of the striatal neurons, express DARPP32 and Calr and arise from the ventral LGE (vLGE) [13;14].

Cholinergic neurons in the telencephalon (both *interneurons* and *projection neurons*) are generated in the MGE. First, cholinergic projection neurons are produced by vMGE, followed by the production of cholinergic interneurons from dMGE, at later time points. Cholinergic interneurons populate the striatum; cholinergic projection neurons populate the pallidum and the septum and project mainly to neocortex and hippocampus, respectively [15].

3. Stages in telencephalic development

A fundamental feature of the nervous system development is the precise temporal sequence of cell type generation. The first neural cells, **neuroepithelial (NE) cells**, arise from the pluripotent stem cells of the early blastocyst that differentiate from the ectoderm towards the neuroectoderm through a process named **neural induction** [16;17].

Morphologically, NE cells are columnar epithelial cells which form the neural plate and later on the ventricular zone (VZ) of the neural tube. They are considered to be primordial neural stem cells that give rise to various types of neurons, followed by glial cells [18-20]. The elaborated process by which NE cells progress towards telencephalic neurons can be divided into several discrete stages:

1. **Early anterior/posterior (A/P) patterning.** The NE cells in the neural plate acquire an A/P identity; the anterior ones give rise to the telencephalic primordium.
2. **Dorsal/ventral (D/V) patterning.** Once the neural tube is formed and the telencephalic primordium is established, it is subdivided into discrete territories where the NE cells proliferate and transform into neural progenitor (NP) cells that reside in the adjacent newly-formed subventricular zone (SVZ). In the dorsal telencephalon, the NP cells are radial glia and basal (or intermediate) progenitors [5;21-23]. Different progenitor domains are formed in the ventral telencephalon: MGE, LGE and CGE.
3. **Neuronal specification.** Each of the progenitor domains produces specific types of neurons which further develop different neurotransmitter identities and connectivity patterns.

The **signaling pathways** controlling the neural cell fate specification during these stages have been the focus of intense research in the recent years [4;19;24-27]. Extrinsic factors, named **morphogens,** induce two or more different cell fates in a concentration-dependent manner by modulating the expression and activity of specific **TF.** The TF can in turn modulate the secretion of morphogens. The combinatorial expression of these TF instructs each unique NP population to generate progenies that are committed to specific neural fates.

4. Stage-related morphogens in mouse telencephalic neurogenesis

The morphogens known to play a role during telencephalon development are: sonic hedgehog (SHH), fibroblast growth factors (FGFs), bone morphogenetic proteins (BMPs),

Wingless/INT proteins (WNTs), transforming growth factors (TGFs) and retinoic acid (RA). They are secreted from specific centers, named organizers, during early stages of development [28].

Genetic evidence based on loss- and gain-of-function studies have indicated that the role of these morphogens can be rather complex. Depending on the developmental stage it ranges from establishment of general patterning characteristics to neuronal specification [5;21;23;26;29-33].

4.1. Early A/P patterning

A/P patterning starts to emerge in parallel with neural induction, prior to and during gastrulation. At embryonic day (E) 8.5, in regions of the embryo protected from the influence of caudalizing factors, such as WNTs, BMPs, and RA, or where their antagonists are secreted, such as Dickkopf1 (DKK1), an inhibitor of the WNT signaling pathway, and Noggin, an inhibitor of the BMP signaling pathway, the NE cells develop an anterior character and form the prospective forebrain (future telencephalon and diencephalon) [28;33-35]. FGFs (e.g. FGF8, FGF15, FGF3) are expressed early on at the anterior tip of the neural plate and then maintained in the anterior limit of the neural tube [32]. Although not a primary inducer of the telencephalic fate, FGF signaling influences the telencephalic gene expression [32;36].

4.2. D/V patterning

With regard to the location and timing of telencephalic progenitor generation, different extrinsic factors are involved in their patterning and self-renewal. WNTs and BMPs pattern the telencephalic progenitors dorsally, while SHH patterns them ventrally. BMPs are expressed dorso-medially and are required for the formation of the choroid plaque and the cortical hem [31;37;38]. WNTs are secreted from the cortical hem and promote the development of the hippocampus [30]. The expression of SHH is first observed at E8.5 in structures adjacent to the ventral telencephalon, and by E9.5 in the MGE and preoptic regions [29]. SHH promotes the formation of all ventral telencephalic subdivisions [29;39-41]. FGFs are involved in both ventral and dorsal patterning [27;30;32;42;43]. Activin, a TGF-related molecule, acts ventrally in the CGE patterning [44]. RA contributes to the patterning of the lateral telencephalon and participates in setting-up the D/V boundary [45-49].

4.3. Neuronal specification

The balance between the signaling inputs that control NP self-renewal and differentiation is critical for the initiation of the terminal differentiation program. FGFs and SHH, in addition to their patterning activities, promote self-renewal and prevent differentiation, while RA promotes neuronal differentiation [1;47]. Notably, it has been shown that the expression of SHH is required during distinct developmental windows for the specification of neuronal identity [29]. FGF signaling may ultimately influence the generation of cell diversity within the ventral telencephalon [30;50]. WNT promotes neuronal differentiation in different late cortical progenitor cell populations [51]. BMPs inhibit neurogenesis but could participate in late neuronal specification and maturation of different subpopulations [52]. Activin is also a potent neurotrophic factor that induces differentiation of telencephalic neural precursors into calretinin-positive cortical interneurons [44].

5. Stage-related TF in mouse telencephalic neurogenesis

The main TF involved in the early patterning and specification belong to **homeobox domain (HD)** and **basic helix-loop-helix (bHLH)** families, however other TF such as **zinc-finger proteins** also have essential functions.

The main HD containing TF families are: paired-box (e.g. Pax6), forkhead box (e.g. Foxg1), NK2 homeobox (e.g. Nkx2.1, Nkx6.1), orthodenthicle homeobox (e.g. Otx1/2,), sine-oculis homeobox (e.g. Six3), GS homeobox (e.g. Gsh2), distal-less homeobox (e.g. Dlx1-6), LIM homeobox (e.g. Isl1, Lhx2, Lhx6, Lhx8), empty-spiracle homeobox (e.g. Emx1/2), T-box: (e.g. Tbr1/2). Other TF, such as Mash1, Ngn1/2 and Olig2, belong to bHLH class. Gli members are zinc-finger proteins.

5.1. Early A/P patterning

The telencephalic neuroepithelium is first characterized by the expression of **FoxG1** (also named BF1) [53], **Pax6** [54;55] and **Gli3** [56]. The anterior phenotype also expresses **Six3, Otx1** and **Otx2** [57-59].

5.2. Dorsal/ventral patterning

In the mouse **dorsal** embryonic telencephalon, Pax6, Emx1 and Emx2 are specifically expressed in VZ and SVZ progenitor domains (Figure 2A).

Pax6 which is essential for setting up the sharp border between ventral and dorsal telencephalon is mainly expressed in the prospective neocortex, while Emx1 and Emx2 are medially expressed in the archicortex (later hippocampus); Lhx2 is expressed in both regions [30;31;45;60;61], Tbr2 is expressed in the SVZ corresponding to basal progenitor domains [62;63].

Nkx2.1 expression is the hallmark of the MGE development. At E9.5, Nkx2.1 appears within the **ventral** telencephalic domain, defines the MGE at the molecular level and persists in this region throughout development (Figure 2A). Around E10.0 the expression of Gsh2 accompanies the emergence LGE and further to CGE, with a lower expression level in MGE (Figure 2A). Nkx6.2 is expressed along the MGE/LGE sulcus and at high levels in the dMGE [1;64].

The mutual antagonism between Pax6 and Nkx2.1 and later on between Pax6 and Gsh2 is required for the correct positioning of the D/V boundary [65-67]. FoxG1 is involved in both ventral and dorsal patterning [27;30;32;42;43;52].

The central mechanism that determines NP D/V patterning is the activity of the Gli family of transcriptional regulators–Gli1, Gli2, and Gli3. SHH promotes the formation of a ventral telencephalic subdivision by inhibiting the dorsalizing effects of Gli3 [27;35;56;68]. Gli3 is highly expressed dorsally, with lower expression in the LGE and MGE. Gli1 is expressed ventrally, at high levels in the progenitor domain of the dMGE and vLGE, whereas Gli2 is highly expressed in the progenitor domain of the dorsal telencephalon, with a lower expression in the LGE (Figure 2B).

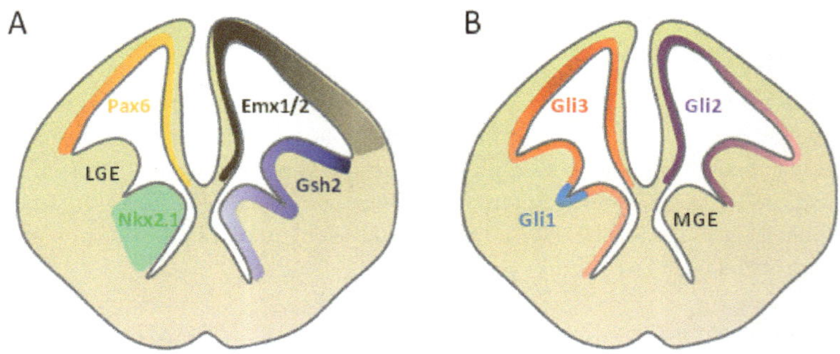

Figure 2. The domains of the main transcription factors implied in dorsal-ventral patterning in mouse embryonic telencephalon.

5.3. Neuronal specification

The mechanisms of neuronal specification in the dorsal telencephalon have been extensively studied in the context of cerebral cortex development. The dorsal progenitors produce neurons, in a tightly controlled temporal order from E10.5 to E17.5. Pax6, Ngn1 and Ngn2 instruct **glutamatergic** identity and inhibit astroglial differentiation [69-72]. The differentiation by Ngns involves the sequential activation of the expression of other TF such as NeuroD, Tbr1 and Tbr2 [69]. NeuroD has been implicated in the terminal differentiation of the hippocampus [73]. The differentiation of specific populations of projection neurons is controlled by neuronal subtype-specific genes, which have only begun to be identified. The timing of cortical neurogenesis is encoded within lineages of individual progenitor cells, with different locations [74].

The earliest born neurons form a layered structure termed the preplate, which is later split into the superficial marginal zone and the deeply located subplate. The cortical plate, which will give rise to six-layered neocortex, begins to develop between these two layers. The later born neurons arriving at the cortical plate migrate past earlier born neurons [5;74]. During development, neurons in different layers are generated in an inside-first, outside-last order, and newly postmitotic neurons are specified to adopt the laminar positions characteristic of their birthdays [5;24;75].

Mash1 is the main neurogenic TF in the ventral telencephalon and is involved also in the neurotransmitter identity specification, being a selective instructor of **GABAergic** identity [70;76-82]. Olig1/2 can promote both neuronal and oligodendroglial fates while inhibiting astrogliogeneis [83].

Dlx genes (Dlx1, 2, 5 and 6) are expressed in ventral progenitors and neurons in MGE, LGE and CGE, and are likely to play a role in neural specification [78;84;85].

Interestingly, MGE, LGE and CGE progenitor domains do not give rise to homogeneous populations of neurons, which is most likely due to a further subdivision of these domains into regions with spatially restricted expression of specific TF.

There is also a temporal control of the specification of various neuronal subtypes; as a general pattern, the earlier- born ventral cells give rise to projection neurons while the more dorsally positioned later-born cells generate interneurons [24;82;86-88].

MGE is characterized by the early production of cholinergic projection neurons from its ventral part, followed by the late production of GABAergic and cholinergic interneurons from the dorsal domains. Two TF are detected at E12.5 exclusively in the MGE: Lhx6 and Lhx8 (or Lhx7) [89], suggesting a role in the specification of MGE-derived neurons. Lhx6-expressing neurons have the characteristics of proto-GABAergic neurons with dual differentiation potential, while Lhx8 seems to be involved in the differentiation of specific cholinergic neurons [15;90]. The differentiation of a common proto-GABAergic precursor into mature subtypes is regulated by the combinatorial activity of the Lhx6, Lhx8 and Isl1. Those proto-GABAergic neurons that maintain the expression of Lhx6 differentiate into mature GABAergic striatal interneurons. By contrast, induction of Isl1 and the combined activity of Lhx7/8 and Isl1 results in down-regulation of Lhx6 and commitment along the cholinergic interneuron sublineage [90-92]. Thus, it appears that a LIM HD transcriptional code determines cell-fate specification and neurotransmitter identity in neuronal subpopulations of the ventral telencephalon.

Ventral LGE generate GABAergic projection neurons that also express Isl1 during early specification, followed by the expression of other striatal-specific TF such as FoxP1, FoxP2, and Ctip2 [93-95]. Later in development, dLGE generates interneurons that migrate to the olfactory bulbs [13;95].

6. Telencephalic neurons generated from mouse ES cells

Mouse ES (mES) cells have emerged as a powerful tool for developmental biology. Several studies have focused on mES-derived telencephalic progenitors and the specific neuronal populations they generate *in vitro* and *in vivo* [3;96-101].

6.1. Early A/P patterning

After the first generation of defined telencephalic precursors from mES cells based on studies of forebrain development [101], significant improvements regarding the success of neural induction and telencephalic patterning have been reported during the following years [96;100].

Blocking the WNTs and BMPs pathways by applying the antagonists DKK1 and BMPR1A-FC, respectively, cause neural induction in more than 90% of mES cells and maintained around 35% of the progenitors as telencephalic, expressing FoxG1 [101]. Other following studies has reported a massive FoxG1 expressing telencephalic progenitor generation in serum-free, RA-free conditions [96-98;100], while using a RA treatment, FoxG1 expression has not been detected [98].

6.2. Dorsal/ventral patterning

SHH or a Hh agonist treatment on telencephalic progenitors suppresses the dorsal marker Pax6 and induced the ventral marker Nkx2.1. SHH application does not cause substantial difference in the level of Gsh2 expression [100;101].

The majority of mES cell-derived progenitors exhibit by default a ventral phenotype which has been attributed to the high level of endogenous SHH signaling. Blocking the Hh signaling converts most of the ventral telencephalic precursors into dorsal progenitors, with the majority expressing typical markers of the dorsal telencephalon: Pax6 and Emx1/2 [3;97;99].

6.3. Neuronal specification

The telencephalic progenitors derived from mES cells can be directed to neurons that express the excitatory neurotransmitter glutamate and the inhibitory neurotransmitter GABA [3;102-106].

The dorsal progenitors have been shown to produce mature neurons with many features of cortical pyramidal neurons in a temporal manner similar with *in vivo* corticogenesis. The first neurons generated in these cultures are reelin-positive Cajal-Retzius-like and subplate-like neurons expressing Tbr1, followed by the glutamatergic neurons generated in an inside-first, outside-last manner. The majority of the cells generated by Gaspard *et al.* express markers of deep cortical layer V and VI neurons, like Tbr1, Otx1, Ctip2 and FoxP2 [102]. Eiraku *et al.* have also generated deep layer neurons, positive for Ctip2 and Emx1 in the first 9 days of neuronal differentiation of dorsalized progenitors [96].

By transplantation of dorsally patterned progenitors into postnatal murine cerebral cortex, the production of cortical projection neurons with the correct morphology and axonal connectivity has been demonstrated [98]. The pyramidal neurons express Otx1, Emx1, and Ctip2, corresponding to deep layers neurons. They integrate and appropriately project long-distance axons to subcortical targets, without forming tumors [98].

Regarding the protocols for ventral neuronal specification, it has been shown that Nkx2.1 and Gsh2 expressing progenitors give rise both to GABAergic and cholinergic neurons [3;100;101].

Furthermore, the use of Lhx6::GFP ES cells has allowed the isolation of cells with potential for developing into ventral telencephalic subpopulations and their follow-up during transplantation into the postnatal brain. Transplanted Lhx6::GFP cells demonstrate the ability to retain migratory capacity and neuronal commitment without forming tumors and exhibit cortical interneuron characteristics [100].

7. Telencephalic neurons generated from human ES cells

Neural induction takes place in human ES (hES) cells similar to mES cells, however with a different timing. Under serum-free conditions, without adding known morphogens [3;101;105-110], by co-culture with stromal cells [111;112] or by using a recently defined protocol with dual-SMAD-inhibition [113], it has been demonstrated that hES cells differentiate into a synchronized population of NE cells organized into neural-tube-like rosettes within 2 weeks, a time corresponding to the development of the neural plate/tube in a human embryo. Around day 8-10, the primitive NE cells express PAX6, and the neural fate is consolidated by SOX1 expression around day 14 [3;100;105;106;108-110].

7.1. Early anterior/posterior patterning

In the absence of exogenous morphogens, hES cells differentiate into progenitors that uniformly expressed anterior TF, including FOXG1, OTX2, SIX3, LHX2 but not posterior TF [3;107;106;109]. Even when the neural induction is performed by co-culturing with stromal cells, a large population of neural progenitors exhibit anterior characteristics [112]. FOXG1 appears at approximately day 10 and it is still expressed at day 24 and even in postmitotic neurons, 1 month after differentiation. PAX6 is co-expressed in nearly all of the FOXG1 telencephalic progenitors (95% of all cells) one month after differentiation, in the absence of growth factors or morphogens [3;106;114].

7.2. Dorsal/ventral patterning

WNT proteins and their downstream molecules have been found to be highly expressed right after the generation of NE cells. In minimal medium and in the absence of known morphogens, hES cell-derived telencephalic progenitors exhibit a dorsal telencephalic trait, which has been attributed to endogenous WNT signaling [115]. The activation of SHH and/or inhibition of WNT permitts the specification of ventral telencephalic progenitors.

At the lower dosage, SHH reduces the PAX6-expressing cell population and increases the NKX2.1 cell population. At the higher dosage, SHH almost completely eliminates the PAX6-expressing cells, while increasing the NKX2.1 ventral progenitors. The combination of DKK1 and SHH at the lower dosage significantly increases NKX2.1 and decreases PAX6 and GLI3 expression. High concentrations of SHH significantly inhibits GLI3 expression compared with low concentrations of SHH. The specification of dorsal-ventral progenitors by WNT and/or SHH has been partially achieved through differentially regulating the expression of active and repressive forms of GLI3. Using of a low concentration of SHH alone results in the differentiation of both LGE and MGE progenitors, whereas additional WNT inhibition (by DKK1) further ventralizes the human neural progenitors, resulting in a predominant population of NKX2.1 expressing MGE progenitors [115]. Aubry *et al.* have patterned the telencephalic progenitors by SHH and DKK1 treatment for 12 days in adherent culture and have found a significant up-regulation of the LGE markers GSH2 and DLX2 [111].

7.3. Neuronal specification

The regionalized dorsal and ventral human telencephalic progenitors further differentiate into functional cortical glutamatergic neurons and telencephalic GABAergic neurons, respectively.

Cortical glutamatergic neurons have been efficiently generated in the absence of morphogens. This indicates the intrinsic tendency of hES cells to generate cortical neural cells [3;109]. Neurons differentiated from dorsal progenitors in the absence of exogenous morphogens for 6 weeks exhibits a pyramidal morphology, with extensive neurite outgrowth, and expressed TBR1 and CTIP2 [96, 115].

Ventral telencephalic GABAergic neurons have been induced with a high concentration of SHH, a low dose of SHH together with WNT inhibitors [115] or by using SHH agonists [3].

Additionally, Aubry *et al.* have focused to the characterization of the striatal-like progenitors, showing that more than a half of the specified neurons were DARPP32 and Calr positive, exhibiting phenotypic features of MSN. Transplantation of the LGE-patterned progenitors in quinolinic acid–lesioned rats (a model for Huntington disease) has confirmed the *in vivo* specification toward striatal MSN [111].

Human ES cell-derived telencephalic glutamatergic and GABAergic neurons have been reported to be electro-physiologically active [111;115;116] and also to integrate in the mature telencephalon after transplantation [117].

8. Modulation of Hh signaling pathway in telencephalic cells generated from mouse and human ES cells

We recently proposed a novel model system in which the *in vitro* differentiation of hES and mES cells are temporally aligned to each other and compared with mouse telencephalic neurogenesis *in vivo*. In this comparative model system, we tested the *in vitro* role of Hh signaling for ES cell-derived telencephalic differentiation (Figure 3) [3].

Neural differentiation of 2 lines of mES cells and 2 lines of hES cells was studied under identical, defined conditions, but following different time-schedules for mouse and human cell cultures. The *in vitro* time schedules were based on data from *in vivo* development as a reference for the stages of neural induction, neural patterning, and neuronal specification. In addition, we developed a specific profile of marker genes, which was derived from *in vivo* studies.

Our results demonstrated that neural differentiation took place in mES cell-derived cultures resulting in the generation of neural progenitors and neurons in a time-frame which mirrors telencephalic neurogenesis *in vivo*. The expression levels of telencephalic markers were comparable between *in vivo* and *in vitro* differentiated populations. We demonstrated that the neural differentiation in human cells can be temporally aligned with mouse cells in the proposed neurogenic time-windows. Thus, our temporally aligned, comparative cell culture model offered a novel platform for analyzing the effect of signaling molecules on the generation of specific telencephalic populations in mouse and human cell cultures.

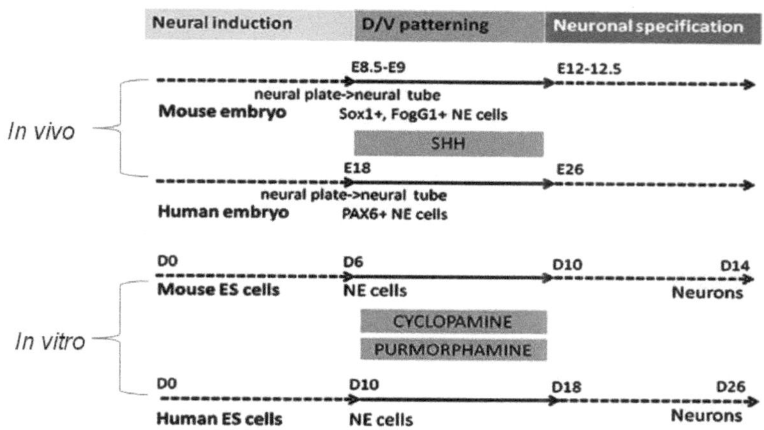

Figure 3. Hh signaling for modulation of dorsal ventral patterning in mouse and human telencephalon in vivo and in vitro, in ES stem cell-derived cell cultures (modified from Nat et al 2012 [3]).

To exemplify the value of this approach we analyzed in greater detail a single process, the step of D/V telencephalic patterning. Thus, we monitored the effect of pharmacological modulators of the Hh signaling pathway, purmorphamine—an agonist and cyclopamine—an antagonist acting on the Smoothened receptor (Smo), regarding the expression of region-specific TFs and signaling molecules relevant for telencephalic development *in vivo*.

Purmorphamine strongly up-regulated the expression of telencephalic ventral markers Nkx2.1, Nkx6.2, Lhx6, and Lhx8 in mouse and human cells, thus reflecting the *in vivo* process of the MGE patterning and specification. Cyclopamine up-regulated the expression of telencephalic dorsal markers, but at lower levels in human compared with mouse cells. Interestingly, the modulation of Smo *in vitro* differentially affected the expression of molecules of the Hh pathway, especially the Gli1 and Gli3 effectors and Ptch receptors, in mouse *vs* human cells.

We additionally examined how the SHH expression itself was modulated by Smo agonist or antagonist treatment. We reported that SHH expression is regulated in a very dynamic way by Hh pathway modulation, both in mES and hES cell-derived models. In particular, a very robust up-regulation of SHH by purmorphamine was observed in the human model, where SHH was not expressed in untreated controls. Shh was expressed in both progenitor cells and neurons in our cultures. This might be explained by the non-cell autonomous mechanisms recently described in the mouse embryonic telencephalon, where both Lhx8 and Lhx6 genes controlled the expression of Shh in the mantle zone of the MGE, corresponding to early-born neurons [118]. Thus, Lhx6 and Lhx8 appear to regulate MGE development by promoting Shh expression in MGE neurons, which, in turn, promotes the developmental program of the dMGE.

The activation of Hh signaling *via* Smo with purmorphamine converts the primitive dorsal telencephalic precursors to ventral progenitors. These progenitors differentiate into neuronal subtypes including GABAergic and cholinergic neurons.

Our results provided evidence for the different default telencephalic differentiation of mouse and human ES cells: ventral and dorsal, respectively. Additionally, it proved the utility of the comparative system for optimizing the directed differentiation of human pluripotent stem cells.

9. Conclusion

Recent studies have shown that both mES cells and hES cells differentiate into region specific progenitors, following the same developmental principles that have been identified by studying mouse CNS development. Together with previous findings, our own data support the model in which the human neural progenitors in culture develop a reverse default D/V phenotype compared with mouse. However, early human NE cells can be efficiently differentiated into dorsal and ventral telencephalic progenitors *via* modulating similar molecular pathways as described in rodents.

Therefore, mES and hES cell-derived models, directly compared in parallel experiments and temporally aligned to *in vivo* telencephalic development, offer a platform for testing the effect of morphogens, growth factors, and pharmacological substances for the generation of specific neuronal subtypes.

Additionally, telencephalic progenitors and neurons generated *in vitro* from human pluripotent cells provide a unique paradigm to study the human telencephalic development.

Even more importantly, the telencephalic differentiation of human induced PS (IPS) cells has recently been reported [119;120].

The application of optimized telencephalic differentiation protocols to IPS cell cultures derived from patients with neurodegenerative or neurogenetic diseases will provide unique new opportunities to develop *in vitro* models of human diseases such as Alzheimer's disease, Huntington's disease, epilepsy, and neuropsychiatric disorders. These models, based on human neurons in culture, will critically complement existing animal models, which do not fully reflect important features specific for the normal and pathological human brain.

Acknowledgements

This work was supported by SPIN FWF W1206-B05, Austria.

Author details

Roxana Nat, Galina Apostolova and Georg Dechant

Institute for Neuroscience, Innsbruck Medical University, Innsbruck, Austria

References

[1] Corbin,J.G., and Butt,S.J. 2011. Developmental mechanisms for the generation of telencephalic interneurons. *Dev. Neurobiol.* 20:947-958.

[2] Nat,R., and Dechant,G. 2011. Milestones of Directed Differentiation of Mouse and Human Embryonic Stem Cells into Telencephalic Neurons Based on Neural Development In Vivo. *Stem Cells Dev.*

[3] Nat,R., Salti,A., Suciu,L., Strom,S., and Dechant,G. 2012. Pharmacological modulation of the Hedgehog pathway differentially affects dorsal/ventral patterning in mouse and human embryonic stem cell models of telencephalic development. *Stem Cells Dev.* 21:1016-1046.

[4] Arlotta,P., Molyneaux,B.J., Chen,J., Inoue,J., Kominami,R., and Macklis,J.D. 2005. Neuronal subtype-specific genes that control corticospinal motor neuron development in vivo. *Neuron* 45:207-221.

[5] Molyneaux,B.J., Arlotta,P., Menezes,J.R., and Macklis,J.D. 2007. Neuronal subtype specification in the cerebral cortex. *Nat. Rev. Neurosci.* 8:427-437.

[6] Hevner,R.F., Neogi,T., Englund,C., Daza,R.A., and Fink,A. 2003. Cajal-Retzius cells in the mouse: transcription factors, neurotransmitters, and birthdays suggest a pallial origin. *Brain Res. Dev. Brain Res.* 141:39-53.

[7] Flames,N., Pla,R., Gelman,D.M., Rubenstein,J.L.R., Puelles,L., and Marin,O. 2007. Delineation of multiple subpallial progenitor domains by the combinatorial expression of transcriptional codes *Journal of Neuroscience* 27:9682-9695.

[8] Wonders,C.P., Taylor,L., Welagen,J., Mbata,I.C., Xiang,J.Z., and Anderson,S.A. 2008. A spatial bias for the origins of interneuron subgroups within the medial ganglionic eminence. *Dev. Biol.* 314:127-136.

[9] Wichterle,H., Turnbull,D.H., Nery,S., Fishell,G., and Alvarez-Buylla,A. 2001. In utero fate mapping reveals distinct migratory pathways and fates of neurons born in the mammalian basal forebrain. *Development* 128:3759-3771.

[10] Wonders,C.P., and Anderson,S.A. 2006. The origin and specification of cortical interneurons. *Nat. Rev. Neurosci.* 7:687-696.

[11] Miyoshi,G., Hjerling-Leffler,J., Karayannis,T., Sousa,V.H., Butt,S.J., Battiste,J., Johnson,J.E., Machold,R.P., and Fishell,G. 2010. Genetic fate mapping reveals that the caudal ganglionic eminence produces a large and diverse population of superficial cortical interneurons. *J. Neurosci.* 30:1582-1594.

[12] Nery,S., Fishell,G., and Corbin,J.G. 2002. The caudal ganglionic eminence is a source of distinct cortical and subcortical cell populations. *Nat. Neurosci.* 5:1279-1287.

[13] Stenman,J., Toresson,H., and Campbell,K. 2003. Identification of two distinct progenitor populations in the lateral ganglionic eminence: implications for striatal and olfactory bulb neurogenesis. *J. Neurosci.* 23:167-174.

[14] Olsson,M., Bjorklund,A., and Campbell,K. 1998. Early specification of striatal projection neurons and interneuronal subtypes in the lateral and medial ganglionic eminence. *Neuroscience* 84:867-876.

[15] Zhao,Y., Marin,O., Hermesz,E., Powell,A., Flames,N., Palkovits,M., Rubenstein,J.L., and Westphal,H. 2003. The LIM-homeobox gene Lhx8 is required for the development of many cholinergic neurons in the mouse forebrain. *Proc. Natl. Acad. Sci. U. S. A* 100:9005-9010.

[16] Levine,A.J., and Brivanlou,A.H. 2007. Proposal of a model of mammalian neural induction. *Dev. Biol.* 308:247-256.

[17] Wilson,S.W., and Houart,C. 2004. Early steps in the development of the forebrain. *Dev. Cell* 6:167-181.

[18] Gotz,M., and Huttner,W.B. 2005. The cell biology of neurogenesis. *Nat. Rev. Mol. Cell Biol.* 6:777-788.

[19] Guillemot,F. 2007. Cell fate specification in the mammalian telencephalon. *Prog. Neurobiol.* 83:37-52.

[20] Sauvageot,C.M., and Stiles,C.D. 2002. Molecular mechanisms controlling cortical gliogenesis. *Curr. Opin. Neurobiol.* 12:244-249.

[21] Anthony,T.E., Klein,C., Fishell,G., and Heintz,N. 2004. Radial glia serve as neuronal progenitors in all regions of the central nervous system. *Neuron* 41:881-890.

[22] Gotz,M., Hartfuss,E., and Malatesta,P. 2002. Radial glial cells as neuronal precursors: a new perspective on the correlation of morphology and lineage restriction in the developing cerebral cortex of mice. *Brain Res. Bull.* 57:777-788.

[23] Pontious,A., Kowalczyk,T., Englund,C., and Hevner,R.F. 2008. Role of intermediate progenitor cells in cerebral cortex development. *Dev. Neurosci.* 30:24-32.

[24] Campbell,K. 2005. Cortical neuron specification: it has its time and place. *Neuron* 46:373-376.

[25] Guillemot,F. 2005. Cellular and molecular control of neurogenesis in the mammalian telencephalon. *Curr. Opin. Cell Biol.* 17:639-647.

[26] Hebert,J.M. 2005. Unraveling the molecular pathways that regulate early telencephalon development. *Curr. Top. Dev. Biol.* 69:17-37.

[27] Hebert,J.M., and Fishell,G. 2008. The genetics of early telencephalon patterning: some assembly required. *Nat. Rev. Neurosci.* 9:678-685.

[28] Stern,C.D. 2001. Initial patterning of the central nervous system: how many organizers? *Nat. Rev. Neurosci.* 2:92-98.

[29] Fuccillo,M., Rallu,M., McMahon,A.P., and Fishell,G. 2004. Temporal requirement for hedgehog signaling in ventral telencephalic patterning. *Development* 131:5031-5040.

[30] Gunhaga,L., Marklund,M., Sjodal,M., Hsieh,J.C., Jessell,T.M., and Edlund,T. 2003. Specification of dorsal telencephalic character by sequential Wnt and FGF signaling. *Nat. Neurosci.* 6:701-707.

[31] Hebert,J.M., Mishina,Y., and McConnell,S.K. 2002. BMP signaling is required locally to pattern the dorsal telencephalic midline. *Neuron* 35:1029-1041.

[32] Iwata,T., and Hevner,R.F. 2009. Fibroblast growth factor signaling in development of the cerebral cortex. *Dev. Growth Differ.* 51:299-323.

[33] Kudoh,T., Wilson,S.W., and Dawid,I.B. 2002. Distinct roles for Fgf, Wnt and retinoic acid in posteriorizing the neural ectoderm. *Development* 129:4335-4346.

[34] Patthey,C., Gunhaga,L., and Edlund,T. 2008. Early development of the central and peripheral nervous systems is coordinated by Wnt and BMP signals. *PLoS One.* 3:e1625.

[35] Rallu,M., Corbin,J.G., and Fishell,G. 2002. Parsing the prosencephalon. *Nat. Rev. Neurosci.* 3:943-951.

[36] Na,E., McCarthy,M., Neyt,C., Lai,E., and Fishell,G. 1998. Telencephalic progenitors maintain anteroposterior identities cell autonomously. *Curr. Biol.* 8:987-990.

[37] Fernandes,M., Gutin,G., Alcorn,H., McConnell,S.K., and Hebert,J.M. 2007. Mutations in the BMP pathway in mice support the existence of two molecular classes of holoprosencephaly. *Development* 134:3789-3794.

[38] Hebert,J.M., Hayhurst,M., Marks,M.E., Kulessa,H., Hogan,B.L., and McConnell,S.K. 2003. BMP ligands act redundantly to pattern the dorsal telencephalic midline. *Genesis.* 35:214-219.

[39] Chiang,C., Litingtung,Y., Lee,E., Young,K.E., Corden,J.L., Westphal,H., and Beachy,P.A. 1996. Cyclopia and defective axial patterning in mice lacking Sonic hedgehog gene function. *Nature* 383:407-413.

[40] Gunhaga,L., Jessell,T.M., and Edlund,T. 2000. Sonic hedgehog signaling at gastrula stages specifies ventral telencephalic cells in the chick embryo. *Development* 127:3283-3293.

[41] Xu,Q., Guo,L., Moore,H., Waclaw,R.R., Campbell,K., and Anderson,S.A. 2010. Sonic hedgehog signaling confers ventral telencephalic progenitors with distinct cortical interneuron fates. *Neuron* 65:328-340.

[42] Fasano,C.A., Phoenix,T.N., Kokovay,E., Lowry,N., Elkabetz,Y., Dimos,J.T., Lemischka,I.R., Studer,L., and Temple,S. 2009. Bmi-1 cooperates with Foxg1 to maintain neural stem cell self-renewal in the forebrain. *Genes Dev.* 23:561-574.

[43] Manuel,M., Martynoga,B., Yu,T., West,J.D., Mason,J.O., and Price,D.J. 2010. The transcription factor Foxg1 regulates the competence of telencephalic cells to adopt subpallial fates in mice. *Development* 137:487-497.

[44] Cambray,S., Arber,C., Little,G., Dougalis,A.G., de,P., V, Ungless,M.A., Li,M., and Rodriguez,T.A. 2012. Activin induces cortical interneuron identity and differentiation in embryonic stem cell-derived telencephalic neural precursors. *Nat. Commun.* 3:841.

[45] Campbell,K. 2003. Dorsal-ventral patterning in the mammalian telencephalon. *Curr. Opin. Neurobiol.* 13:50-56.

[46] Marklund,M., Sjodal,M., Beehler,B.C., Jessell,T.M., Edlund,T., and Gunhaga,L. 2004. Retinoic acid signalling specifies intermediate character in the developing telencephalon. *Development* 131:4323-4332.

[47] Patani,R., Hollins,A.J., Wishart,T.M., Puddifoot,C.A., Alvarez,S., de Lera,A.R., Wyllie,D.J., Compston,D.A., Pedersen,R.A., Gillingwater,T.H. et al 2011. Retinoid-independent motor neurogenesis from human embryonic stem cells reveals a medial columnar ground state. *Nat. Commun.* 2:214.

[48] Toresson,H., Parmar,M., and Campbell,K. 2000. Expression of Meis and Pbx genes and their protein products in the developing telencephalon: implications for regional differentiation. *Mech. Dev.* 94:183-187.

[49] Waclaw,R.R., Wang,B., and Campbell,K. 2004. The homeobox gene Gsh2 is required for retinoid production in the embryonic mouse telencephalon. *Development* 131:4013-4020.

[50] Machon,O., Backman,M., Machonova,O., Kozmik,Z., Vacik,T., Andersen,L., and Krauss,S. 2007. A dynamic gradient of Wnt signaling controls initiation of neurogenesis in the mammalian cortex and cellular specification in the hippocampus. *Dev. Biol.* 311:223-237.

[51] Panchision,D.M., Pickel,J.M., Studer,L., Lee,S.H., Turner,P.A., Hazel,T.G., and McKay,R.D. 2001. Sequential actions of BMP receptors control neural precursor cell production and fate. *Genes Dev.* 15:2094-2110.

[52] Gutin,G., Fernandes,M., Palazzolo,L., Paek,H., Yu,K., Ornitz,D.M., McConnell,S.K., and Hebert,J.M. 2006. FGF signalling generates ventral telencephalic cells independently of SHH. *Development* 133:2937-2946.

[53] Tao,W., and Lai,E. 1992. Telencephalon-restricted expression of BF-1, a new member of the HNF-3/fork head gene family, in the developing rat brain. *Neuron* 8:957-966.

[54] Haubst,N., Berger,J., Radjendirane,V., Graw,J., Favor,J., Saunders,G.F., Stoykova,A., and Gotz,M. 2004. Molecular dissection of Pax6 function: the specific roles of the paired domain and homeodomain in brain development. *Development* 131:6131-6140.

[55] Holm,P.C., Mader,M.T., Haubst,N., Wizenmann,A., Sigvardsson,M., and Gotz,M. 2007. Loss- and gain-of-function analyses reveal targets of Pax6 in the developing mouse telencephalon. *Mol. Cell Neurosci.* 34:99-119.

[56] Aoto,K., Nishimura,T., Eto,K., and Motoyama,J. 2002. Mouse GLI3 regulates Fgf8 expression and apoptosis in the developing neural tube, face, and limb bud. *Dev. Biol.* 251:320-332.

[57] Acampora,D., Barone,P., and Simeone,A. 1999. Otx genes in corticogenesis and brain development. *Cereb. Cortex* 9:533-542.

[58] Appolloni,I., Calzolari,F., Corte,G., Perris,R., and Malatesta,P. 2008. Six3 controls the neural progenitor status in the murine CNS. *Cereb. Cortex* 18:553-562.

[59] Simeone,A., Puelles,E., and Acampora,D. 2002. The Otx family. *Curr. Opin. Genet. Dev.* 12:409-415.

[60] Furuta,Y., Piston,D.W., and Hogan,B.L. 1997. Bone morphogenetic proteins (BMPs) as regulators of dorsal forebrain development. *Development* 124:2203-2212.

[61] Quinn,J.C., Molinek,M., Martynoga,B.S., Zaki,P.A., Faedo,A., Bulfone,A., Hevner,R.F., West,J.D., and Price,D.J. 2007. Pax6 controls cerebral cortical cell number by regulating exit from the cell cycle and specifies cortical cell identity by a cell autonomous mechanism. *Dev. Biol.* 302:50-65.

[62] Englund,C., Fink,A., Lau,C., Pham,D., Daza,R.A., Bulfone,A., Kowalczyk,T., and Hevner,R.F. 2005. Pax6, Tbr2, and Tbr1 are expressed sequentially by radial glia, intermediate progenitor cells, and postmitotic neurons in developing neocortex. *J. Neurosci.* 25:247-251.

[63] Nieto,M., Monuki,E.S., Tang,H., Imitola,J., Haubst,N., Khoury,S.J., Cunningham,J., Gotz,M., and Walsh,C.A. 2004. Expression of Cux-1 and Cux-2 in the subventricular zone and upper layers II-IV of the cerebral cortex. *J. Comp Neurol.* 479:168-180.

[64] Welagen,J., and Anderson,S. 2011. Origins of neocortical interneurons in mice. *Dev. Neurobiol.* 71:10-17.

[65] Carney,R.S., Cocas,L.A., Hirata,T., Mansfield,K., and Corbin,J.G. 2009. Differential regulation of telencephalic pallial-subpallial boundary patterning by Pax6 and Gsh2. *Cereb. Cortex* 19:745-759.

[66] Corbin,J.G., Rutlin,M., Gaiano,N., and Fishell,G. 2003. Combinatorial function of the homeodomain proteins Nkx2.1 and Gsh2 in ventral telencephalic patterning. *Development* 130:4895-4906.

[67] Toresson,H., Potter,S.S., and Campbell,K. 2000. Genetic control of dorsal-ventral identity in the telencephalon: opposing roles for Pax6 and Gsh2. *Development* 127:4361-4371.

[68] Yu,W., Wang,Y., McDonnell,K., Stephen,D., and Bai,C.B. 2009. Patterning of ventral telencephalon requires positive function of Gli transcription factors. *Dev. Biol.* 334:264-275.

[69] Mattar,P., Britz,O., Johannes,C., Nieto,M., Ma,L., Rebeyka,A., Klenin,N., Polleux,F., Guillemot,F., and Schuurmans,C. 2004. A screen for downstream effectors of Neurogenin2 in the embryonic neocortex. *Dev. Biol.* 273:373-389.

[70] Parras,C.M., Schuurmans,C., Scardigli,R., Kim,J., Anderson,D.J., and Guillemot,F. 2002. Divergent functions of the proneural genes Mash1 and Ngn2 in the specification of neuronal subtype identity. *Genes Dev.* 16:324-338.

[71] Schuurmans,C., and Guillemot,F. 2002. Molecular mechanisms underlying cell fate specification in the developing telencephalon. *Curr. Opin. Neurobiol.* 12:26-34.

[72] Schuurmans,C., Armant,O., Nieto,M., Stenman,J.M., Britz,O., Klenin,N., Brown,C., Langevin,L.M., Seibt,J., Tang,H. et al 2004. Sequential phases of cortical specification involve Neurogenin-dependent and -independent pathways. *EMBO J.* 23:2892-2902.

[73] Galichet,C., Guillemot,F., and Parras,C.M. 2008. Neurogenin 2 has an essential role in development of the dentate gyrus. *Development* 135:2031-2041.

[74] Shen,Q., Wang,Y., Dimos,J.T., Fasano,C.A., Phoenix,T.N., Lemischka,I.R., Ivanova,N.B., Stifani,S., Morrisey,E.E., and Temple,S. 2006. The timing of cortical neurogenesis is encoded within lineages of individual progenitor cells. *Nat. Neurosci.* 9:743-751.

[75] McConnell,S.K. 1995. Constructing the cerebral cortex: neurogenesis and fate determination. *Neuron* 15:761-768.

[76] Casarosa,S., Fode,C., and Guillemot,F. 1999. Mash1 regulates neurogenesis in the ventral telencephalon. *Development* 126:525-534.

[77] Hanashima,C., Fernandes,M., Hebert,J.M., and Fishell,G. 2007. The role of Foxg1 and dorsal midline signaling in the generation of Cajal-Retzius subtypes. *J. Neurosci.* 27:11103-11111.

[78] Long,J.E., Cobos,I., Potter,G.B., and Rubenstein,J.L. 2009. Dlx1&2 and Mash1 transcription factors control MGE and CGE patterning and differentiation through parallel and overlapping pathways. *Cereb. Cortex* 19 Suppl 1:i96-106.

[79] Muzio,L., and Mallamaci,A. 2005. Foxg1 confines Cajal-Retzius neuronogenesis and hippocampal morphogenesis to the dorsomedial pallium. *J. Neurosci.* 25:4435-4441.

[80] Oishi,K., Watatani,K., Itoh,Y., Okano,H., Guillemot,F., Nakajima,K., and Gotoh,Y. 2009. Selective induction of neocortical GABAergic neurons by the PDK1-Akt pathway through activation of Mash1. *Proc. Natl. Acad. Sci. U. S. A* 106:13064-13069.

[81] Parras,C.M., Galli,R., Britz,O., Soares,S., Galichet,C., Battiste,J., Johnson,J.E., Nakafuku,M., Vescovi,A., and Guillemot,F. 2004. Mash1 specifies neurons and oligodendrocytes in the postnatal brain. *EMBO J.* 23:4495-4505.

[82] Wang,B., Waclaw,R.R., Allen,Z.J., Guillemot,F., and Campbell,K. 2009. Ascl1 is a required downstream effector of Gsx gene function in the embryonic mouse telencephalon. *Neural Dev.* 4:5.

[83] Ross,S.E., Greenberg,M.E., and Stiles,C.D. 2003. Basic helix-loop-helix factors in cortical development. *Neuron* 39:13-25.

[84] Panganiban,G., and Rubenstein,J.L. 2002. Developmental functions of the Distal-less/Dlx homeobox genes. *Development* 129:4371-4386.

[85] Petryniak,M.A., Potter,G.B., Rowitch,D.H., and Rubenstein,J.L. 2007. Dlx1 and Dlx2 control neuronal versus oligodendroglial cell fate acquisition in the developing forebrain. *Neuron* 55:417-433.

[86] Butt,S.J., Fuccillo,M., Nery,S., Noctor,S., Kriegstein,A., Corbin,J.G., and Fishell,G. 2005. The temporal and spatial origins of cortical interneurons predict their physiological subtype. *Neuron* 48:591-604.

[87] Butt,S.J., Sousa,V.H., Fuccillo,M.V., Hjerling-Leffler,J., Miyoshi,G., Kimura,S., and Fishell,G. 2008. The requirement of Nkx2-1 in the temporal specification of cortical interneuron subtypes. *Neuron* 59:722-732.

[88] Waclaw,R.R., and Campbell,K. 2009. Regional control of cortical lamination. *Nat. Neurosci.* 12:1211-1212.

[89] Grigoriou,M., Tucker,A.S., Sharpe,P.T., and Pachnis,V. 1998. Expression and regulation of Lhx6 and Lhx7, a novel subfamily of LIM homeodomain encoding genes, suggests a role in mammalian head development. *Development* 125:2063-2074.

[90] Fragkouli,A., van Wijk,N.V., Lopes,R., Kessaris,N., and Pachnis,V. 2009. LIM homeodomain transcription factor-dependent specification of bipotential MGE progenitors into cholinergic and GABAergic striatal interneurons. *Development* 136:3841-3851.

[91] Fragkouli,A., Hearn,C., Errington,M., Cooke,S., Grigoriou,M., Bliss,T., Stylianopoulou,F., and Pachnis,V. 2005. Loss of forebrain cholinergic neurons and impairment in spatial learning and memory in LHX7-deficient mice. *Eur. J. Neurosci.* 21:2923-2938.

[92] Liodis,P., Denaxa,M., Grigoriou,M., Akufo-Addo,C., Yanagawa,Y., and Pachnis,V. 2007. Lhx6 activity is required for the normal migration and specification of cortical interneuron subtypes. *J. Neurosci.* 27:3078-3089.

[93] Arlotta,P., Molyneaux,B.J., Jabaudon,D., Yoshida,Y., and Macklis,J.D. 2008. Ctip2 controls the differentiation of medium spiny neurons and the establishment of the cellular architecture of the striatum. *J. Neurosci.* 28:622-632.

[94] Tamura,S., Morikawa,Y., Iwanishi,H., Hisaoka,T., and Senba,E. 2004. Foxp1 gene expression in projection neurons of the mouse striatum. *Neuroscience* 124:261-267.

[95] Waclaw,R.R., Wang,B., Pei,Z., Ehrman,L.A., and Campbell,K. 2009. Distinct temporal requirements for the homeobox gene Gsx2 in specifying striatal and olfactory bulb neuronal fates. *Neuron* 63:451-465.

[96] Eiraku,M., Watanabe,K., Matsuo-Takasaki,M., Kawada,M., Yonemura,S., Matsumura,M., Wataya,T., Nishiyama,A., Muguruma,K., and Sasai,Y. 2008. Self-organized formation of polarized cortical tissues from ESCs and its active manipulation by extrinsic signals. *Cell Stem Cell* 3:519-532.

[97] Gaspard,N., Bouschet,T., Herpoel,A., Naeije,G., van den,A.J., and Vanderhaeghen,P. 2009. Generation of cortical neurons from mouse embryonic stem cells. *Nat. Protoc.* 4:1454-1463.

[98] Ideguchi,M., Palmer,T.D., Recht,L.D., and Weimann,J.M. 2010. Murine embryonic stem cell-derived pyramidal neurons integrate into the cerebral cortex and appropriately project axons to subcortical targets. *J. Neurosci.* 30:894-904.

[99] Jing,Y., Machon,O., Hampl,A., Dvorak,P., Xing,Y., and Krauss,S. 2011. In vitro differentiation of mouse embryonic stem cells into neurons of the dorsal forebrain. *Cell Mol. Neurobiol.* 31:715-727.

[100] Maroof,A.M., Brown,K., Shi,S.H., Studer,L., and Anderson,S.A. 2010. Prospective isolation of cortical interneuron precursors from mouse embryonic stem cells. *J. Neurosci.* 30:4667-4675.

[101] Watanabe,K., Kamiya,D., Nishiyama,A., Katayama,T., Nozaki,S., Kawasaki,H., Watanabe,Y., Mizuseki,K., and Sasai,Y. 2005. Directed differentiation of telencephalic precursors from embryonic stem cells. *Nat. Neurosci.* 8:288-296.

[102] Gaspard,N., Bouschet,T., Hourez,R., Dimidschstein,J., Naeije,G., van den,A.J., Espuny-Camacho,I., Herpoel,A., Passante,L., Schiffmann,S.N. et al 2008. An intrinsic mechanism of corticogenesis from embryonic stem cells. *Nature* 455:351-357.

[103] Eiraku,M., Watanabe,K., Matsuo-Takasaki,M., Kawada,M., Yonemura,S., Matsumura,M., Wataya,T., Nishiyama,A., Muguruma,K., and Sasai,Y. 2008. Self-organized formation of polarized cortical tissues from ESCs and its active manipulation by extrinsic signals. *Cell Stem Cell* 3:519-532.

[104] Ying,Q.L., Stavridis,M., Griffiths,D., Li,M., and Smith,A. 2003. Conversion of embryonic stem cells into neuroectodermal precursors in adherent monoculture. *Nat. Biotechnol.* 21:183-186.

[105] Joannides,A.J., Fiore-Heriche,C., Battersby,A.A., Athauda-Arachchi,P., Bouhon,I.A., Williams,L., Westmore,K., Kemp,P.J., Compston,A., Allen,N.D. et al 2007. A scaleable and defined system for generating neural stem cells from human embryonic stem cells. *Stem Cells* 25:731-737.

[106] Kirkeby,A., Grealish,S., Wolf,D.A., Nelander,J., Wood,J., Lundblad,M., Lindvall,O., and Parmar,M. 2012. Generation of Regionally Specified Neural Progenitors and Functional Neurons from Human Embryonic Stem Cells under Defined Conditions. *Cell Rep.* 1:703-714.

[107] Lavaute,T.M., Yoo,Y.D., Pankratz,M.T., Weick,J.P., Gerstner,J.R., and Zhang,S.C. 2009. Regulation of neural specification from human embryonic stem cells by BMP and FGF. *Stem Cells* 27:1741-1749.

[108] Nat,R., Nilbratt,M., Narkilahti,S., Winblad,B., Hovatta,O., and Nordberg,A. 2007. Neurogenic neuroepithelial and radial glial cells generated from six human embryonic stem cell lines in serum-free suspension and adherent cultures. *Glia* 55:385-399.

[109] Pankratz,M.T., Li,X.J., Lavaute,T.M., Lyons,E.A., Chen,X., and Zhang,S.C. 2007. Directed neural differentiation of human embryonic stem cells via an obligated primitive anterior stage. *Stem Cells* 25:1511-1520.

[110] Zhang,S.C., Wernig,M., Duncan,I.D., Brustle,O., and Thomson,J.A. 2001. In vitro differentiation of transplantable neural precursors from human embryonic stem cells. *Nat. Biotechnol.* 19:1129-1133.

[111] Aubry,L., Bugi,A., Lefort,N., Rousseau,F., Peschanski,M., and Perrier,A.L. 2008. Striatal progenitors derived from human ES cells mature into DARPP32 neurons in vitro and in quinolinic acid-lesioned rats. *Proc. Natl. Acad. Sci. U. S. A* 105:16707-16712.

[112] Elkabetz,Y., Panagiotakos,G., Al Shamy,G., Socci,N.D., Tabar,V., and Studer,L. 2008. Human ES cell-derived neural rosettes reveal a functionally distinct early neural stem cell stage. *Genes Dev.* 22:152-165.

[113] Chambers,S.M., Fasano,C.A., Papapetrou,E.P., Tomishima,M., Sadelain,M., and Studer,L. 2009. Highly efficient neural conversion of human ES and iPS cells by dual inhibition of SMAD signaling. *Nat. Biotechnol.* 27:275-280.

[114] Watanabe,K., Ueno,M., Kamiya,D., Nishiyama,A., Matsumura,M., Wataya,T., Takahashi,J.B., Nishikawa,S., Nishikawa,S., Muguruma,K. et al 2007. A ROCK inhibitor permits survival of dissociated human embryonic stem cells. *Nat. Biotechnol.* 25:681-686.

[115] Li,X.J., Zhang,X., Johnson,M.A., Wang,Z.B., Lavaute,T., and Zhang,S.C. 2009. Coordination of sonic hedgehog and Wnt signaling determines ventral and dorsal telencephalic neuron types from human embryonic stem cells. *Development* 136:4055-4063.

[116] Johnson,M.A., Weick,J.P., Pearce,R.A., and Zhang,S.C. 2007. Functional neural development from human embryonic stem cells: accelerated synaptic activity via astrocyte coculture. *J. Neurosci.* 27:3069-3077.

[117] Denham,M., Parish,C.L., Leaw,B., Wright,J., Reid,C.A., Petrou,S., Dottori,M., and Thompson,L.H. 2012. Neurons derived from human embryonic stem cells extend long-distance axonal projections through growth along host white matter tracts after intra-cerebral transplantation. *Front Cell Neurosci.* 6:11.

[118] Flandin,P., Zhao,Y., Vogt,D., Jeong,J., Long,J., Potter,G., Westphal,H., and Rubenstein,J.L. 2011. Lhx6 and Lhx8 coordinately induce neuronal expression of Shh that controls the generation of interneuron progenitors. *Neuron* 70:939-950.

[119] Liu,H., and Zhang,S.C. 2011. Specification of neuronal and glial subtypes from human pluripotent stem cells. *Cell Mol. Life Sci.* 68:3995-4008.

[120] Zeng,H., Guo,M., Martins-Taylor,K., Wang,X., Zhang,Z., Park,J.W., Zhan,S., Kronenberg,M.S., Lichtler,A., Liu,H.X. et al 2010. Specification of region-specific neurons including forebrain glutamatergic neurons from human induced pluripotent stem cells. *PLoS. One.* 5:e11853.

Chapter 11

Neural Stem/Progenitor Cells for Spinal Cord Regeneration

Ryan Salewski, Hamideh Emrani and Michael G. Fehlings

Additional information is available at the end of the chapter

1. Introduction

Central nervous system (CNS) repair and regeneration following traumatic injury or disease pathology is a widely studied and widely debated field. This book chapter will outline the pathology of spinal cord injury (SCI) with particular focus on how it lends itself to cell-based intervention. Next, we will outline the different populations of cells proposed for SCI treatment, including neural stem/progenitor cells (NSPC), and methods of generating clinically relevant NSPCs from adult tissue, embryonic stem (ES) cells and induce pluripotent stem (iPS) sources. Lastly, we will examine the use of NSPCs in SCI models with a specific focus on how the environment affects the transplanted population and how the transplanted cells modulate the spinal cord niche.

2. Pathology of spinal cord injury

Spinal cord injury (SCI) is a devastating event that significantly affects the morbidity and quality of life in adults (Average age of patients at the time of injury is 38.0 years old). [1] The prevalence of traumatic SCI worldwide is approximately 750 per million with an increasing annual incidence. [2] In order to be able to develop effective treatments for SCI, it is necessary to have a detailed understanding of the pathophysiological events that happen during SCI in the body and how they interact with each other to cause the functional deficits seen in patients. These events have complicated roles post-SCI. For example, the inflammatory response and reactive astrogliosis that are seen post-SCI have damaging *and* neuroprotective and –restorative effects. [3]

The pathophysiology of SCI is biphasic; it consists of a "primary" and a "secondary" stage. The primary injury is the result of an initial mechanical insult, which is followed by a series of cellular and molecular events that, in turn, lead to further destruction of the spinal cord tissue. It is well known that the mechanical injury seldom results in complete transection of the spinal cord. Most fracture dislocations or burst fractures of the spine result in disc displacement into and laceration or compression of the cord resulting in blood vessel, axonal and cellular membrane disruption.

Decreased blood supply to the tissue and cells of the spinal cord results in nutrient and oxygen deficiency in the injured tissue, which in turn is followed by a cascade of biochemical or "secondary" events that eventually lead to further tissue necrosis. [3-5] Thus, the primary insult precedes sequential pathological changes such as further vascular dysfunction and hemorrhage, edema, ischemia, excitotoxicity, electrolyte shifts, free radical production, inflammation, axonal and neuronal necrosis, demyelination, cyst formation and infarction. [5] The events will be discussed in further detail in following sections and are summarized in Figure 1.

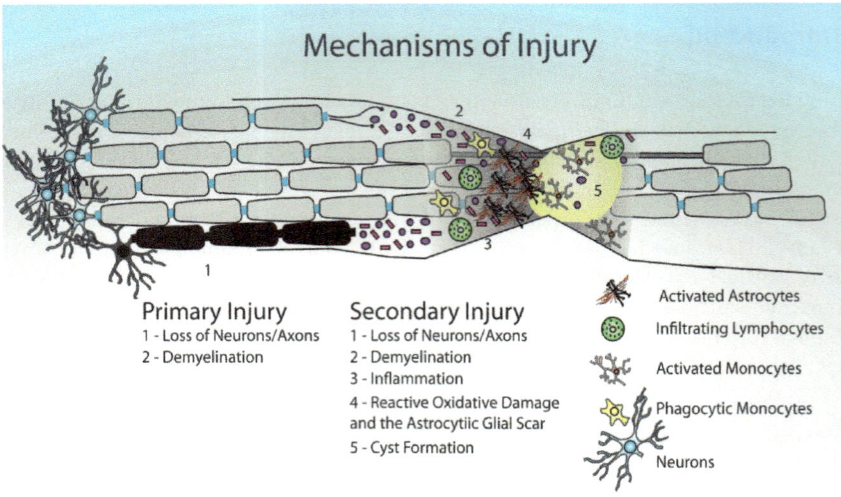

Figure 1. Mechanisms of Injury in SCI. SCI pathology results from several mechanisms occurring both concurrently and in sequence. Primary mechanical insult results in initial loss of axons (1) and demyelination (2). Subsequent secondary injury is characterized by further neuronal/axonal cell death (1) and myelin degradation (2), usually due to secondary inflammation from infiltrating lymphocytes and monocytes (3) and also reactive oxygen species secreted by activated astrocytes composing the glial scar (4). Both the glial scar (4) and post-traumatic cyst or syrinx formation (5) pro- vide physical impediments to regeneration, and cyst formation can further damage neurons by exerting physical pressure on their damaged axons. * from *Ruff and Fehlings. (2010). Panminerva Med 52:125-147, with permission*

SCI is a complex set of damaging events that occur at the cellular level and it can be divided into four main stages: the immediate, acute, intermediate, and chronic phase of SCI.[3] The first two hours post-SCI is the immediate stage during which the body is going through processes as a result of the primary injury itself. Severing of axons, neural and glial death, and spinal shock, all instantly result in loss of function below and at the level of the injury. The spinal cord becomes swollen which is accompanied by hemorrhage into the grey matter, cellular necrosis, vascular disruption and ischemia. Vascular disruption leads to further hemorrhage into the white matter and, as a result of the combined effect of edema and hemorrhage, many segments of the spinal cord, rostral and caudal to the site of injury, become ischemic. [6] Even though gross histopathological changes may not be visible at this stage, many pathophysiological events have already started. For example, activation of microglial cells and an instantaneous increase in pro-inflammatory cytokines TNFand IL and excitotoxic levels of extracellular glutamate can be detected within minutes of an injury. [3, 7, 8]

2.1. Stages SCI progression

2.1.1. Acute stage

During the acute stage of the SCI, the events of the secondary injury prevail. This is subdivided into early acute (2-48 hours) and subacute (2 days-2weeks). Vascular disruption, hemorrhage, and the resulting ischemia are central constituents of the early acute stage [5, 7], which result in the loss of normal autoregulatory mechanisms. The loss of ionic homeostasis immediately following SCI and excitotoxicity are closely related processes that each significantly contribute to the propagation of cellular injury after SCI. The ionic deregulation plays an important role in increasing necrosis and cell death following SCI. For instance, irregularity of Ca2+ concentration initiates activation of calpains and caspase cascades which in turn cause further cellular apoptosis. [9] Additionally, activated microglia express FAS ligand receptors and signaling through the p75 neurotrophin receptors that initiate the caspase and calpain cascade leading to proteolysis and DNA cleavage by effector caspases and trigger even further apoptotic cell death. [10] As a result of these events, a large number of cells, including oligodendrocytes, die. In addition to death of the neural cells, loss of calcium, sodium and potassium ionic channel homeostasis, and demyelination disrupt signal transduction in the spinal cord and result in sensorimotor inactivity and paralysis. [3-5]

The extracellular levels of glutamate rise rapidly due to direct injury to cells and failure of energy-dependent transporters, notably the Na+K+ adenosine triphosphatase membrane transporter that normally functions to regulate extracellular concentrations of ions, glutamate, and other molecules. [11] Excessive activation of glutamate receptors leads to an increase in the influx of Na+ and Ca2+ through the NMDA and alpha-amino-3-hydroxy-5-methyl-isoxazoleproprionate/kainate receptors and excitotoxicity. [12] This causes further neural and glial death.

Reactive oxygen (O2) species (ROS) is at detectable levels 12 hours after SCI and remains elevated for almost one week, returning to preinjury levels 4-5 weeks post-injury. The increased amount of ROS leads to increased membrane lipid oxidation and an increase in cellular lysis, organelle damage and Ca2+ ion concentration irregularities. [13, 14] It has been shown that Peroxynitrite, which is generated through reaction of ROS and nitric acid, is directly involved in the induction of neural apoptosis in rat SCI. [13]

The brain blood barrier (BBB) is a highly selective endothelial filter for transport of compounds in and out of the central nervous system. This becomes highly permeable as a result of the primary mechanical insult to the cord and presence of inflammatory mediators. It has been shown that peak BBB permeability occurs at 24 hours following injury in the rat and returns control levels by 2 weeks. [15] Two inflammatory mediators – TNF and IL-1 - are known to increase vascular permeability. In addition, other compounds released by glial cells or invading immune cells which are believed to play a role in increasing BBB permeability include ROS, nitric oxide, histamine, matrix metalloproteinases, and elastase. [3, 13] Additionally, disruption of the vasculature following SCI results in the breakage of the BBB, leading to an inflammatory response and infiltration of astrocytes, microglia, T cells, neutrophils, and invading monocytes. Invasion of macrophages and neutrophils to the site of injury increases cellular disruption and causes further inflammatory-triggered necrosis. Inflammation then results in activation of microglia which, together with leukocytes, cause malfunction of oxidative metabolism in demyelinated axons and proliferation of astrocytes as well as increased expression of glial fibrillary acid protein (GFAP) and the formation of a glial or astrocytic scar. [2-4] Further to this, a multitude of noncellular mediators, including TNF, interferons, and ILs play important roles.

The inflammatory response in SCI is a highly complex event with a dual nature. Some aspects of the inflammatory response further advance the secondary injury phase, while others are beneficial in removing cellular debris and starting the regenerative process [16]. For instance, TNF plays an important role in cellular death post-SCI and its inhibition has been shown to result in functional neurological recovery after SCI. However, it has also been shown to have a neuroprotective role in *in vitro* and murine models of SCI. [17, 18]

2.1.2. Subacute phase

The subacute phase lasts from 2 days to 2 weeks after the initial injury. This is the stage where it is hoped that therapeutic strategies currently in development, including cellular treatments and strategies, will be helpful. For instance, we have shown in our lab that transplantation of adult murine neural precursor cells at 2 weeks post-injury promotes remyelination and functional recovery. Such effects were not seen when the cells were transplanted at later time points or during the chronic stage of the injury. [19] Keirstead et al, have also reported the failure of transplanted human ESC-derived oligodendrocyte progenitor cells to survive, migrate and promote functional recovery when they were injected to the site of injury either at the time of injury or after the subacute phase. [20]

During the initial hours to days following SCI, astrocytes undergo cytotoxic edema and necrotic cellular death; however, a second delayed astrocytic response happens during the subacute phase. During this stage, there is a significant increase in the astrocytic intermediate filament GFAP as a result of the proliferative and hypertrophic activity of astrocytes. These reactive astrocytes form the astrocytic (gliotic) scar through their interweaving cytoplasmic processes, which becomes a physical and chemical barrier to axonal regeneration. It is important to note that in humans, there is significantly less astroglial scarring observed than is observed in rodent SCI models. [21] Other than scar formation, astrocytes also promote the reestablishment of ionic homeostasis and the integrity of the BBB, which is beneficial in decreasing edema and immune cell infiltration. [22]

During the subacute stage of the injury, there is a significantly higher phagocytic response observed in the CNS compared to the PNS. While this could partly account for the lack of regenerative ability seen in the CNS, the phagocytic response is believed to be efficient in cell debris removal and, to some extent, in promotion of axonal growth inside the lesion. [13]

2.1.3. Intermediate phase

The intermediate phase starts at two weeks and continues to 6 months post-injury. Main characteristics of this stage are continuous maturation of the gliotic scar and the start of axonal regeneration. Regenerative axonal sprouting has been observed in corticospinal tract axons in rat models of contusive SCI from 3 weeks to 3 months following injury, and reticulospinal fibers have been observed from 3 to 8 months post injury. [23] It is encouraging to observe that regenerative potential still exists in adult spinal cord, however, these regenerations have not been able to produce significant functional recovery in severe SCI.

2.1.4. Chronic phase

The chronic phase starts about 6 months after the initial SCI and lasts throughout the lifetime of the SCI patient. Further gliotic scar formation, development of cysts and syrinxes within the lesion, and continuous Wallerian degeneration of severed and injured axons are the main characteristics of this stage. [3, 23-25] Two to three years post-injury, the lesion has usually stabilized and is characterized by formation of a cyst cavity and mayelomalacia, which is the final stage of necrotic death. [26] Treatment strategies at this stage focus on rehabilitative approaches to promote plasticity, regeneration and remyelination of injured axons. Unfortunately, to date there has not been any report of the application of stem cells at this stage resulting in any significant functional improvement.

2.2. Cell-based approaches in SCI

As explained in the previous section, in the pathophysiology of SCI, some processes can be considered to be double-edged swords with both positive and negative effects and interations., These are not yet completely understood. One example of such an interaction is the astrocytic response which, on one hand results in the development of astrocytic scar limiting axonal regeneration and functional recovery, and on the other results in reestablishment of the BBB, ionic homeostasis, and decreased immune cell infiltration. What makes the pathophysiology of SCI and the translation of treatment strategies into the clinic even more complicated is its variance and uniqueness among different patients with different cases of injury. Experimental SCI models, which are mostly rodent models, consist of a homogeneous population, in contrast to the vastly heterogeneous human SCI population.

Two main aims of cell-based treatment for SCI are replacing lost or injured cells such as oligodendrocytes and neurons, or providing the cells with a microenvironment that supports or enhances the neuroprotective and regenerative ability of cells within the lesion. Stem and progenitor cells, and Schwann cells are examples of cells that are being used in studies to replace lost cells. Additionally, many studies have shown that these cells have the ability to remyelinate axons in the injury site while also providing them with supportive growth and neuroprotective factors. [1, 19, 27-29]

3. Cell populations for SCI treatment

Even though modern surgical and medical treatment approaches have dramatically decreased mortality rate due to SCI, current clinical techniques provide only modest efficacy in improving outcomes for patients, especially during the chronic stages of the disease. Thus, there is a need for new techniques that could improve recovery for SCI patients. Cell replacement strategies use stem cells because of their long-term proliferative abilities and the trophic support they provide to the regenerating tissue. In the following sections we will briefly review different types of stem cells that are being investigated as cell sources in therapeutic approaches for SCI.

3.1 Cell types used in SCI therapy

3.1.1. Mesenchymal stem cells

Multipotent mesenchymal stem cells (MSCs) are non-hematopoietic multipotential progenitor cells that were initially characterized by Caplan as cells with self-renewing capacity that can give rise to skeleton and other lineages of the mesenchyme through the mesengenic process [30, 31]. However, with the exception of a few stem cells, which are progenitors with "clonal self-renewal and multilineage potential", MSCs represent a non-homogenous population of cells and not all of the cells have the same potential for differentiation. Therefore, the International Society for Cellular Therapy (ISCT), suggests usage of the term, "Multipotent mesenchymal stromal cells", for the plastic adherent population of cells isolated from stromal tissue of bone. [32] Additionally, in 2006 Dominici et al., from the International Society for Cellular Therapy, defined a minimum set of criteria for MSCs some of which include lacking hematopoietic cell surface markers such as CD34 (endothelial marker) and CD45 (pan-leukocyte marker), and containing cell surface markers such as CD105 (endoglin), CD90 (Thy-1), and CD73 (ecto 5′ nucleotidase) and to be able to generate at least three lineages of the mesenchyme [33]. MSCs are primarily isolated from bone in adults but they also reside in adipose tissue, cartilage, synovium, periosteum, muscles and fetal tissue such as placenta and umbilical cord.

There are many studies on the application of MSCs to SCI models with variable reports on the ability of the cells to survive, integrate, and differentiate into neuronal lineages. [34] MSCs from both rats and humans have been shown to be capable of generating neural morphology and expressing neural and astrocytic markers *in vitro*. However, they have similar differentiation profiles only when transplanted into an embryonic or developing CNS. When transplanted into adult rat CNS, neither rat nor human MSCs were able to differentiate into neuronal cells. Mostly, they generated perivascular macrophages in the rat brain. [35-37]

There are other studies in which transplanted MSCs were tracked in rat or mouse injury models through GFP or electromagnetic tagging coupled with immunochemistry and MR imaging. Even though both types of studies report functional improvements, only a fraction of cells are reported to show expression of neuronal or astrocytic markers and only a very small number of cells are reported as having differentiated into neurons. [37-39] There are differing reports on the extent of MSC transplantation benefits in functional recovery. MSCs have shown to be effective at 4 weeks up to 1 year after the injury [41], depending on the timing of transplantation from the time of injury [40] to 1 week [37, 38, 41], or 3 months post injury [42]. Other studies show lack of any functional benefit observable through the Basso Beattie Bresnahan (BBB) open field locomotor scoring system. [43] However, all of the mentioned studies report on the ability of MSC transplants to preserve the injured tissue, both gray and white matter, and to provide micro environmental cues supportive of axonal growth, rather than replacing lost cells. [42, 43] Given the inconsistency seen in the results of transplanting MSCs into SCI models in rats, mice and primates, it is necessary to have a better understanding of the type of cells in the MSC population that are being transplanted[44] and investigate all the possible mechanisms behind the functional recovery observed in these models.

3.1.2. Schwann cells

Schwann cells are the myelinating cells in the peripheral nervous system. Since the first transplantation of SCs into SCI by Duncan et al. in 1981 [34], these cells have been used in many different SCI models and have been shown to be able to remyelinate axons and provide a permissive environment for them to regenerate and grow. Binge et al. [45] showed that SCs also have a small but significant effect on increasing functional recovery. However, their remyelinating and regenerating ability does not go beyond the growth-permissive surface, which explains why there is only a slight improvement in functional recovery. [3, 44-46] Additionally, it has been shown that axons in the corticospinal tract (CST) remain unaffected by SC transplants. [34] Also, they have been shown to generate a more active astrocytic response compared to other cell types such as NPCs which results in less efficient integration of these cells into the injured spinal cord. [34] As a result, the clinical application of SCs alone for SCI treatment appears extremely limited.

To overcome this limitation, many combinatorial strategies have evolved which associate SCs with growth factors or bioengineering scaffolds and other cells types to enhance recovery. [4, 47-50] Additionally, new sources for SCs are being investigated such as skin derived precursor cells from the dermis of the skin [51-54] and MSCs. [55-58] However, it is yet to be proven whether these cells hold any advantage in treating SCI compared with SCs that are derived from the PNS.

3.1.3. Olfactory ensheathing cells

OECs are glial cells derived from the olfactory bulb or lamina propria of the olfactory mucosa and are termed olfactory nerve Schwann cells due to morphological similarities to SCs. Having a lifelong capacity to proliferate and being able to facilitate passage of new axons from regenerating receptor neurons in the PNS in the olfactory mucosa to the target neurons in the CNS in the olfactory bulb glomeruli, has made them an excellent candidate for cell treatment strategies in SCI. [58, 59] They may be specifically advantageous when co-transplanted with SCs, since they can overcome SCs' limitations in passing the transplant graft and entering the injured CNS environment to produce functional synapses. [3, 60, 61]

OECs create a permissive environment for axonal growth and regeneration by interacting with the astrocytes in the glial scar and promoting angiogenesis. [62] This neuroprotective effect has led to their use in numerous clinical trials outside North America. However, they all report mixed results with none showing a significant benefit. [3, 27] Additionally, there are numerous axonal regeneration claims seen in OEC literature, which have not been confirmed by other studies and there are inconsistent reports on their regenerative capacity *in vivo*. The reasons for such discrepancies are not completely understood but could be attributed to variability in cell sources, cultures, and injury models studied. [63, 64] Thus, there is a need for further studies on the biology of OECs and more refined criteria set for isolation of these cells in order for their translation into the clinic to be feasible. [34]

3.1.4. Neural stem/progenitor cells

Neural Stem/Progenitor Cells (NSPCs) are multipotent stem cells that self-renew and differentiate into lineage-specific neural precursor cells, which can give rise to neurons, astrocytes, and oligodendrocytes through asymmetric cell division. [30] Indeed, neural precursor cells and oligodendroglial precursor cells have been shown to replace damaged cells, secrete trophic factors, regulate gliosis and scar formation, reduce cystic cavity size and axonal destruction, as well as to remyelinate axons.[3, 27, 65] However, the scarcity of adult NSPCs limits the clinical translation of transplanting these cells in injured tissue. Therefore, alternative routes to derive NSPCs have been studied.

4. Generation of NSPC from various sources

4.1. Adult tissue derived NSPCs

NSPCs can be derived from various regions along the neuroaxis during embryonic development and in adult life [66, 67]. These cells retain their mulipotentiality and can generate neural cells in culture. NPSCs have been isolated from the subependymal zone of the adult mammalian brain and from ependymal and non-ependymal regions of the adult mammalian spinal cord. [68-70] Single adult NPSCs can be isolated *in vitro* in the presence of growth factors (epithelial growth factor, EGF; fibroblast growth factor, FGF) that enable the proliferation and formation of clonally-derived free-floating colonies. The differentiation and survival of cellular subpopulations can be promoted *in vitro* by exposure to bone morphogenetic proteins (BMPs) to produce astrocytes [71, 72], insulin-like growth factor (IGF)-I, interleukin-1 (IL-1), Neuregulin-1 (Nrg-1) to generate oligodendrocyte [73, 74], and neurogenin-2 to produce neurons [75, 76].

For experimental purposes neurospheres can be generated from the germinal zone of the adult mouse brain, according to well-established techniques [77, 78]. Briefly, the subventricular zone

(SVZ) of the forebrain of mice can be dissected and transferred to a low calcium aCSF solution. Cells are plated on uncoated tissue culture flasks in serum free medium containing FGF2 and EGF for 7 days. The neurospheres are passaged weekly by mechanical dissociation in the same medium. This method of generating NSPCs has obvious clinical limitations as it requires brain tissue to generate the renewable cell population.

4.2. Embryonic stem cell (ESC) derived-NSPCs

The first isolation of a pluripotent population of cells from the mouse embryo over 30 years ago revolutionized the emerging field of regenerative medicine. [79, 80] Once a similar population of cells were identified and isolated from a human source, [81] the possibilities and potential for clinical application for the derivatives of these cells became limitless. Neurons and glial cells were among the first differentiated cells to be generated from these pluripotent cells. Although there are some differences between human and murine ES cells, such as LIF responsiveness *in vitro* [82], many of the neural differentiation protocols established for mouse ES cells have been adapted for use with human ES cells. There are multiple strategies that are implemented to generate neural cells from ES cells with varying degrees of cell homogeneity, differentiation potential, efficiency and time requirements. In general, two strategies exist to direct ES cells to NSPC: the first uses embryoid body (EB) formation to mimic the physiological neurodevelopment of the embryo and the second involves removal of all cues that would direct the cells to a non-ectoderm lineage by limiting cell-cell interactions with low cell density culture and environmental signals, with serum-free media.

4.2.1. NSPC generation with EB intermediate

Using EB intermediates to generate NSPCs and their differentiated products mimics the physiological environment that produces neuroectoderm. [83, 84] In brief, the ES cells are transferred from their expansion conditions on feeder cells to a suspension culture and allowed to form aggregates. Within a few days, the EBs formed resemble an anterior pre-streak stage embryo with an epiblast-like core. [85] At this stage the cells are still able to form cells from all three germ layers. Next conditions are such that they drive the neuroectoderm lineage while inhibiting the endoderm and mesoderm fates concentrating the NSPC population and thus yield cells that can differentiate to neurons and glial cells.

The use of retinoic acid (RA) with the EB based neuralization protocols can vastly improve the neural lineage cells produced. [86, 87] Many studies have shown that RA plays a key role during neurogenesis, both *in vitro* conditions as well as physiologically. RA treatment directs cell towards those of the posterior CNS. [88] The general culturing process involves EB formation, as described above, for 4 days, followed by RA treatment (4-/4+) and then 1 week of adherent conditions. A high proportion of the differentiated cells have neural properties, with positive identification for both glutamatergic and motor neurons. [88, 89]

Other neuralization protocols that use an EB intermediate, such as culturing with carcinoma or stromal cell-line conditioned media or via selection in defined media conditions, can be used to generate NSPCs with relatively high efficiency. [90, 91] However, a key limitation with NSPCs generated from EB intermediates exists; despite success with these approaches, concerns related to the restricted potential of NSPCs remain. The involvement of EB formation creates a risk for the persistence of non-neural cells in the final population. This has been associated with teratoma formation and increase tumorigenicity. The persistence of non-neural cell can be traced back to the non-specific differentiation pattern associated with the initial aggregation of EB.

4.2.2. NSPC generation from default pathway

In order to circumvent EB intermediates, and its limitations, during neuralization of pluripotent cells, our lab has opted to use the default pathways to direct ES cells to a neural lineage. ([92]; Figure 2) This pathway relies on the fact that, in the absence of extrinsic signaling to form non-ectoderm lineage, the cells will adopt a neuroectoderm fate. [93, 94] The default mechanism is based on studies that showed the inhibition of BMP signaling by protein inhibitors or by gene expression manipulation leads to neural lineage commitment. A small percentage (0.2%) of single ESCs cultured under serum-free, low cell density condition proliferate in the presence of LIF to form floating neurospheres of cells that express the neuroepithelial markers Nestin and Sox1, but downregulate the ES cell markers Oct4 and SSEA1. [93, 94] Moreover, a small proportion of cells derived from primary neurospheres can generate secondary colonies when subcloned, which are independent of LIF, but are dependent on FGF2. These cells have been termed definitive (dNSPC). [94]

In order to assess the clinical potential of the NSPCs generated by this method, with specific focus on SCI, our lab has extensively characterized the ES-derived dNSPCs *in vitro*. [92] In brief, ES cells were directed to primitive and definitive NSPC fates. Their mRNA profile was evaluated using RT-PCR and *in vitro* differentiation patterns were quantified and compared to aNSPCs populations isolated from the SVZ. The ES-dNSPC populations were similar to aNPCs analyzed at the mRNA level with a significant decrease in pluripotency (*Nanog, Oct4*) and stemness (*Tdgf1, Dnmt3b, Gaf3*) markers with increased transcription of neural-specific markers (*Pax6, Nestin, Olig2, Synaphysin*). The pNSPC retained many of the pluripotency and stem markers associated with undifferentiated ES cells reflecting the importance of driving the NSPC to a definitive state. To assess the *in vitro* differentiation pattern of the ES-derived NSPCs and aNSPC controls, the cells were cultured on matrigel for one week with 1% FBS media. The cells were immunolabelled for NSPCs (Nestin), neurons (BetaIII Tubulin), astrocytes (GFAP), and oligodendrocytes (Olig2, PDGFRa, CNPase). Both ES-dNSPCs and aNSPCs yielded primarily differentiated neural cells with the majority being astrocytes (~65%). The largest proportion of cells from the ES-pNSPCs were undefined or retained the NSPC marker Nestin. Although astrocytic differentiation may not be the desired cell, this differentiation into astrocytic cells demonstrates that the *in vitro* environment is very different from the *in vivo* niche.

The potential of these cells to survive, integrate, and differentiate *in vivo* is critical to evaluating their role in regenerative medicine applications. Since remyelination following SCI is a likely potential mechanism of recovery, our lab uses a dysmyelinated *Shiverer* mouse to assess the *in vivo* potential of our ES-dNSPC. *Shiverer* mice lack compact myelin basic protein (MBP) and therefore are an ideal candidate to evaluate the myelination ability of these cells. [95] In general, the Shiverer mouse, under isoflurane anaesthesia, received a T6-T7 laminectomy followed by 4 intraspinal injections of ES-dNSPC (100,000 in 2ul of media). The mice were immune suppressed with continued cyclosporine A treatment. Six weeks following transplantation the animals were perfused and spinal tissue was fixed with 4% PFA. Cryosections of tissue were immunohistochemically labeled for neural cell markers. The ES-dNSPCs were able to survive and integrate into the host tissue in a similar pattern to that previously described with aNPCs. The transplanted cells preferentially migrated to the white matter tracts and differentiated to oligodendrocytes with multiple processes that expressed MBP. The quantification of the differentiation pattern showed that the transplanted cells become primary mature APC+ oligodendrocytes with limited astroglial and neuronal fates. The variability between *in vivo* and *in vitro* differentiation potential can be attributed to the instructive nature of the spinal cord niche. The *Shiverer* spinal cord has been shown to have greater amounts of NG2-expressing oligodendrocyte progenitors. [96] The environment that leads to the excess of these progenitors is also acting on the transplanted cells. This instructive/permissive niche could be a result of signaling molecules such as GRO-1 [97] and neuregulin (NGR) [98], both of which are released by astrocytes and neurons.

ES cells are the most defined source of readily available pluripotent cells that can be used in cell-based treatment for SCI. Although, they have some safety and ethical concerns, this population will remain extremely relevant in the future of spinal cord regeneration.

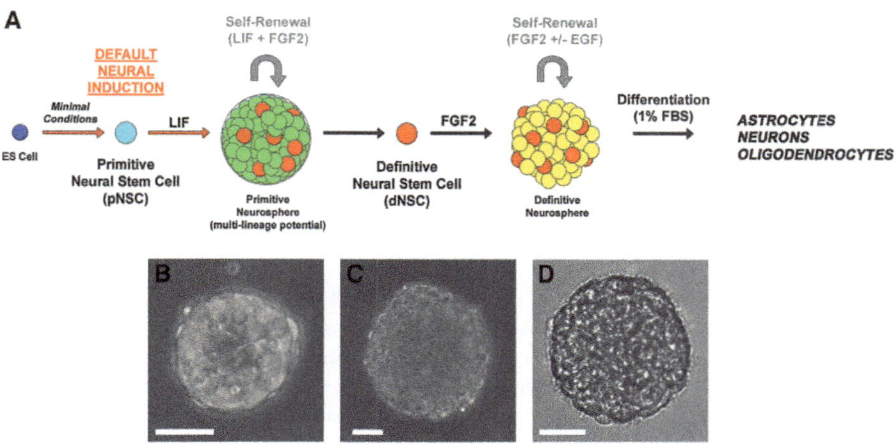

Figure 2. Default neural differentiation of embryonic stem cells. (A) Schematic representation of neural induction of ESCs through the default pathway: Individual ESCs when cultured at low density in minimal serum-free media containing LIF acquire a neural identity through a default mechanism. These neural stem cells colonies are termed pNSPCs, are LIF- dependent, and divide to form clonally-produced floating neurosphere colonies. pNSPC-derived neurospheres can be dissociated into single cells and passaged indefinitely in serum-free media containing LIF or can be passaged into serum-free media containing FGF2 to produce a distinct population of FGF2-dependent cells termed dNSPCs that also divide to form clonally-produced neurospheres. These spheres can also be passaged indefinitely and when differentiated produce all three cell types of the neural lineage. (B) Phase-contrast image of a neurosphere colony generated by a pNSPC. (C) Phase-contrast image of a neurosphere colony generated by a dNSPC. (D) Phase-contrast image of a neurosphere generated by adult neural stem cells derived from the subependymal layer of the adult mouse forebrain. For B–D, bar equals 50 mm. ESCs, embryonic stem cells; LIF, leukemia inhibitory factor; dNSPC, definitve neural stem cell; pNSPC, primitive neural stem cell; FGF2, basic fibroblast growth factor; Olig2, oligodendrocyte transcription factor 2. *from *Rowland et al., 2011, Stem cell and Develop. 20(11); 1829-1845, with permission.*

4.3. Induced pluripotent stem cells (IPSC) derived NSPCs

Given the aforementioned concerns with ES cells combined with the immunogenicity that arises from allograft transplantation, the search for a patient-specific and accessible cell source has been a principle endeavor of regenerative medicine. Historically, many techniques and strategies have been developed to accomplish this aim, most notably somatic cell nuclear transfers (SCNT). SCNT is the process by which the nucleus of the somatic cell being reprogrammed is transferred to an enucleated ooctye [99]. This technique became famous in the late 1990s when Dr. Ian Wilmut cloned the first mammal, a sheep named "Dolly". [100] Although there is no obvious mechanism that would preclude SCNT from reprogramming human cells, this technique has yet to be successfully applied in human cells. Furthermore, the requirement for donor ooctyes, combined with an inefficient and technically difficult processes makes SCNT unlikely to be a viable option for clinical application even in the most ideal circumstances.

The discovery of IPS cell technology has made a significant stride towards realizing the promise of patient-specific regenerative medicine. IPS cells are somatic cells that have been reprogrammed to ectopically express certain transcription factors that induce an ES cell-like state, in terms of their differentiation potential and response to *in vitro* culture conditions. [28] This technology allows for a constant and relatively easy method of generating cells for autologous transplantation from readily available cell sources such as skin cells. In 2006, Takahashi and Yamanaka used retrovirus transfected with 24 transcription factors in mouse embryonic fibroblasts (MEF). [101] Through careful elimination they were able to reduce the required genes to four: OCT4, Sox2, KLF4 and c-myc. The expression of these four genes was sufficient to revert the MEFs to an undifferentiated, pluripotent state that was verified using teratoma formation and contribution to a chimeric mouse. Since the initial characterization of the iPS cells there has been a tremendous amount of research further expand and refine the technology. The Yamanaka factors have been used to reprogrammed various cells from tissues from a variety of species including mice [101], rats [102], rhesus monkeys [103], and humans [104-107].

The first generation of iPS cell technology is not without its shortcomings and clinical obstacles. The process of reprogramming can be slow and inefficient and includes oncogenic potential of the factors themselves, insertion mutatgenesis, and the risks associated with the use of viral vectors. All of this can contribute to limited clinical translational potential. Fortunately, substantial research has rapidly developed iPS techniques that are viral vector and mutation free. For example, piggyBac transposition is a viral-free system that can be used to deliver the reprogramming factors in both human and mice fibroblasts [108, 109]. A single transposon containing all four iPS transcription factors is introduced to the cells and reprogrammed colonies are selected. IPS cell lines with a single insertion site are identified and transposon is seamlessly excised yielding stable, reprogrammed cell lines that are do not contain any exogenous DNA or have any insertion mutation. Other viral-free and mutation-free methods exist including using lentiviruses [110, 111],an episomal system [112], and the use of recombinant proteins [113], to generate more clinically relevant iPS cells.

Even with the advancement in iPS cell generation, intrinsic differences between ES and iPS cells exist. IPS and ES are often described as "indistinguishable", however, key differences have been identified. The initial characterization of the iPS cells from Takahashi and Yamanaka noted variation in global gene expression as well as differences in epigenetic characters, specifically histone methylation.[101] Epigenetic memory of iPS cells can influence the differentiation potential and the differentiation of the iPS cells, favouring the identity of the tissue of origin. [114] The impact of epigenetic variability still remains an area of debate and methods to optimize iPS cells are underway.

4.3.1. Neuralization of IPS cells

The conceptual outline of how iPS cells may be used in the treatment of SCI is described in figure 3. [28] Many of the *in vitro* neuralization protocols outlined above for generating NSPCs and terminally differentiated neural cells, neurons, astroglia and oligodendrocyte, from ES cells can be applied to iPS cells. iPS cell have been used in models of Parkinson's [110, 115], spinal muscular atrophy (SMA) [116], amyotrophic lateral sclerosis (ALS) [117], and SCI [118]. Although there have been positive results using iPS-derived neural cells for cell-based treatment, the variation in iPS cells has resulted in variability in the safety and neuralization of these cells. A comprehensive evaluation of NSPCs from mouse iPS cell lines generated from various tissue sources and reprogramming methods has shown differences in tumorigenesis between iPS cell lines compared to NSPCs from ES cell lines. [119]

4.3.2. Improving the IPS neuralization using NOTCH pathway agonism

The variation in neuralization potential between iPS cell lines and their ES cell counterparts represents an area of regenerative medicine that, if not addressed, could be an obstacle to clinical translation. Our lab specifically examined the difference in neuralization potential of multiple iPS cells lines. [120] We used iPS cells generated using piggyBac transposon technology to eliminate variation that could be attributed to the resurgence of the silenced transgenes or due to insertion mutations. [108, 109] Furthermore, the default pathway of neuralization was utilized to avoid issues associated with the EB formation as an intermediate step in generating NSPCs from a pluripotent cell source. Even with the additional precautions to help generate safe and clinically-relevant cells, there was retention of plurioptency markers as well as persistence of non-ectoderm lineage markers. In order for the potential for iPS technology to be realized, methods to effectively and consistently generate definitive cells must be developed.

We examined the role of BMP antagonism during the initial neuralization of the pluripotent IPS cells. We identited this as a possible area where IPS cell neuralization could be improved. Noggin, a BMP antagonist, has previously been shown to increase the number of neurospheres generated using the default pathway and ESCs.[94] BMPs are involved in directing pluripotent cells to an endoderm lineage fate. Although the inclusion of Noggin during the *in vitro* culture of primary primitive NSPCs did increase the number of neurospheres, it did not affect the character of the NSPCs as determined by a battery of gene markers analyzed by RT-PCR. Furthermore, there was no difference on the subsequent mRNA profile between definitive NSPCs with or without Noggin treatment. These data led us to conclusion that the variability in the PB-IPS cells' response to the default pathway is not a result of poor initial neuralization but likely due to incomplete transition from primitive NSPC to definitive NSPCs state.

The NOTCH pathway has been shown to be involved in many aspects of neurodevelopment and its role persists in the adult CNS. [121, 122] Disruption in NOTCH signaling leads to a reduction in NSPCs while conversely the induction of this pathway promotes NSPCs *in vivo.* [123, 124] The NSPC niche of the SVZ expresses receptors and ligands of the NOTCH pathway. [125] Delta-like ligands (DLL) or Jagged are the principle ligands of the NOTCH pathway, and interact with the membrane-bound NOTCH receptor. The NOTCH intracellular domain (NICD) is cleaved by gamme-sectrase. NICD is translocated to the nucleus to facilitate the transcription of targets such as Hair and enhancer of split, HES genes. [126] Furthermore, NOTCH appears to play a critical role in transition from primitive to definitive neural state. Primitive NSPCs were readily generated in LIF-dependent culture conditions from ES cells as well as NSPCs isolated from E7.5 embyros from NOTCH-deficient sources. However, passage of these cells to a definitive state was disrupted indicating a crucial role for NOTCH. [124, 127] Using these data we hypothesized that agonizing the NOTCH pathway during the neuralization of PB-iPSs would improve the neural character of the definitive NSPCs generated and thus, improve the clinical relevance and translation potential of the cells.

We demonstrated that the addition of recombinant mouse DLL4 to the definitive culture conditions of the default pathway of neuralization improved the generation of definitive NSPCs compare to those cells grown in parallel using standard default conditions. [120] DLL4 was selected to this pathway since DLL4 is most avid ligand for the NOTCH1 receptor.[128] The definitive neurospheres treated with DLL4 produced a greater number of spheres that retained a free-floating phenotype while untreated spheres showed extensive adhesion and signs of differentiation. Also, the mRNA profile of the DLL4 treated dNSPC showed a reduction in pluripotency markers *(Lin28, Nanog, Oct3/4)* as well as reduction or elimination of endodermal markers (*Gata6, Afp*) compared to control cells. This pattern was confirmed at the protein level with immuncytochemistry. The dNSPCs were also cultured in chamberslides matrigel in SFM containing 1% FBS to induce the differentiation of the cells. The differentiation profile of the DLL4-treated definitive NSPCs reflected the ES-derived dNSPCs as well as aNSPCs. Primarily differentiated neural cells were identified following 1 week of differentiation with mostly GFAP+ astrocytes in the iPS-dNSPC(+DLL4) group compared to non-treated iPS-dNSPCs that were primarily positive for the undifferentiated NSPC marker Nestin or were not labeled by any of the neural markers used. Lastly, the neurons, oligodendrocytes and astrocytes from DLL4-treated dNSPCs were shown to be electrophysiologically functional.

In addition to the NOTCH pathway, Sonic Hedgehog (SHH) and WNT signaling are both known to play roles in neurodevelopment. These pathways have been shown to have independent and interconnected mechanisms of action and there is evidence of considerable crosstalk with NOTCH signaling. SHH expression can be up-regulated in a time dependent profile with the Jagged1 in NSPCs *in vitro.* [125] WNT signaling has been shown to influence the transition of primitive NSPCs to definitive state through the manipulation of *Hes* expression. [129, 130]

iPS cell technology combined with the default pathway of neuralization has tremendous potential to revolutionize the treatment of SCI. Patients could someday use their own skin cells to regenerate and repair their injury (Figure 3).

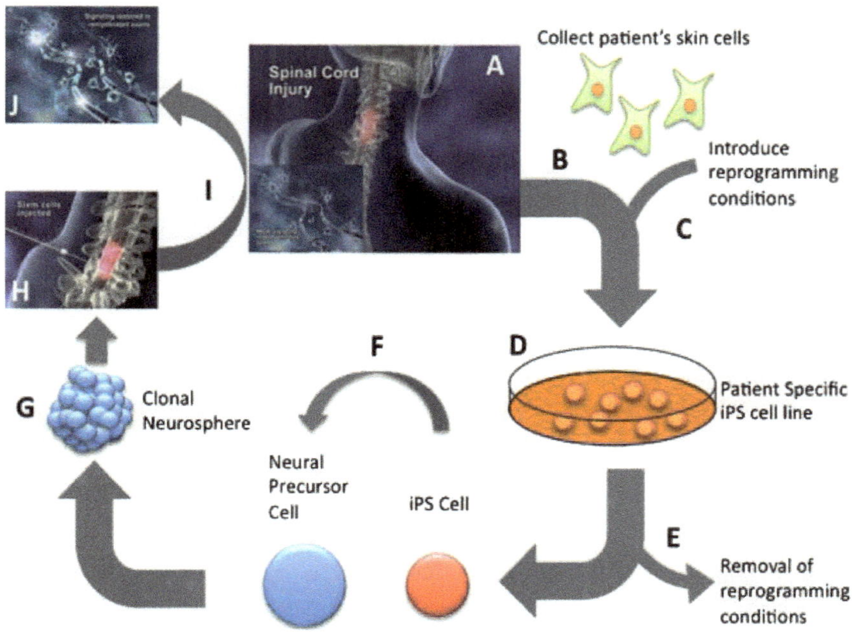

Figure 3. A general schematic representation of the generation of iPS cells, the promotion of neural precursor cells, and their use in spinal cord remyelination. A: Following a spinal cord injury, demyelination occurs resulting in vulnerable axons and impaired CNS function. B: The patient's fibroblasts, or skin cells, are harvested. C: Reprogramming conditions/factors are introduced to induce self-renewal and pluripotency properties. D: The cells are now iPS cells. E: When full and independent reprogramming is achieved, reprogramming condition/factors are removed. F: Neuralization of the iPS cell to NPCs under minimal conditions. G: Growth factors (i.e., FGF) further differentiate the cells to become definitive neurospheres. H: iPS cell-derived neural stem/precursor cells can be injected into the injured spinal cord. I: Once transplanted, these cells can differentiate CNS cells such as myelinating oligodendrocytes. J: iPS-NPC-mediated remyelination, or by some unidentified neuroprotective effect, can result in functional recovery following spinal cord injury. * from *Salewski et al., 2010, J. Cell Physiol. 222; 515-521, with permission*

5. Transplantation of neural stem/progenitor cells into the injured spinal cord

5.1. Model of SCI and NSPC transplantation

The *in vivo* regenerative and neuroprotective effect of the cell-based treatments must be evaluated in preclinical animal models. The rodent clip compression model of SCI developed in our lab mimics injuries observed in human SCI, in terms of primary and secondary injury processes and, in particular, with regards to lesion and cavity formation. This creates a situation where we can optimize the cell culture and transplantation paradigm while extensively characterizing and evaluating the safety and efficiency of our NSPCs in a clinically relevant small animal model prior to their implementation into larger animal models or a clinical trial.

In general, our SCI model involves injured rats that receive a clip compression injury of spinal cord either at the cervical or thoracic level. [19, 65] The model characteristics, histopathology, assessment of axonal integrity, molecular examination of axonal structure, and behavioural assessment have been extensively characterized. [131-134] This model of moderately severe SCI, results in a central cavitation and loss of 80% of axons in the spinal cord white matter, demyelination of the surviving axons in the residual subpial rim and spastic paraparesis. Following acute (2 week) or chronic (6 weeks) SCI, we have administered four intraspinal injections of aNSPCs in growth media to the rats at locations 2mm caudal and 2mm rostral to the injury site. To enhance the survival of the transplanted cells, growth factors [PDGF-AA bFGF and EGF] in a solution containing aCSF, BSA (100 μg/ml) and gentamycine (50 μg/ml) has been infused intrathecally to the area of transplantation for 7 days using a microcatheter connected to an osmotic minipump. A battery of behavioural tests, histological outcomes and electrophysiological measures are used to determine the therapeutic effect aNPC transplantation.

5.2. Effect of transplant on subacute and chronic injury

In our study of subacute intervention following SCI, transplantation was delayed to two weeks following injury. [19] The animals were examined using a number of measures of locomotor function, including the BBB scale, ladder walk analysis and gait/coordination assessment, for eight weeks post-SCI. At the eight week endpoint of the experiment, the animals were euthanized and their tissue collected for histological and electron microscopy.

The transplanted NSPCs had substantial survival (~40%) in the spinal cord when the growth factor mini osmotic pump was used and these cells demonstrated multipotency. In contrast to their *in vitro* differentiation profile, the transplanted cells mostly became oligodendrocytes in the injured spinal cord. In fact, the cells preferentially migrated to the white matter tract and showed extensive myelination. ([19]; Figure 4) The role of myelination will be fully addressed when we discuss potential mechanisms of neuroprotection/neurorepair. Behavioral and functional benefits from aNSPC engraftment were observed. There was significant locomotor recovery compared to the injured control groups. The BBB is a 21 point scale that is used to evaluate hindlimb locomotion in an open field. [43] Immediately following the SCI, all rats were fully paraplegic and exhibited no hindlimb function. The control rats were able to recover to a BBB score of 8, denoting plantar placement of the paw without weight support. The experimental group that received the aNSPC treatment was able to reach a score of 10 on the BBB. Although a 2-point increase may seem negligible, the BBB is a non-linear scale and these animals show occasional weight supported plantar stepping which is a substantial functional improvement. Furthermore, the animals that received the transplanted cells show improvement on other independent behavioral tests including grid walk and footprint tests. Our results show that the improved recovery of locomotor function in the transplanted groups was a result of the effects of the aNPCs since there was no significant difference in the walking ability of the plain injured or sham controls in all behavioral tests used.

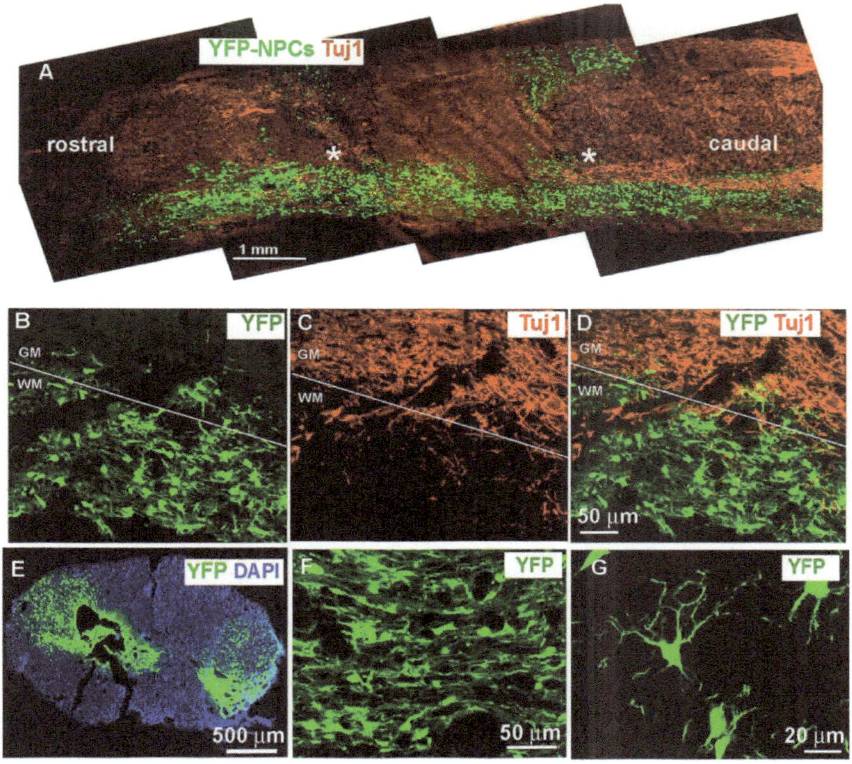

Figure 4. YFP-NPCs in the spinal cord of a subacutely injured rat 8 weeks after transplantation. A, A confocal image from a longitudinal section of an injured spinal cord taken from the dorsal spinal cord of a transplanted rat above the central cavity. A low-magnified image shows the extent of YFP-NPC survival within the injured spinal cord 8 weeks after transplantation. Grafted YFP-NPCs (green) were dispersed along the rostrocaudal axis of the spinal cord 5 mm away from the implantation sites (*). YFP-NPCs also migrated to the contralateral site of the spinal cord to a lesser extent. Double labeling with the neuronal marker betaIII tubulin (Tuj1) showed that YFP-NPCs reside predominantly in the white-matter area (A–D). Our histological data showed no signs of tumor formation in the spinal cord. E, Confocal image of a transverse section of the spinal cord from a transplanted rat (8 weeks after transplantation) showing the distribution of YFP-NPCs in the lateral columns. F, G, YFP cells mainly showed multipolar morphology and extended numerous branches in the white-matter tissue along the length of axons. WM, White matter; GM, gray matter. * from *Karimi-Abdolrezaee et al, 2006, J Neurosci 26:3377-3389, with permission*

The successful implementation of the NSPC therapy in the subacute model is a key step forward in spinal cord regenerative medicine. It has a relevant therapeutic window, although narrow, and requires intervention shortly after the initial injury. The chronic injured population represents a large section of the SCI community and currently many of the proposed treatments cannot be used to repair their injuries. The chronic injured environment is characterized by many additional challenges including cell loss, a cystic cavity and the inhibitory influences of the glial scar. [65]

We noted that when aNSPCs were transplanted at 6 weeks post-SCI, the chronically injured spinal cord was not an hospitable environment. To address this, we examined methods to modify the SCI environment to create a permissive environment. Our data suggested that expression of chondroitin sulfate proteoglycans (CSPG) reduces the survival and thus, the therapeutic potential of our aNPC treatment. [65] Chondroitinase ABC (ChABC) was administered to the chronic SCI environment to breakdown CSPGs that were upregulated as a result of the injury. We then analyzed the synergistic effect of the transplanted aNSPCs with ChABC and growth factor pump on the repair and plasticity of the chronically injured spinal cord. Survival, integration and migration of the transplanted cells in the chronic SCI with ChABC was extensive compare to treatment without ChABC and growth factors where survival was low and the transplanted cells remained at the injection site. ([65]; Figure 5) The differentiation potential of the aNSPCs was similar to that observed in the subacute injury/transplanted paradigm with the majority of cells displaying oligodendrocyte markers. There was also improvement observed at the functional locomotor level. The animals that received the combinatorial treatment of ChABC followed by aNSPCs and GF pump had a significant improvement on the BBB scale as well as with ladder-walk analysis. These behavioral improvements were also linked to neuroanatomical changes associated with the aNPC therapy. This is the first successful application of an aNSPC-based treatment for chronic SCI and represents a critical step forward improving the lives of patient currently living with SCI.

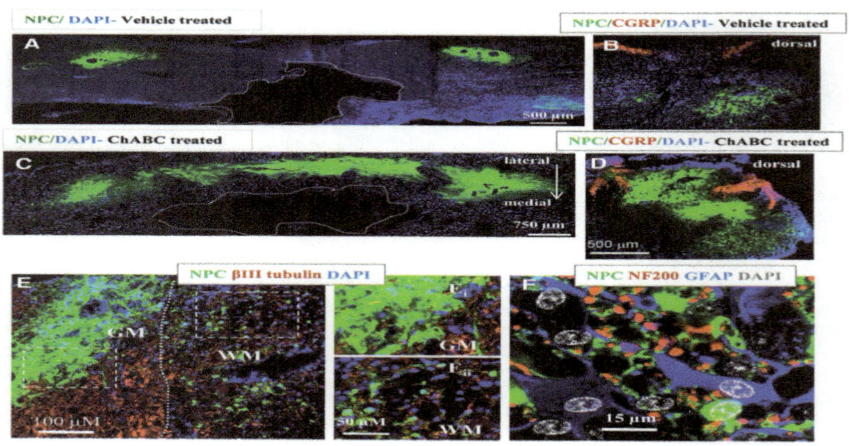

Figure 5. ChABC treatment greatly optimizes NPC transplantation in the chronically injured spinal cord. A–D, Confocal images of longitudinal and cross sections of chronically injured spinal cord transplanted with NPCs at 9 weeks after transplantation show a significant increase in the number of surviving NPCs (green) in ChABC-treated spinal cord (C,D) compared to the vehicle-treated spinal cords (A, B). D, The majority of NPCs integrated within white matter areas including dorsal, lateral, and ventral columns. Quantification of transplant volume revealed a 6.2-fold increase in ChABC-treated rats (n6, 3.70.79mm3) compared to vehicle-treated rats (n6, 0.60.24mm3) (p0.01, Student's t test). NPC cell survival analysis also showed a 5.7-fold increase in number of surviving NPCs (YFP/DAPI-positive cells) in ChABC-treated rats (28.256.77%) relative to the vehicle-treated ones (4.91.96%) (p0.01, Student's t test). ChABC treatment resulted in a significant increase in rostral and caudal migration of NPCs from the injection sites (4.20.50mm)

compared to vehicle treatment (1.40.4mm)(p0.001, Student's t test). We also found a 4.6-fold increase in the total length of rostrocaudal distribution of NPCs in ChABC-treated rats (13.02mmin the best case, average 8.321.5 mm) compared to vehicle-treated rats (2.24mminthe best case, average 1.820.5mm)(p0.005, Student's t test). * *from Karimi-Abdolrezaee et al, 2010, J Neurosci 30:1657-1676., with permission*

5.3. Possible mechanism of neurorepair/neuroprotection

Although our lab and others have clearly shown that cell-based therapies for SCI can be beneficial, the mechanisms by which the benefits are achieved still remains an area of debate. Trophic factor support [40, 135-137] and remyelination [19, 27, 65] as well as other mechanisms including plasticity and axon integrity have been suggested as possible mechanisms of recovery with cell-based treatments for SCI.

5.3.1. Trophic factor support

Trophin delivery as a potential mechanism of benefit in cell-based treatments, such as the use of bone marrow stromal cells (BMSC) following trauma, was first proposed in response to evidence that there was a degree of neuroprotection despite a lack of survival of transplanted cells. [40, 135-137] Trophic factors have been shown to have apoptotic effects[138], enhance axonal regrowth[139], promote endogenous remyelination[140, 141], and neuronal plasticity[142, 143]. BMSCs as well as aNSPCs have been shown by our lab and others to produces these trophic factors *in vitro*, however little evidence to show their involvement *in vivo* has been shown. [144]

To study trophin production and involvement *in vivo*, we examine both brain- and spinal-derived NPCs, compared them to BMSCs, and transplanted them into injured rat spinal cords. [145] Candidate trophic factor (NGF, BDNF, NT-3, NT-4/5, GDNF, CNTF, PDGF-A, EGF, bFGF, LIF, IGF-1, GGF2, TGF-b1, VEGF-A) expression was examined in spinal tissue homogenates as well as specifically in the transplanted cell population by FAC sorting for the eGFP labeled cells. The neurotrophin levels were increased following SCI and the transplantation of aNSPC with GF pump further elevated specific trophic factors, in particular, GDNF, LIF and bFGF. Furthermore, the analysis of the FAC sorted transplanted population of aNSPC showed increased neurotrophin production, specifically CNTF, EGF and bFGF. The study was the first to shown that both changes in the host tissue as well as the transplanted aNSPCs can influence trophic factor levels *in vivo*. Although further research is required to determine if trophic factor support is the sole mechanism that conveys neuro-protection or neuro-repair, our research does shows that it is a likely contributing factor to the functional improvements observed.

5.3.2. Remyelination

Myelin is a critical component of the CNS and is required for its proper functioning. Myelin is needed for the precise molecular organization of the axon, particularly with regards to nodal architecture. The arrangement of Na+ channels, K+ channels and contactin-associated protein at and around the nodes of Ranvier is closely linked to myelin, and a disruption in myelination results in loss of nodal organization. Furthermore, following SCI there is extensive loss of white matter and often otherwise functional axons are bare and rendered useless. In this situation, restoring the myelination of these axons can have large effects on the overall outcome and locomotor function since relatively few spared axons can have a tremendous effect on improving neural outcomes.

These data suggest that the remyelination could be the mechanism by which aNSPC transplantation is able to repair the injured spinal cord. Following our subacute intervention as well as chronic injury with combinatorial therapy, we observed migration of engrafted cells to white matter tracts, mature oligodendrocytic differentiation and expression of myelin basic protein (MBP) by these cells associated with axons. ([19]; Figure 6) Furthermore, the exogenous myelination was confirmed by electron microscopy to form multilayer compact myelin around axons and to restore the nodal architecture as shown by immune labeling for Kv1.2 and panKa.

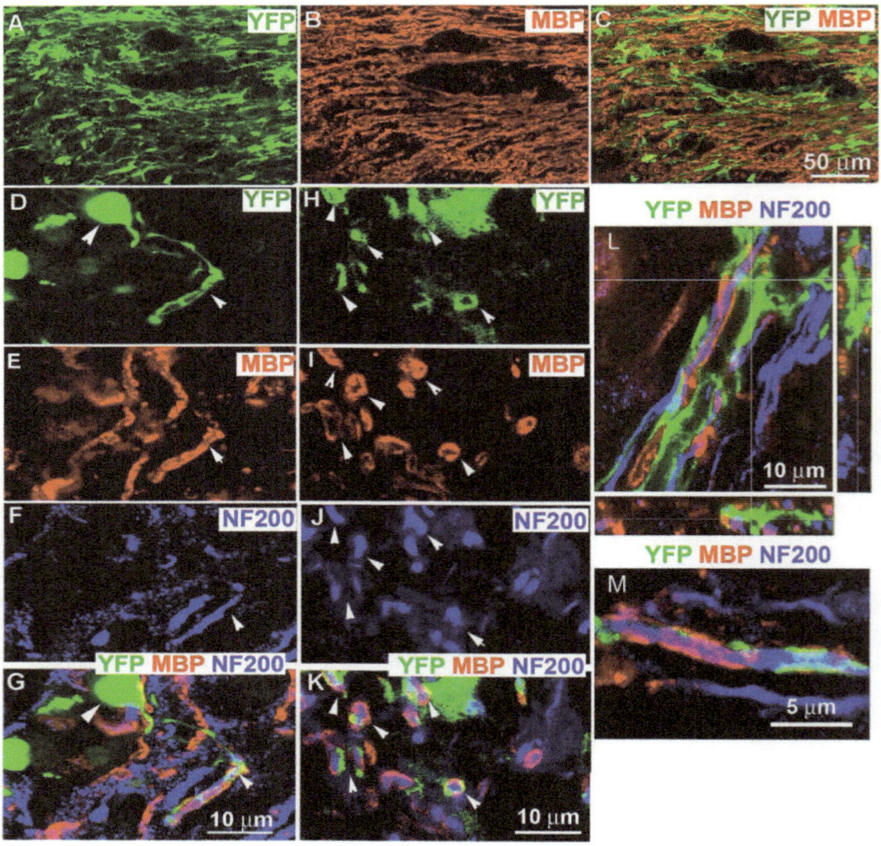

Figure 6. Exogenous remyelination following subscute SCI with aNSPC transplantation: YFP-NPC-derived oligodendrocytes generate MBP and ensheath the injured axons of the spinal cord. A–C, Confocal images of longitudinal sections of an injured spinal cord 8 weeks after transplantation. The area grafted with YFP-NPCs (green) displays a

robust expression of MBP (red) in the white matter of an injured spinal cord. Cell bodies of donor cells are surrounded with MBP. Triple-labeling experiments on longitudinal (D–G) and cross (H–K) sections of spinal cord white matter showed that MBP-expressing YFP-NPCs ensheathed the injured axons (identified by NF200; blue). These images (D–G) clearly show the oligodendrocyte morphology of one grafted YFP cell (arrowheads) that extends its processes and expresses MBP around an injured axon and the close proximity of these cells with newly myelinated axons. L, M, Images taken by deconvolution confocal microscopy show a higher-magnification image confirming axonal ensheathment of MBP-expressing YFP-NPCs around the injured axons. *from *Karimi-Abdolrezaee et al, 2006, J Neurosci 26:3377-3389, with permission*

Although exogenous myelination has been proposed as a mechanism for aNSPC-mediated recovery, potential endogenous myelination cannot be ruled out. There is still extensive research required to delineate the precise role of remyelination and specifically the role of remyelination induced by transplanted cells.

5.3.3. Other mechanisms

In addition to the roles of trophic support and myelination, other mechanisms have been proposed. It is possible that effects on axon integrity and neuronal plasticity play key roles in SCI recovery. We noted positive effects in these areas following our combinatorial strategy of ChABC and aNSPC in the chronically injured spinal cord.[65] Cortiospinal tract (CST) labeling using PKC-g and anterograde tracing showed evidence of enhanced axonal integrity and collateral spouting. This phenomena was seen only at the local level with long-distance CST regeneration beyond the lesion not observed. Promotion of plasticity of serontonergic (5HT) fibers was observed with ChABC and aNSPC therapy as noted by a significant increase in its immunointensity rostral to the injury epicenter. The 5HT positive fibers were observed in areas of aNSPC engraftment. Many mechanisms are likely working in concert to elicit the behavioral and functional outcomes observed by our lab and others after application of aNSPC therapy.

6. Conclusions

Spinal cord injury pathology creates a situation where cell-based interventions are attractive as potential treatments to promote repair and regeneration. There are a variety of cell sources available for this aim, however, in our research experience, NSPCs are the most likely to provide lasting and appropriate neurological recovery. Both adult brain and spinal tissue are sources of NSPCs for transplantation along with the pluripotent cells (ESC and iPSC) when differentiated *in vitro* to a restricted NSPC identity. Once transplanted into the injured spinal cord, the spinal niche directs the NSPCs to terminally differentiated neural cell types, both neuronal and glial. Our work suggests remyelination via oligodendrocytes is the principal mechanism of recovery although trophic support as well as neuronal lineages that are created are other possible mechanisms by which NSPC treatment is beneficial in SCI. Our results with chronic SCI, which is characterized by cavitation and glial scarring, has shown that stem cell therapy alone may be of limited benefit. Thus, combinatorial stem cell approaches with bioengineered strategies, such as use of chondroitinase, will be a key area of future research in the field of neuro-regenerative medicine.

Author details

Ryan Salewski[1], Hamideh Emrani[1] and Michael G. Fehlings[2]

1 Toronto Western Research Institute, University Health Network, Toronto Western Hospital, Canada

2 Division of Neurosurgery and Spinal Program University of Toronto; Krembil Neuroscience Centre, UHN, Toronto Western Hospital, Canada

References

[1] Eftekharpour E, S Karimi-Abdolrezaee and MG Fehlings. (2008). Current status of experimental cell replacement approaches to spinal cord injury. Neurosurg Focus 24:E19.

[2] Wyndaele M and JJ Wyndaele. (2006). Incidence, prevalence and epidemiology of spinal cord injury: what learns a worldwide literature survey? Spinal Cord 44:523-529.

[3] Rowland JW, GW Hawryluk, B Kwon and MG Fehlings. (2008). Current status of acute spinal cord injury pathophysiology and emerging therapies: promise on the horizon. Neurosurg Focus 25:E2.

[4] Ruff CA and MG Fehlings. (2010). Neural stem cells in regenerative medicine: bridging the gap. Panminerva Med 52:125-147.

[5] Tator CH and MG Fehlings. (1991). Review of the secondary injury theory of acute spinal cord trauma with emphasis on vascular mechanisms. J Neurosurg 75:15-26.

[6] Kakulas BA. (2004). Neuropathology: the foundation for new treatments in spinal cord injury. Spinal Cord 42:549-563.

[7] Tator CH and I Koyanagi. (1997). Vascular mechanisms in the pathophysiology of human spinal cord injury. J Neurosurg 86:483-492.

[8] Pineau I and S Lacroix. (2007). Proinflammatory cytokine synthesis in the injured mouse spinal cord: multiphasic expression pattern and identification of the cell types involved. J Comp Neurol 500:267-285.

[9] Schanne FA, AB Kane, EE Young and JL Farber. (1979). Calcium dependence of toxic cell death: a final common pathway. Science 206:700-702.

[10] Nagata S and P Golstein. (1995). The Fas death factor. Science 267:1449-1456.

[11] Lipton SA and PA Rosenberg. (1994). Excitatory amino acids as a final common pathway for neurologic disorders. N Engl J Med 330:613-622.

[12] Park E, AA Velumian and MG Fehlings. (2004). The role of excitotoxicity in secondary mechanisms of spinal cord injury: a review with an emphasis on the implications for white matter degeneration. J Neurotrauma 21:754-774.

[13] Donnelly DJ and PG Popovich. (2008). Inflammation and its role in neuroprotection, axonal regeneration and functional recovery after spinal cord injury. Exp Neurol 209:378-388.

[14] Xiong Y, AG Rabchevsky and ED Hall. (2007). Role of peroxynitrite in secondary oxidative damage after spinal cord injury. J Neurochem 100:639-649.

[15] Noble LJ and JR Wrathall. (1989). Distribution and time course of protein extravasation in the rat spinal cord after contusive injury. Brain Res 482:57-66.

[16] Fleming JC, MD Norenberg, DA Ramsay, GA Dekaban, AE Marcillo, AD Saenz, M Pasquale-Styles, WD Dietrich and LC Weaver. (2006). The cellular inflammatory response in human spinal cords after injury. Brain 129:3249-3269.

[17] Cheng B, S Christakos and MP Mattson. (1994). Tumor necrosis factors protect neurons against metabolic-excitotoxic insults and promote maintenance of calcium homeostasis. Neuron 12:139-153.

[18] Kim GM, J Xu, SK Song, P Yan, G Ku, XM Xu and CY Hsu. (2001). Tumor necrosis factor receptor deletion reduces nuclear factor-kappaB activation, cellular inhibitor of apoptosis protein 2 expression, and functional recovery after traumatic spinal cord injury. J Neurosci 21:6617-6625.

[19] Karimi-Abdolrezaee S, E Eftekharpour, J Wang, CM Morshead and MG Fehlings. (2006). Delayed transplantation of adult neural precursor cells promotes remyelination and functional neurological recovery after spinal cord injury. J Neurosci 26:3377-3389.

[20] Keirstead HS, G Nistor, G Bernal, M Totoiu, F Cloutier, K Sharp and O Steward. (2005). Human embryonic stem cell-derived oligodendrocyte progenitor cell transplants remyelinate and restore locomotion after spinal cord injury. J Neurosci 25:4694-4705.

[21] Hagg T and M Oudega. (2006). Degenerative and spontaneous regenerative processes after spinal cord injury. J Neurotrauma 23:264-280.

[22] Herrmann JE, T Imura, B Song, J Qi, Y Ao, TK Nguyen, RA Korsak, K Takeda, S Akira and MV Sofroniew. (2008). STAT3 is a critical regulator of astrogliosis and scar formation after spinal cord injury. J Neurosci 28:7231-7243.

[23] Hill CE, MS Beattie and JC Bresnahan. (2001). Degeneration and sprouting of identified descending supraspinal axons after contusive spinal cord injury in the rat. Exp Neurol 171:153-169.

[24] Ehlers MD. (2004). Deconstructing the axon: Wallerian degeneration and the ubiquitin-proteasome system. Trends Neurosci 27:3-6.

[25] Coleman MP and VH Perry. (2002). Axon pathology in neurological disease: a neglected therapeutic target. Trends Neurosci 25:532-537.

[26] McDonald JW, D Becker, CL Sadowsky, JA Jane, Sr., TE Conturo and LM Schultz. (2002). Late recovery following spinal cord injury. Case report and review of the literature. J Neurosurg 97:252-265.

[27] Eftekharpour E, S Karimi-Abdolrezaee, J Wang, H El Beheiry, C Morshead and MG Fehlings. (2007). Myelination of congenitally dysmyelinated spinal cord axons by adult neural precursor cells results in formation of nodes of Ranvier and improved axonal conduction. J Neurosci 27:3416-3428.

[28] Salewski RP, E Eftekharpour and MG Fehlings. (2010). Are induced pluripotent stem cells the future of cell-based regenerative therapies for spinal cord injury? J Cell Physiol 222:515-521.

[29] Hawryluk GW, J Rowland, BK Kwon and MG Fehlings. (2008). Protection and repair of the injured spinal cord: a review of completed, ongoing, and planned clinical trials for acute spinal cord injury. Neurosurg Focus 25:E14.

[30] Caplan AI. (1991). Mesenchymal stem cells. J Orthop Res 9:641-650.

[31] Caplan AI. (1994). The mesengenic process. Clin Plast Surg 21:429-435.

[32] Horwitz EM, K Le Blanc, M Dominici, I Mueller, I Slaper-Cortenbach, FC Marini, RJ Deans, DS Krause and A Keating. (2005). Clarification of the nomenclature for MSC: The International Society for Cellular Therapy position statement. Cytotherapy 7:393-395.

[33] Dominici M, K Le Blanc, I Mueller, I Slaper-Cortenbach, F Marini, D Krause, R Deans, A Keating, D Prockop and E Horwitz. (2006). Minimal criteria for defining multipotent mesenchymal stromal cells. The International Society for Cellular Therapy position statement. Cytotherapy 8:315-317.

[34] Tetzlaff W, EB Okon, S Karimi-Abdolrezaee, CE Hill, JS Sparling, JR Plemel, WT Plunet, EC Tsai, D Baptiste, LJ Smithson, MD Kawaja, MG Fehlings and BK Kwon. (2011). A systematic review of cellular transplantation therapies for spinal cord injury. J Neurotrauma 28:1611-1682.

[35] Vallieres L and PE Sawchenko. (2003). Bone marrow-derived cells that populate the adult mouse brain preserve their hematopoietic identity. J Neurosci 23:5197-5207.

[36] Massengale M, AJ Wagers, H Vogel and IL Weissman. (2005). Hematopoietic cells maintain hematopoietic fates upon entering the brain. J Exp Med 201:1579-1589.

[37] Parr AM, CH Tator and A Keating. (2007). Bone marrow-derived mesenchymal stromal cells for the repair of central nervous system injury. Bone Marrow Transplant 40:609-619.

[38] Lee J, S Kuroda, H Shichinohe, J Ikeda, T Seki, K Hida, M Tada, K Sawada and Y Iwasaki. (2003). Migration and differentiation of nuclear fluorescence-labeled bone marrow stromal cells after transplantation into cerebral infarct and spinal cord injury in mice. Neuropathology 23:169-180.

[39] Koda M, S Okada, T Nakayama, S Koshizuka, T Kamada, Y Nishio, Y Someya, K Yoshinaga, A Okawa, H Moriya and M Yamazaki. (2005). Hematopoietic stem cell and marrow stromal cell for spinal cord injury in mice. Neuroreport 16:1763-1767.

[40] Wu S, Y Suzuki, Y Ejiri, T Noda, H Bai, M Kitada, K Kataoka, M Ohta, H Chou and C Ide. (2003). Bone marrow stromal cells enhance differentiation of cocultured neurosphere cells and promote regeneration of injured spinal cord. J Neurosci Res 72:343-351.

[41] Hofstetter CP, EJ Schwarz, D Hess, J Widenfalk, A El Manira, DJ Prockop and L Olson. (2002). Marrow stromal cells form guiding strands in the injured spinal cord and promote recovery. Proc Natl Acad Sci U S A 99:2199-2204.

[42] Zurita M and J Vaquero. (2006). Bone marrow stromal cells can achieve cure of chronic paraplegic rats: functional and morphological outcome one year after transplantation. Neurosci Lett 402:51-56.

[43] Basso DM, MS Beattie and JC Bresnahan. (1995). A sensitive and reliable locomotor rating scale for open field testing in rats. J Neurotrauma 12:1-21.

[44] Pinzon A, B Calancie, M Oudega and BR Noga. (2001). Conduction of impulses by axons regenerated in a Schwann cell graft in the transected adult rat thoracic spinal cord. J Neurosci Res 64:533-541.

[45] Xu XM, V Guenard, N Kleitman and MB Bunge. (1995). Axonal regeneration into Schwann cell-seeded guidance channels grafted into transected adult rat spinal cord. J Comp Neurol 351:145-160.

[46] Pearse DD, AR Sanchez, FC Pereira, CM Andrade, R Puzis, Y Pressman, K Golden, BM Kitay, B Blits, PM Wood and MB Bunge. (2007). Transplantation of Schwann cells and/or olfactory ensheathing glia into the contused spinal cord: Survival, migration, axon association, and functional recovery. Glia 55:976-1000.

[47] Tom VJ and JD Houle. (2008). Intraspinal microinjection of chondroitinase ABC following injury promotes axonal regeneration out of a peripheral nerve graft bridge. Exp Neurol 211:315-319.

[48] Houle JD, VJ Tom, D Mayes, G Wagoner, N Phillips and J Silver. (2006). Combining an autologous peripheral nervous system "bridge" and matrix modification by chon-

droitinase allows robust, functional regeneration beyond a hemisection lesion of the adult rat spinal cord. J Neurosci 26:7405-7415.

[49] Fouad K, L Schnell, MB Bunge, ME Schwab, T Liebscher and DD Pearse. (2005). Combining Schwann cell bridges and olfactory-ensheathing glia grafts with chondroitinase promotes locomotor recovery after complete transection of the spinal cord. J Neurosci 25:1169-1178.

[50] Lavdas AA, J Chen, F Papastefanaki, S Chen, M Schachner, R Matsas and D Thomaidou. (2010). Schwann cells engineered to express the cell adhesion molecule L1 accelerate myelination and motor recovery after spinal cord injury. Exp Neurol 221:206-216.

[51] Toma JG, M Akhavan, KJ Fernandes, F Barnabe-Heider, A Sadikot, DR Kaplan and FD Miller. (2001). Isolation of multipotent adult stem cells from the dermis of mammalian skin. Nat Cell Biol 3:778-784.

[52] Toma JG, IA McKenzie, D Bagli and FD Miller. (2005). Isolation and characterization of multipotent skin-derived precursors from human skin. Stem Cells 23:727-737.

[53] Biernaskie J, JS Sparling, J Liu, CP Shannon, JR Plemel, Y Xie, FD Miller and W Tetzlaff. (2007). Skin-derived precursors generate myelinating Schwann cells that promote remyelination and functional recovery after contusion spinal cord injury. J Neurosci 27:9545-9559.

[54] McKenzie IA, J Biernaskie, JG Toma, R Midha and FD Miller. (2006). Skin-derived precursors generate myelinating Schwann cells for the injured and dysmyelinated nervous system. J Neurosci 26:6651-6660.

[55] Kamada T, M Koda, M Dezawa, K Yoshinaga, M Hashimoto, S Koshizuka, Y Nishio, H Moriya and M Yamazaki. (2005). Transplantation of bone marrow stromal cell-derived Schwann cells promotes axonal regeneration and functional recovery after complete transection of adult rat spinal cord. J Neuropathol Exp Neurol 64:37-45.

[56] Wakao S, T Hayashi, M Kitada, M Kohama, D Matsue, N Teramoto, T Ose, Y Itokazu, K Koshino, H Watabe, H Iida, T Takamoto, Y Tabata and M Dezawa. (2010). Long-term observation of auto-cell transplantation in non-human primate reveals safety and efficiency of bone marrow stromal cell-derived Schwann cells in peripheral nerve regeneration. Exp Neurol 223:537-547.

[57] Park HW, MJ Lim, H Jung, SP Lee, KS Paik and MS Chang. (2010). Human mesenchymal stem cell-derived Schwann cell-like cells exhibit neurotrophic effects, via distinct growth factor production, in a model of spinal cord injury. Glia 58:1118-1132.

[58] Ruff CA, JT Wilcox and MG Fehlings. (2011). Cell-based transplantation strategies to promote plasticity following spinal cord injury. Exp Neurol 235:78-90.

[59] Doucette R. (1991). PNS-CNS transitional zone of the first cranial nerve. J Comp Neurol 312:451-466.

[60] Ramon-Cueto A, MI Cordero, FF Santos-Benito and J Avila. (2000). Functional recovery of paraplegic rats and motor axon regeneration in their spinal cords by olfactory ensheathing glia. Neuron 25:425-435.

[61] Ramon-Cueto A, GW Plant, J Avila and MB Bunge. (1998). Long-distance axonal regeneration in the transected adult rat spinal cord is promoted by olfactory ensheathing glia transplants. J Neurosci 18:3803-3815.

[62] Richter MW and AJ Roskams. (2008). Olfactory ensheathing cell transplantation following spinal cord injury: hype or hope? Exp Neurol 209:353-367.

[63] Au E, MW Richter, AJ Vincent, W Tetzlaff, R Aebersold, EH Sage and AJ Roskams. (2007). SPARC from olfactory ensheathing cells stimulates Schwann cells to promote neurite outgrowth and enhances spinal cord repair. J Neurosci 27:7208-7221.

[64] Richter MW, PA Fletcher, J Liu, W Tetzlaff and AJ Roskams. (2005). Lamina propria and olfactory bulb ensheathing cells exhibit differential integration and migration and promote differential axon sprouting in the lesioned spinal cord. J Neurosci 25:10700-10711.

[65] Karimi-Abdolrezaee S, E Eftekharpour, J Wang, D Schut and MG Fehlings. (2010). Synergistic effects of transplanted adult neural stem/progenitor cells, chondroitinase, and growth factors promote functional repair and plasticity of the chronically injured spinal cord. J Neurosci 30:1657-1676.

[66] Morshead CM, BA Reynolds, CG Craig, MW McBurney, WA Staines, D Morassutti, S Weiss and D van der Kooy. (1994). Neural stem cells in the adult mammalian forebrain: a relatively quiescent subpopulation of subependymal cells. Neuron 13:1071-1082.

[67] Weiss S, C Dunne, J Hewson, C Wohl, M Wheatley, AC Peterson and BA Reynolds. (1996). Multipotent CNS stem cells are present in the adult mammalian spinal cord and ventricular neuroaxis. J Neurosci 16:7599-7609.

[68] Weiss S, BA Reynolds, AL Vescovi, C Morshead, CG Craig and D van der Kooy. (1996). Is there a neural stem cell in the mammalian forebrain? Trends Neurosci 19:387-393.

[69] Martens DJ, V Tropepe and D van Der Kooy. (2000). Separate proliferation kinetics of fibroblast growth factor-responsive and epidermal growth factor-responsive neural stem cells within the embryonic forebrain germinal zone. J Neurosci 20:1085-1095.

[70] Yamamoto S, N Yamamoto, T Kitamura, K Nakamura and M Nakafuku. (2001). Proliferation of parenchymal neural progenitors in response to injury in the adult rat spinal cord. Exp Neurol 172:115-127.

[71] Gross RE, MF Mehler, PC Mabie, Z Zang, L Santschi and JA Kessler. (1996). Bone morphogenetic proteins promote astroglial lineage commitment by mammalian subventricular zone progenitor cells. Neuron 17:595-606.

[72] Weissman IL, DJ Anderson and F Gage. (2001). Stem and progenitor cells: origins, phenotypes, lineage commitments, and transdifferentiations. Annu Rev Cell Dev Biol 17:387-403.

[73] Calaora V, B Rogister, K Bismuth, K Murray, H Brandt, P Leprince, M Marchionni and M Dubois-Dalcq. (2001). Neuregulin signaling regulates neural precursor growth and the generation of oligodendrocytes in vitro. J Neurosci 21:4740-4751.

[74] Hsieh J, JB Aimone, BK Kaspar, T Kuwabara, K Nakashima and FH Gage. (2004). IGF-I instructs multipotent adult neural progenitor cells to become oligodendrocytes. J Cell Biol 164:111-122.

[75] Falk A, N Holmstrom, M Carlen, R Cassidy, C Lundberg and J Frisen. (2002). Gene delivery to adult neural stem cells. Exp Cell Res 279:34-39.

[76] Hofstetter CP, NA Holmstrom, JA Lilja, P Schweinhardt, J Hao, C Spenger, Z Wiesenfeld-Hallin, SN Kurpad, J Frisen and L Olson. (2005). Allodynia limits the usefulness of intraspinal neural stem cell grafts; directed differentiation improves outcome. Nat Neurosci 8:346-353.

[77] Chiasson BJ, V Tropepe, CM Morshead and D van der Kooy. (1999). Adult mammalian forebrain ependymal and subependymal cells demonstrate proliferative potential, but only subependymal cells have neural stem cell characteristics. J Neurosci 19:4462-4471.

[78] Craig CG, R D'sa, CM Morshead, A Roach and D van der Kooy. (1999). Migrational analysis of the constitutively proliferating subependyma population in adult mouse forebrain. Neuroscience 93:1197-1206.

[79] Evans MJ and MH Kaufman. (1981). Establishment in culture of pluripotential cells from mouse embryos. Nature 292:154-156.

[80] Martin GR. (1981). Isolation of a pluripotent cell line from early mouse embryos cultured in medium conditioned by teratocarcinoma stem cells. Proc Natl Acad Sci U S A 78:7634-7638.

[81] Thomson JA, J Itskovitz-Eldor, SS Shapiro, MA Waknitz, JJ Swiergiel, VS Marshall and JM Jones. (1998). Embryonic stem cell lines derived from human blastocysts. Science 282:1145-1147.

[82] Brons IG, LE Smithers, MW Trotter, P Rugg-Gunn, B Sun, SM Chuva de Sousa Lopes, SK Howlett, A Clarkson, L Ahrlund-Richter, RA Pedersen and L Vallier. (2007). Derivation of pluripotent epiblast stem cells from mammalian embryos. Nature 448:191-195.

[83] Pierce GB and FJ Dixon, Jr. (1959). Testicular teratomas. I. Demonstration of teratogenesis by metamorphosis of multipotential cells. Cancer 12:573-583.

[84] Martin GR, LM Wiley and I Damjanov. (1977). The development of cystic embryoid bodies in vitro from clonal teratocarcinoma stem cells. Dev Biol 61:230-244.

[85] Keller G. (2005). Embryonic stem cell differentiation: emergence of a new era in biology and medicine. Genes Dev 19:1129-1155.

[86] McDonald JW, XZ Liu, Y Qu, S Liu, SK Mickey, D Turetsky, DI Gottlieb and DW Choi. (1999). Transplanted embryonic stem cells survive, differentiate and promote recovery in injured rat spinal cord. Nat Med 5:1410-1412.

[87] Bain G, D Kitchens, M Yao, JE Huettner and DI Gottlieb. (1995). Embryonic stem cells express neuronal properties in vitro. Dev Biol 168:342-357.

[88] Li XJ, ZW Du, ED Zarnowska, M Pankratz, LO Hansen, RA Pearce and SC Zhang. (2005). Specification of motoneurons from human embryonic stem cells. Nat Biotechnol 23:215-221.

[89] Bibel M, J Richter, K Schrenk, KL Tucker, V Staiger, M Korte, M Goetz and YA Barde. (2004). Differentiation of mouse embryonic stem cells into a defined neuronal lineage. Nat Neurosci 7:1003-1009.

[90] Rathjen J, JA Lake, MD Bettess, JM Washington, G Chapman and PD Rathjen. (1999). Formation of a primitive ectoderm like cell population, EPL cells, from ES cells in response to biologically derived factors. J Cell Sci 112 (Pt 5):601-612.

[91] Lee H, GA Shamy, Y Elkabetz, CM Schofield, NL Harrsion, G Panagiotakos, ND Socci, V Tabar and L Studer. (2007). Directed differentiation and transplantation of human embryonic stem cell-derived motoneurons. Stem Cells 25:1931-1939.

[92] Rowland JW, JJ Lee, RP Salewski, E Eftekharpour, D van der Kooy and MG Fehlings. (2011). Generation of neural stem cells from embryonic stem cells using the default mechanism: in vitro and in vivo characterization. Stem Cells Dev 20:1829-1845.

[93] Tropepe V, S Hitoshi, C Sirard, TW Mak, J Rossant and D van der Kooy. (2001). Direct neural fate specification from embryonic stem cells: a primitive mammalian neural stem cell stage acquired through a default mechanism. Neuron 30:65-78.

[94] Smukler SR, SB Runciman, S Xu and D van der Kooy. (2006). Embryonic stem cells assume a primitive neural stem cell fate in the absence of extrinsic influences. J Cell Biol 172:79-90.

[95] Chernoff GF. (1981). Shiverer: an autosomal recessive mutant mouse with myelin deficiency. J Hered 72:128.

[96] Bu J, A Banki, Q Wu and A Nishiyama. (2004). Increased NG2(+) glial cell proliferation and oligodendrocyte generation in the hypomyelinating mutant shiverer. Glia 48:51-63.

[97] Wu Q, RH Miller, RM Ransohoff, S Robinson, J Bu and A Nishiyama. (2000). Elevated levels of the chemokine GRO-1 correlate with elevated oligodendrocyte progenitor proliferation in the jimpy mutant. J Neurosci 20:2609-2617.

[98] Canoll PD, JM Musacchio, R Hardy, R Reynolds, MA Marchionni and JL Salzer. (1996). GGF/neuregulin is a neuronal signal that promotes the proliferation and survival and inhibits the differentiation of oligodendrocyte progenitors. Neuron 17:229-243.

[99] Hochedlinger K and R Jaenisch. (2006). Nuclear reprogramming and pluripotency. Nature 441:1061-1067.

[100] Campbell KH, J McWhir, WA Ritchie and I Wilmut. (1996). Sheep cloned by nuclear transfer from a cultured cell line. Nature 380:64-66.

[101] Takahashi K and S Yamanaka. (2006). Induction of pluripotent stem cells from mouse embryonic and adult fibroblast cultures by defined factors. Cell 126:663-676.

[102] Liu H, F Zhu, J Yong, P Zhang, P Hou, H Li, W Jiang, J Cai, M Liu, K Cui, X Qu, T Xiang, D Lu, X Chi, G Gao, W Ji, M Ding and H Deng. (2008). Generation of induced pluripotent stem cells from adult rhesus monkey fibroblasts. Cell Stem Cell 3:587-590.

[103] Liao J, C Cui, S Chen, J Ren, J Chen, Y Gao, H Li, N Jia, L Cheng, H Xiao and L Xiao. (2009). Generation of induced pluripotent stem cell lines from adult rat cells. Cell Stem Cell 4:11-15.

[104] Takahashi K, K Tanabe, M Ohnuki, M Narita, T Ichisaka, K Tomoda and S Yamanaka. (2007). Induction of pluripotent stem cells from adult human fibroblasts by defined factors. Cell 131:861-872.

[105] Yu J, MA Vodyanik, K Smuga-Otto, J Antosiewicz-Bourget, JL Frane, S Tian, J Nie, GA Jonsdottir, V Ruotti, R Stewart, Slukvin, II and JA Thomson. (2007). Induced pluripotent stem cell lines derived from human somatic cells. Science 318:1917-1920.

[106] Lowry WE, L Richter, R Yachechko, AD Pyle, J Tchieu, R Sridharan, AT Clark and K Plath. (2008). Generation of human induced pluripotent stem cells from dermal fibroblasts. Proc Natl Acad Sci U S A 105:2883-2888.

[107] Park IH, R Zhao, JA West, A Yabuuchi, H Huo, TA Ince, PH Lerou, MW Lensch and GQ Daley. (2008). Reprogramming of human somatic cells to pluripotency with defined factors. Nature 451:141-146.

[108] Kaji K, K Norrby, A Paca, M Mileikovsky, P Mohseni and K Woltjen. (2009). Virus-free induction of pluripotency and subsequent excision of reprogramming factors. Nature 458:771-775.

[109] Woltjen K, IP Michael, P Mohseni, R Desai, M Mileikovsky, R Hamalainen, R Cowling, W Wang, P Liu, M Gertsenstein, K Kaji, HK Sung and A Nagy. (2009). piggyBac

transposition reprograms fibroblasts to induced pluripotent stem cells. Nature 458:766-770.

[110] Soldner F, D Hockemeyer, C Beard, Q Gao, GW Bell, EG Cook, G Hargus, A Blak, O Cooper, M Mitalipova, O Isacson and R Jaenisch. (2009). Parkinson's disease patient-derived induced pluripotent stem cells free of viral reprogramming factors. Cell 136:964-977.

[111] Sommer CA, M Stadtfeld, GJ Murphy, K Hochedlinger, DN Kotton and G Mostoslavsky. (2009). Induced pluripotent stem cell generation using a single lentiviral stem cell cassette. Stem Cells 27:543-549.

[112] Yu J, K Hu, K Smuga-Otto, S Tian, R Stewart, Slukvin, II and JA Thomson. (2009). Human induced pluripotent stem cells free of vector and transgene sequences. Science 324:797-801.

[113] Zhou H, S Wu, JY Joo, S Zhu, DW Han, T Lin, S Trauger, G Bien, S Yao, Y Zhu, G Siuzdak, HR Scholer, L Duan and S Ding. (2009). Generation of induced pluripotent stem cells using recombinant proteins. Cell Stem Cell 4:381-384.

[114] Kim K, A Doi, B Wen, K Ng, R Zhao, P Cahan, J Kim, MJ Aryee, H Ji, LI Ehrlich, A Yabuuchi, A Takeuchi, KC Cunniff, H Hongguang, S McKinney-Freeman, O Naveiras, TJ Yoon, RA Irizarry, N Jung, J Seita, J Hanna, P Murakami, R Jaenisch, R Weissleder, SH Orkin, IL Weissman, AP Feinberg and GQ Daley. (2010). Epigenetic memory in induced pluripotent stem cells. Nature 467:285-290.

[115] Wernig M, JP Zhao, J Pruszak, E Hedlund, D Fu, F Soldner, V Broccoli, M Constantine-Paton, O Isacson and R Jaenisch. (2008). Neurons derived from reprogrammed fibroblasts functionally integrate into the fetal brain and improve symptoms of rats with Parkinson's disease. Proc Natl Acad Sci U S A 105:5856-5861.

[116] Ebert AD, J Yu, FF Rose, Jr., VB Mattis, CL Lorson, JA Thomson and CN Svendsen. (2009). Induced pluripotent stem cells from a spinal muscular atrophy patient. Nature 457:277-280.

[117] Dimos JT, KT Rodolfa, KK Niakan, LM Weisenthal, H Mitsumoto, W Chung, GF Croft, G Saphier, R Leibel, R Goland, H Wichterle, CE Henderson and K Eggan. (2008). Induced pluripotent stem cells generated from patients with ALS can be differentiated into motor neurons. Science 321:1218-1221.

[118] Tsuji O, K Miura, Y Okada, K Fujiyoshi, M Mukaino, N Nagoshi, K Kitamura, G Kumagai, M Nishino, S Tomisato, H Higashi, T Nagai, H Katoh, K Kohda, Y Matsuzaki, M Yuzaki, E Ikeda, Y Toyama, M Nakamura, S Yamanaka and H Okano. (2010). Therapeutic potential of appropriately evaluated safe-induced pluripotent stem cells for spinal cord injury. Proc Natl Acad Sci U S A 107:12704-12709.

[119] Miura K, Y Okada, T Aoi, A Okada, K Takahashi, K Okita, M Nakagawa, M Koyanagi, K Tanabe, M Ohnuki, D Ogawa, E Ikeda, H Okano and S Yamanaka. (2009). Variation in the safety of induced pluripotent stem cell lines. Nat Biotechnol 27:743-745.

[120] Salewski RP, J Buttigieg, RA Mitchell, D van der Kooy, A Nagy and MG Fehlings. (2012). The Generation of Definitive Neural Stem Cells from PiggyBac Transposon-Induced Pluripotent Stem Cells Can Be Enhanced by Induction of the NOTCH Signaling Pathway. Stem Cells Dev.

[121] Yoon K and N Gaiano. (2005). Notch signaling in the mammalian central nervous system: insights from mouse mutants. Nat Neurosci 8:709-715.

[122] Louvi A and S Artavanis-Tsakonas. (2006). Notch signalling in vertebrate neural development. Nat Rev Neurosci 7:93-102.

[123] Nakamura Y, S Sakakibara, T Miyata, M Ogawa, T Shimazaki, S Weiss, R Kageyama and H Okano. (2000). The bHLH gene hes1 as a repressor of the neuronal commitment of CNS stem cells. J Neurosci 20:283-293.

[124] Hitoshi S, T Alexson, V Tropepe, D Donoviel, AJ Elia, JS Nye, RA Conlon, TW Mak, A Bernstein and D van der Kooy. (2002). Notch pathway molecules are essential for the maintenance, but not the generation, of mammalian neural stem cells. Genes Dev 16:846-858.

[125] Androutsellis-Theotokis A, RR Leker, F Soldner, DJ Hoeppner, R Ravin, SW Poser, MA Rueger, SK Bae, R Kittappa and RD McKay. (2006). Notch signalling regulates stem cell numbers in vitro and in vivo. Nature 442:823-826.

[126] Ables JL, JJ Breunig, AJ Eisch and P Rakic. (2011). Not(ch) just development: Notch signalling in the adult brain. Nat Rev Neurosci 12:269-283.

[127] Hitoshi S, RM Seaberg, C Koscik, T Alexson, S Kusunoki, I Kanazawa, S Tsuji and D van der Kooy. (2004). Primitive neural stem cells from the mammalian epiblast differentiate to definitive neural stem cells under the control of Notch signaling. Genes Dev 18:1806-1811.

[128] D'Souza B, L Meloty-Kapella and G Weinmaster. (2010). Canonical and non-canonical Notch ligands. Curr Top Dev Biol 92:73-129.

[129] Dang LT and V Tropepe. (2010). FGF dependent regulation of Zfhx1b gene expression promotes the formation of definitive neural stem cells in the mouse anterior neurectoderm. Neural Dev 5.

[130] Hirsch C, LM Campano, S Wohrle and A Hecht. (2007). Canonical Wnt signaling transiently stimulates proliferation and enhances neurogenesis in neonatal neural progenitor cultures. Exp Cell Res 313:572-587.

[131] Fehlings MG and CH Tator. (1995). The relationships among the severity of spinal cord injury, residual neurological function, axon counts, and counts of retrogradely labeled neurons after experimental spinal cord injury. Exp Neurol 132:220-228.

[132] Fehlings MG, CH Tator and RD Linden. (1989). The relationships among the severity of spinal cord injury, motor and somatosensory evoked potentials and spinal cord blood flow. Electroencephalogr Clin Neurophysiol 74:241-259.

[133] Nashmi R and MG Fehlings. (2001). Mechanisms of axonal dysfunction after spinal cord injury: with an emphasis on the role of voltage-gated potassium channels. Brain Res Brain Res Rev 38:165-191.

[134] Nashmi R, OT Jones and MG Fehlings. (2000). Abnormal axonal physiology is associated with altered expression and distribution of Kv1.1 and Kv1.2 K+ channels after chronic spinal cord injury. Eur J Neurosci 12:491-506.

[135] Enzmann GU, RL Benton, JF Talbott, Q Cao and SR Whittemore. (2006). Functional considerations of stem cell transplantation therapy for spinal cord repair. J Neurotrauma 23:479-495.

[136] Koshizuka S, S Okada, A Okawa, M Koda, M Murasawa, M Hashimoto, T Kamada, K Yoshinaga, M Murakami, H Moriya and M Yamazaki. (2004). Transplanted hematopoietic stem cells from bone marrow differentiate into neural lineage cells and promote functional recovery after spinal cord injury in mice. J Neuropathol Exp Neurol 63:64-72.

[137] Ohta M, Y Suzuki, T Noda, Y Ejiri, M Dezawa, K Kataoka, H Chou, N Ishikawa, N Matsumoto, Y Iwashita, E Mizuta, S Kuno and C Ide. (2004). Bone marrow stromal cells infused into the cerebrospinal fluid promote functional recovery of the injured rat spinal cord with reduced cavity formation. Exp Neurol 187:266-278.

[138] Koda M, M Murakami, H Ino, K Yoshinaga, O Ikeda, M Hashimoto, M Yamazaki, C Nakayama and H Moriya. (2002). Brain-derived neurotrophic factor suppresses delayed apoptosis of oligodendrocytes after spinal cord injury in rats. J Neurotrauma 19:777-785.

[139] Neuhuber B, B Timothy Himes, JS Shumsky, G Gallo and I Fischer. (2005). Axon growth and recovery of function supported by human bone marrow stromal cells in the injured spinal cord exhibit donor variations. Brain Res 1035:73-85.

[140] Tolwani RJ, JM Cosgaya, S Varma, R Jacob, LE Kuo and EM Shooter. (2004). BDNF overexpression produces a long-term increase in myelin formation in the peripheral nervous system. J Neurosci Res 77:662-669.

[141] Hempstead BL and JL Salzer. (2002). Neurobiology. A glial spin on neurotrophins. Science 298:1184-1186.

[142] Nakamura M, H Okano, Y Toyama, HN Dai, TP Finn and BS Bregman. (2005). Transplantation of embryonic spinal cord-derived neurospheres support growth of supra-

spinal projections and functional recovery after spinal cord injury in the neonatal rat. J Neurosci Res 81:457-468.

[143] Chen Q, L Zhou and HD Shine. (2006). Expression of neurotrophin-3 promotes axonal plasticity in the acute but not chronic injured spinal cord. J Neurotrauma 23:1254-1260.

[144] Hawryluk GW, AJ Mothe, M Chamankhah, J Wang, C Tator and MG Fehlings. (2010). In vitro characterization of trophic factor expression in neural precursor cells. Stem Cells Dev 21:432-447.

[145] Hawryluk GW, A Mothe, J Wang, S Wang, C Tator and MG Fehlings. (2012). An in vivo characterization of trophic factor production following neural precursor cell or bone marrow stromal cell transplantation for spinal cord injury. Stem Cells Dev 21:2222-2238.

Chapter 12

Epigenetic Regulation of Neural Differentiation from Embryonic Stem Cells

Atsushi Shimomura and Eri Hashino

Additional information is available at the end of the chapter

1. Introduction

During development, ESCs in the inner cell mass of the blastocyst undergo progressive fate restriction and sequentially give rise to tissue-specific multipotent progenitor cells [1-3]. In the nervous system, neural progenitor cells (NPCs) are defined as multipotent cells capable of differentiating into neurons and glia, the latter of which include astrocytes and oligodendrocytes. NPCs undergo sequential fate restriction during nervous system development [4-6]. During early embryonic development, NPCs give rise exclusively to neuronal cell types, however at later stages they differentiate into glial cell types [7, 8]. Understanding how ESCs differentiate into neuronal or glial cell types, thus, constitutes a fundamental aspect of nervous system development.

ESCs possess two cardinal cellular characteristics: self-renewal capacity and pluripotency [2, 3]. ESCs, when undifferentiated, maintain a unique gene expression profile which keeps themselves in a pluripotent state [3, 9-12]. When ESCs begin to differentiate, however, this profile is dramatically altered without changes in the DNA sequence, allowing initial cell lineage specification to take place [11, 13-15]. Studies on lineage choice and differentiation of stem cells suggest that the crosstalk between transcription factors and epigenetic mechanisms plays pivotal roles in maintaining the existing transcriptional profile or changing it into a new transcriptional profile [16, 17].

Chromatin in eukaryotes is organized into arrays of nucleosomes, which are comprised of DNA wrapped around a histone octamer containing 2 copies of individual core histones, H2A, H2B, H3, and H4 [18]. Chromatin can be tightly or loosely packed to alter its accessibility to transcription factors and RNA polymerases, thereby ultimately modulating the efficiency of gene transcription [19-23]. Epigenetic mechanisms act to change this accessibility both locally and globally through modifications of nucleosomes, and by remodeling of nucleosomes [21, 24, 25]. In addition to epigenetic modifications and chromatin remodeling, epigenetic regulators have been recently extended to non-coding RNAs (ncRNAs), because ncRNAs can affect chromatin structure and transcriptional activation by regulating expression of key nucleosome modifiers [26]. These epigenetic controls appear to influence gene expression profiles, which are essential for self-renewal and differentiation capacities of ESCs. Thus, a clear understanding of the epigenetic mechanisms underlying gene expression patterns will provide significant and novel insights into cell fate specification of ESCs directed to differentiate into neurons. Furthermore, the epigenetic mechanisms are believed to be capable of responding to extrinsic signals such as morphogens and cytokines [8]. Therefore, knowledge of the epigenetic mechanisms is also important for our understanding of neural differentiation by extrinsic factors. In this review, we will describe the major epigenetic processes that underlie the acquisition of the NPC fate from ESCs as well as the subsequent neuronal subtype specification. The focus of this review is weighted on neuronal cell lineage specification, and not on glial cell specification.

2. Epigentic mechanisms

2.1. Post-translational modifications of histones

Post-translational chemical modifications of histones in chromatin are diverse and include methylation, acetylation, phosphorylation, sumoylation, ubiquitilation, and ADP-ribosylation [25, 27]. Here, we will focus on histone methylation and acetylation because these modifications are considered to be most important and widespread for influencing biological processes during neural differentiation.

Histone methylation occurs mainly at lysine and arginine residues on the tails of the histone H3 and H4 [28]. Histone methylation is reversible. Methylation at these sites has been associated with not only transcriptional activation and repression [27, 29] but also multiple biological processes, including heterochromatin formation and genomic imprinting [27, 28]. The differences in the effects of methylation depend on the lysine residues. For example, methylation of histone H3 lysine 9 (H3K9), H3K27, or H4K20 is generally linked to formation of gene silencing [30, 31], whereas methylation on H3K4, H3K36, and H3K79 is associated with actively transcribed regions and gene activation [29, 32, 33]. In addition, lysine residues can be mono-(me1), di-(me2), or tri-methylated (me3). These differentially methylated lysine residues lead to different levels of transcriptional activation or repression, resulting in diverse functional outcomes. For example, H4K20me1 plays an important role in transcriptional repression and X inactivation, while H4K20me2 and H4K20me3 are linked to DNA repair of double-stranded DNA damage [34].

All core histones can be dynamically acetylated on lysine residues in their tails and occasionally within the globular core. Histone acetylation removes the positive charge on the histones, thereby weakening the interaction with negatively charged DNA [25, 29]. As a consequence, chromatin is transformed into a more relaxed structure, which is associated with transcriptional activation. Like methylation, histone acetylation is reversible. This reversible acetylation in histones is an important mechanism of controlling gene expression because histone acetylation and deacetylation are linked to transcriptional activation and inactivation, respectively [25, 27].

2.2. DNA methylation

DNA methylation is one of the major repressive epigenetic pathways. Methylation occurs at the cytosine residues followed by a guanine (CpG dinucleotides) in the DNA sequence. CpG DNA methylation of gene promoters is a well-known hallmark for transcriptionally inactive genes, and is generally associated with stable gene silencing, such as genomic imprinting and X chromosome inactivation [35, 36]. The DNA methylation state is established during embryogenesis by several DNA methyltransferases (DNMTs) [35]. In mammals, 2 types of DNMTs have been identified. DNMT3A and DNMT3B establish *de novo* DNA methylation, while DNMT1 maintains DNA methylation patterns during DNA replication [37]. These DNA methylation sites then recruit methyl-CpG-binding proteins, including methyl-CpG-binding domain (MBD) proteins [38, 39], which bind the histone deacetylase (HDAC)-containing repressor complex, and consequently repress transcription [40, 41].

2.3. Chromatin remodeling

Chromatin structure is not static, but subject to change in response to internal and external developmental signals [23]. Dynamic changes in the chromatin structure are regulated by ATP-dependent chromatin remodelers, which allow the transcriptional machinery to access its targets more or less effectively [42-44]. Using energy derived from ATP hydrolysis, ATP-dependent chromatin remodelers relocate nucleosomes either by mobilizing or restructuring nucleosomes [45, 46]. Thus, ATP-dependent chromatin remodelers can function both in transcriptional activation and repression via their nucleosome remodeling activity. Nearly all ATP-dependent chromatin remodelers are multi-protein complexes that contain an ATPase subunit, which belongs to the sucrose non-fermenting 2 (SNF2) family of ATPases. Based on the homology between their ATPase domains, ATP-dependent chromatin remodeling complexes are divided into 4 groups: switch/sucrose non-fermenting (SWI/SNF), imitation switch (ISWI), chromo helicase DNA binding (CHD), and inositol auxotroph 80 (INO80) [42-44].

Genetic and biochemical studies indicate that some ATP-dependent chromatin remodeling complexes contain epigenetic factors such as HDAC and MBD proteins. For example, nucleosome-remodeling deacetylase (NuRD) is a multi-subunit complex that includes a SWI2/SNF2 helicase/ATPase domain-containing Mi2 protein, HDAC1, HDAC2, and MBD3 [47]. The NuRD complexes promote the establishment of a specific chromatin structure at rRNA genes that are transcriptionally inactive but are poised for transcriptional activation and control transcription of these genes [48]. Thus, ATP-dependent chromatin complexes play essential roles in epigenetic regulation of transcription along with several histone-modifying enzymes and/or modified histone codes.

2.4. Non-coding RNAs

Apart from the role of histone modifications and DNA methylation, another form of epigenetic regulation involves non-coding RNAs (ncRNAs). A large variety of ncRNAs can be classified into 2 major classes based on their transcript size: small ncRNAs (less than 200 nucleotides) and long ncRNAs (greater than 200 nucleotides) [49]. Each of these classes can be further divided into subclasses. Micro RNA (miRNA) is a subgroup of small ncRNA molecules ~22 nucleotides in length. miRNAs post-transcriptionally regulate gene expression by binding to complimentary or uncomplimentary sequences on target mRNA transcripts, which results in either mRNA degradation or inhibition of translation [50]. In animal cells, miRNA genes tend to be clustered in the genome, and are widely distributed [51]. Approximately half of the human miRNA genes are located in the introns of protein-coding genes. Expression studies have revealed that the clustered miRNA genes are often co-expressed, suggesting that they are jointly transcribed as a polycistron [52, 53].

3. Transition from ESCS to NPCS

3.1. Histone modifications

Expression of pluripotency genes, such as *OCT4* or *NANOG*, is a hallmark of undifferentiated ESCs. The promoters and/or enhancers of these pluripotency genes are marked by H3K4me3, which is strongly associated with transcriptionally active genes. In contrast, the majority of genes, whose upregulation leads to differentiation, are inactivated or expressed at very low levels [54, 55]. These genes loci are maintained in a transcriptionally competent but inactive state characterized by both active (H3-K4me3) and repressive (H3-K27me3) histone marks, a configuration described as a "bivalent domain" (Figure 1) [54, 55]. Bivalent histone methylation in the promoters of proneural genes, such as Neurogenins (*Ngns*), *Pax6*, and *Mash1*, has been reported in undifferentiated ESCs [56]. H3K27 and H3K4 methylation is catalyzed by Polycomb-group (PcG) and Trithorax-group (TrxG) proteins, respectively [57]. PcG proteins form a complex referred to as the Polycomb Repressor Complex (PRC). PRCs can be biochemically subdivided into 2 groups: PRC1 and PRC2. PRC1 and PRC2 are essential for the repression of key developmental genes and maintenance of pluripotency in ESCs [58, 59]. The PRC2 complexes, which contain Enhancer of Zeste Homolog (EZH), a histone methyltransferase (HMTase), catalyze tri-methylation of H3K27 [60]. This histone mark leads to the recruitment of PRC1, thereby contributing to a repressive chromatin state [61, 62]. Consistent with this, ESCs deficient in a PRC2 component display de-repression of tissue-specific genes, including neural-associated genes [59]. TrxG proteins also act as large multimeric complexes [57]. TrxG complexes possess methyltransferase activity directed specifically towards H3K4, thereby leading to increased levels of H3K4me3 [57]. *Dpy-30* is a mammalian homolog of the *Drosophila* TrxG protein, and a core component of myeloid/lymphoid or mixed-lineage leukemia (MLL) histone methyltransferase complexes. Depletion of *Dpy-30* in ESCs results in a defect in their neural lineage specification through reduced H3K4 methylation at bivalent domains of key developmental loci [63]. Collectively, these findings suggest that the bivalent domain mediated by PcG and TrxG proteins plays a key epigenetic role in maintenance of the undifferentiated state and suppress neural differentiation.

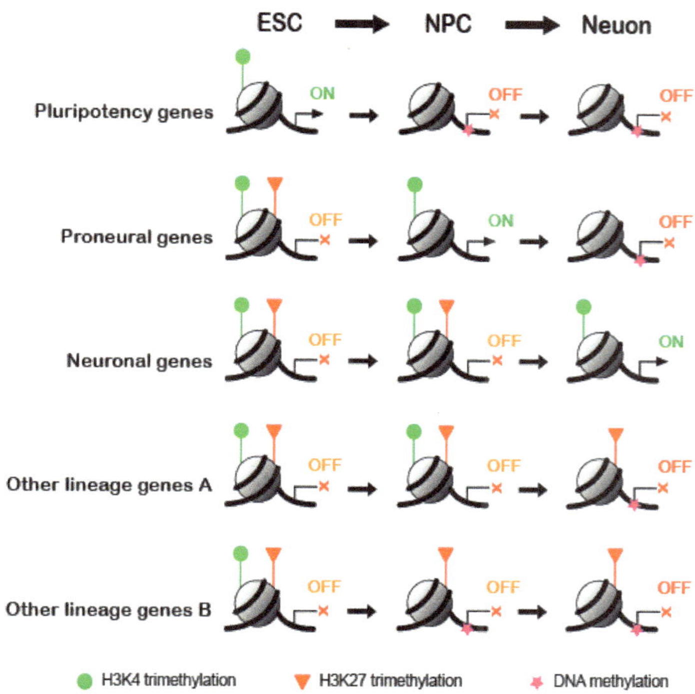

Figure 1. Schematic diagram of transcriptional states during neuronal fate acquisition from ESCs. In ESCs, pluripotency genes are transcriptionally activated (green "ON"). Key developmental genes are transcriptionally silent, yet competent for expression (orange "OFF"). This silencing ensures rapid reactions to extracellular inductive signals. Upon neural lineage choice, the transcriptional states of various developmental genes are altered. Pluripotency genes and genes associated with other lineages become repressed during the transition from ESCs to neurogenic NPCs (red "OFF"). Such a state of transcriptional repression is maintained over a long period. Gene activation and repression correlates with the presence of H3K4 tri-methylation (green flags) and H3K27 tri-methylation (red flags). DNA methylation (shocking pink stars) contributes to repression in combination with H3K27 tri-methylation.

Genome-wide mapping by chromatin immunoprecipitation has revealed that differentiation of ESCs is generally accompanied by global changes in histone methylation [55, 56]. In the course of neural lineage commitment, the promoters of many neural lineage genes have been shown to lose H3K27me3 from the bivalent domain, retain H3K4me3, and become activated. At the same time, the promoter loci of non-neural lineage genes maintain H3K27me3 in the bivalent domain, while removing H3K4me3, which results in a stable silent state. The promoters of some pluripotency genes such as *SOX2*, *POU5F1*, and *NANOG* shift from modification by H3K4me3 alone to neither H3K4 nor H3K27 methylation as they are repressed during differentiation. As ESCs differentiate into NPCs, H3K27 specific demethylase JMJD3 is recruited to and resolves the bivalent domain at the promoters of neuron-specific genes such as nestin [64]. The majority of the JMJD3 target genes are key inducers of neurogenesis, including Pax6 and Sox1. Knockdown of the H3K4me2/3 demethylase *JARID1B* results in upregulation of stem cell-specific genes in ESC-derived NPCs [65]. Furthermore, *JARID1B* knockdown ESCs fail to progress beyond the NPC stage [65]. These results suggest that JARID1B promotes ESCs to differentiate towards a neural lineage by silencing genes associated with pluripotency. Thus, when ESCs are committed to a neural lineage, bivalent domains appear to be resolved in a lineage-specific fashion by leaving methyl marks either being activated or repressed. This mechanism is believed to allow rapid transcription of developmental genes in response to a variety of extrinsic cues.

Other repressive histone marks have also been reported to play important roles during differentiation. A sustained increase in silent chromatin marked by H3K9 methylation is observed in ESC-derived cells undergoing differentiation [66], suggesting that repressive histone marks H3K9me2/3 is essential for promoting differentiation. Additionally, it is possible that H3K9me2/3 marks play an important role in the establishment of an expression profile of neuron specific genes in response to extracellular signals [67]. Ciliary neurotrophic factor (CNTF), an astrocyte differentiation factor, is incapable of inducing expression of glial fibrillary acidic protein (*GFAP*), an astrocytes-specific marker gene, in NPCs, because the *GFAP* promoter is marked by H3K9 methylation. However, fibroblast growth factor 2 (FGF2) confer NPCs with responsiveness to CNTF by adding active H3K4 methylation and removing H3K9 methylation at the GFAP promoter. Thus, H3K9 methylation controls the timing of astrogliogenesis through regulation of CNTF-mediated signaling.

In addition to histone methylation, histone acetylation also appears to be an important epigenetic modification during neural differentiation from ESCs, as ESCs generally undergo striking changes in the global pattern of histone acetylation during neural differentiation [68]. Histone acetylation is catalyzed by histone acetyltransferase (HAT), while histone deacetylation is catalyzed by histone deacetylase (HDAC) [69]. Generally, HATs induce the transcriptional activation of their target genes. However, the 60-kDa HIV-Tat interactive protein (Tip60) histone acetyltransferase has been implicated in both transcriptional repression and activation [70]. Tip60-p400 chromatin remodeling complexes containing Tip60 are necessary to maintain characteristic features of ESCs [71]. Tip60-p400 complexes acetylate histone H4 on the promoters of both activated and repressed genes. Additionally, distribution patterns of p400 in ESCs strongly correlate with H3K4me3 marks on the promoters of both active and inactive genes. These results suggest that Tip60-p400 complex-mediated histone acetylation functions as an active mark in the bivalent domain together with the active H3K4me3 mark in ESCs.

3.2. DNA methylation

Genome-wide mapping of DNA methylation patterns has revealed dynamic DNA methylation states at gene promoters during ESC differentiation (Figure 1) [72, 73]. The most pronounced changes in the DNA methylation state occur during neural lineage commitment [74], suggesting that alterations in the DNA methylation state more strongly correlate with neural lineage commitment and loss of pluripotency than with terminal neural differentiation. The promoters of highly expressed housekeeping and pluripotency genes in ESCs exhibit low methylation levels [75]. By contrast, most key developmental and tissue-specific genes exhibit high methylation levels, and are transcriptionally repressed [75]. As ESCs undergo differentiation, significant changes in DNA methylation patterns are observed. *De novo* methylation occurs on the promoter regions of pluripotency-associated factors [74].

DNA methylation potentially accompanies histone modifications during neural differentiation from ESCs. Cross-referencing DNA methylation patterns with mapping of histone H3K27me3 in ESCs and ESC-derived neurons has revealed that, upon differentiation, the regions marked by H3K27me3 acquire DNA methylation in a sequence-independent manner [74, 75]. H3K27me3 and DNA methylation are compatible throughout most of the genome [76]. Furthermore, deficiency of *DNMT* in ESCs causes widespread H3K27me3 genomic changes [76]. Taken together, these data suggest that DNA methylation, in cooperation with histone modifications, may function as a protective gear by repressing pluripotency and other lineage-specific genes during differentiation.

3.3. Chromatin remodeling

In addition to histone modifications and DNA methylation, the ATP-dependent chromatin remodeling complexes also play a pivotal role in the maintenance of ESC pluripotency. As previously described, Tip60-p400 chromatin remodeling complexes appear to be necessary for the maintenance of ESCs, including pluripotency [71]. Subunits of the NuRD complexes have also been shown to be important for ESC pluripotency and differentiation [77, 78]. Furthermore, ESCs contain another specialized ATP-dependent chromatin remodeling complex: the Brahma-associated factor (BAF) complex. The BAF complexes are characterized by 2 SWI2/SNF2-like ATPases, BRG1 and BRM. The BAF complexes in ESCs have a unique subunit composition (termed esBAF) that is not seen in other tissues, such as NPCs and post-mitotic neurons [79]. This specialized subunit composition is essential for establishment and maintenance of ESCs. The esBAF complexes contain BRG1 but not BRM, and BAF155 but not BAF170 (Figure 2). As ESCs differentiate into NPCs, these complexes undergo several subunit exchanges. The esBAF complexes incorporate BRM and excludes BAF60B, thereby forming the neural progenitor-specific BAF (npBAF) complexes in NPCs. The npBAF complex-specific subunit is necessary and sufficient for amplification of NPCs [80].

3.4. Non-coding RNAs

Increasing evidence demonstrates contributions of specific miRNAs in establishing ESC properties and their transitioning to NPCs. The miR-290-295 cluster codes for miRNAs are the most abundant in mouse ESCs and constitute over 70% of their entire miRNA population [81]. Consistent with their high expression levels, miR-290-295 miRNAs are involved in many functions in ESCs. For example, miR-290-295 miRNAs promote the transition from mitosis to S phase by targeting G1/S transition inhibitors such as Cdkn1a [82]. Furthermore, miR-290-295 miRNAs have been shown to target the *Rbl2* gene, which controls the expression of the DNA methyltransferases, DNMT3A and DNMT3B, thereby establishing *de novo*

DNA methylation in ESCs [83]. miR-9 is gradually upregulated during neural differentiation from ESCs [84, 85]. Furthermore, miR-9 performs diverse functions in different aspects of neuronal differentiation [86]. For example, during neural differentiation of human ESCs, miR-9 expression is not detectable in embryoid bodies, but is turned on in NPCs [84]. Inhibition of miR-9 activity has been found to suppress proliferation and simultaneously promote migration of NPCs [84]. Collectively, miRNAs could regulate multiple developmental processes at the post-transcriptional level.

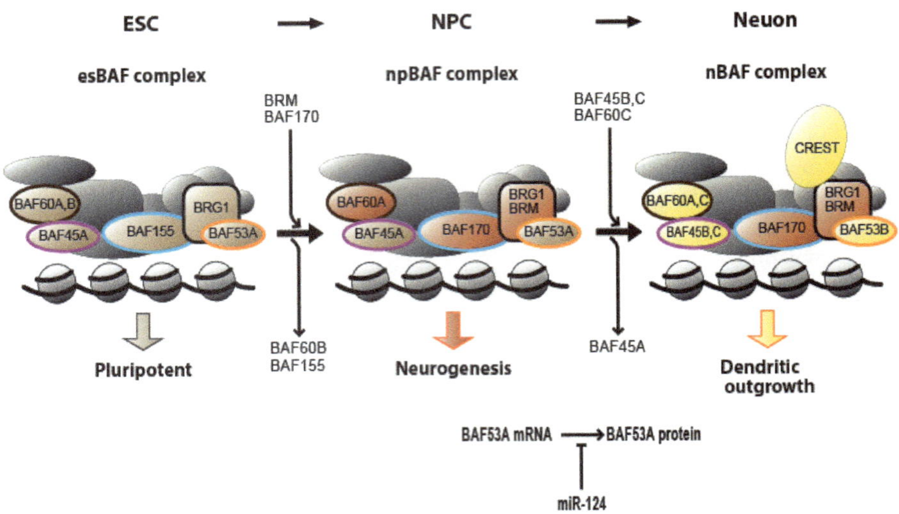

Figure 2. A switch in subunit composition of the BAF complexes during neuronal differentiation from ESCs. The exchange of the components is essential for the transition from ESCs to post-mitotic neurons. The exchangeable subunits are colored as follows: esBAF complex-specific subunit, ocher; npBAF complex-specific subunit, red; and nBAF complex-specific subunit, yellow. Cell type-specific BAF complexes have distinct functions that are indispensable for their properties. The BAF complex in ESCs, NPCs, and neurons are defined as esBAF, npBAF, and nBAF, respectively. The microRNA miR-124, binds to *BAF53A* mRNA transcripts to suppress its expression, thereby facilitating the replacement of BAF53 in the npBAF complexes.

4. Transition from NPCs to neurons

4.1. Histone modifications

After being committed to a neural lineage, NPCs exit the cell cycle and sequentially undergo neural and glial differentiation. Wnt signaling, which plays important roles in the maintenance of embryonic and adult stem cells, promotes differentiation of neurogenic ESCs to neurons, but does not promote differentiation of astrogenic NPCs into neurons [8]. In neurogenic NPCs, one of the target genes for Wnt signaling is the proneural gene *Ngn1*, which promotes neurogenesis and inhibits astrocytic differentiation [87]. During the transition from neurogenic NPCs to astrogenic NPCs, the level of repressive H3K27me3 mark at the promoter of the *Ngn1* gene gradually increases, leading to gene silencing [88]. Therefore, activation of the Wnt signaling does not lead to transactivation of *Ngn1* at later developmental stages. This illustrates how histone methylation can modulate responsiveness of NPCs to extracellular cues, thereby rendering NPCs to switch from neurogenesis to astrogenesis.

CREB-binding protein (CBP), one of the most extensively studied HAT proteins, has been found to play an essential role in motor neuron differentiation by interacting with retinoic acid (RA) signaling [89]. Retinoic acid receptors (RARs) are DNA-binding proteins and form a complex with Neurogenin2 (Ngn2) on the promoter of a motor neuron enhancer gene. Binding of RA to RARs triggers recruitment of CBP on the promoter, which leads to acetylation of core histone proteins and activation of the motor neuron enhancer gene. These results indicate that neuronal subtype specification is regulated, at least in part, by the interplay between intrinsic epigenetic mechanisms and extrinsic cues.

Histone deacetylation by HDACs also plays essential roles in neuronal differentiation, as evidenced by studies using histone deacetylase inhibitors, such as valproic (VP) and trichostatin A (TSA) [90-92]. VPA promotes neuronal differentiation from adult hippocampal NPCs by inducing the proneural genes, *Ngn1, Math1,* and *NeuroD,* and histone H4 acetylation, while inhibiting glial differentiation [92]. A combination of TSA with sonic hedgehog (Shh), fibroblast growth factor 8 (FGF8) and Wnt instructs non-mesencephalic NPCs to give rise to dopaminergic neurons [93]. Inhibiting the activity of all HDAC1, 2, and 3 in NPCs leads to suppression of oligodendrocyte differentiation, while HDAC2 activity alone inhibits astrocyte differentiation. On the other hand, the HDAC1 activity is required for neural differentiation [94]. HDACs are generally present within large multi-subunit protein complexes in the nucleus [69]. Among them in association with neuronal differentiation is the HDAC/CoREST/REST repressor complex. The repressor element 1-silencing transcription factor (REST) is a vertebrate zinc finger transcriptional repressor protein, which plays a fundamental role in neurogenesis [95-97]. REST is expressed in both ESCs and NSCs, but is not expressed in ES-derived neurons [98]. REST binds to an evolutionally conserved DNA motif known as the repressor element 1 (RE1) [96, 97]. REST represses the expression of RE1-containing neuronal genes via recruitment of HDAC/CoREST complexes containing HDAC1 and HDAC 2 [97]. Thus, RE1 motif-associated neuronal genes in ESCs and NPCs appear to be suppressed by REST. This repression could block premature expression of genes associated with terminal differentiation at earlier stages than needed. Recently, a genome-wide binding site analysis revealed the target genes of REST during cholinergic, GABAergic, glutamatergic, and medium spiny projection neuronal specification from NPCs [99]. A large number of the identified REST target genes are unique for each neuronal subtype, strongly suggesting that histone deacetylase plays essential roles in epigenetic control of neuronal subtype specification as well as neuronal lineage commitment.

4.2. DNA methylation

DNA methylation has been shown to suppress astrocyte-specific genes in NPCs during early stages of development. Promoters of many astrocyte-specific genes contain the signal transducer and activator of transcription (STAT) binding elements. With this, astrocyte-specific genes are transcriptionally activated through the Janus kinase (JAK)-STAT pathway, one of whose ligands is the cytokine leukemia inhibitory factor (LIF). However, neurogenic NPCs are not competent to differentiate into astrocytes even when they are grown with LIF, because the STAT-binding elements within astrocyte-specific genes promoters are methylated [100, 101]. This DNA methylation inhibits the association of activated STATs with the promoter of astrocyte-specific genes, thereby repressing their transcription. Conditional deletion of *DNMT1* in embryonic NPCs results in DNA hypomethylation and alteration of the timing of astrocytogenesis [101]. In addition, knockdown of *DNMT3B* in ESCs alters the timing of their neural differentiation [102]. These findings suggest that DNA methylation controls the timing and developmental switch from neurogenesis to astrogliogenesis of NPCs by altering responsiveness to their extracellular developmental cues.

4.3. Chromatin remodeling

As NPCs exit the cell cycle and differentiate into mature neurons, BAF60C is incorporated into the npBAF complexes [80, 103]. BAF45A and BAF53A in the complexes give way to BAF45B/C and BAF53B, respectively (Figure 2) [80, 103], establishing the post-mitotic neuron-specific nBAF complexes. Preventing the exchange of npBAF and nBAF components impairs neuronal differentiation, indicating that a switch in subunit composition of the BAF complexes is required for the transition from pluripotent ESCs to post-mitotic neurons [80, 103]. The nBAF complexes, along with Ca^{2+}-responsive dendritic regulator CREST, also play a role in regulating the activation of genes essential for activity-dependent dendritic outgrowth, suggesting that the nBAF complexes are required for morphological/synaptic development of neurons [103, 104].

The BAF complexes incorporate the BAF57 subunit containing DNA-binding HMG-box domains [105]. In addition, the BAF complex subunits contain motifs known to bind to modified histones, including chromo-, bromo-, and PHD domains [103]. The bromodomain can bind acetylated histones [106]. The chromo- and PHD domains function as lysine-methylated histone-binding domains [106]. The esBAF and npBAF complexes contain different chromodomain proteins (BAF155 or BAF170) [103], whereas the npBAF and nBAF complexes contain different PHD domain proteins (BAF45a or BAF45b) [80, 103]. Thus, changes in subunit composition could alter targets of the BAF complexes, thereby causing changes in gene expression patterns during neuronal differentiation.

4.4. Non-coding RNAs

A number of miRNAs involved in cell fate decision during stem cell differentiation is also highly expressed in the nervous systems. Among these is miR-9, which is expressed specifically in neurogenic areas of the embryonic and adult brains [107, 108]. TLX, an orphan nuclear receptor, is essential for maintaining a self-renewable and undifferentiated state [109], as well as cell cycle progression [110] of NPCs in the developing brain. TLX is highly expressed in NPCs, but its expression is down-regulated upon neural differentiation [111]. Conversely, miR-9 expression increases during neural differentiation [111]. Furthermore, miR-9 has been shown to negatively regulate NPC proliferation and accelerate differentiation through targeting *TLX* transcription [111]. These findings suggest that miR-9 can switch from undifferentiated to differentiated state of NPCs by downregulating *TLX* expression. Another miRNA, miR-124, has been reported to promote neuronal differentiation by targeting several genes involved in selection of non-neuronal cell fates. For example, miR-124 regulates the BAF complex subunit composition during differentiation from NPCs to neurons (Figure 2) by binding and thus suppressing *BAF53A* mRNA transcripts, which allows facilitation of a switch between BAF53 subunits [112]. These studies indicate that miRNA expression should be strictly controlled to ensure proper differentiation of ESCs into neurons. Consistent with this assumption, miR-124 is expressed in neurons, but not in astrocytes [113], and the miR-124 level increases during neural differentiation [84]. Remarkably, the control of miR-124 expression itself is mediated by an epigenetic mechanism. The promoter of the *miR-124* gene contains a functional RE1 site. In ESCs and NPCs, REST occupies the miR-124 gene locus and represses its expression [114], allowing persistent expression of non-neuronal mRNAs. However, once NPCs start to differentiate into neurons, REST is downregulated, thereby disinhibiting miR-124 expression. miR-124 then triggers degradation of non-neuronal mRNA transcripts, which promotes differentiation towards a neuronal lineage. One of the known target genes for miR-124 is C-terminal domain phosphatase 1 (*SCP1*), which represses transcription of RE1-containing neuronal genes by REST, thereby preventing cells from adopting a neuronal lineage and producing non-neural tissues [115]. Together, *miR-124* is a target for REST, but at the same token also targets the REST co-repressor. This represents the presence of a negative feedback loop between miRNA and a REST silencing complex, and such a mechanism may be broadly used to ensure proper cell fate transitions during development.

Neurons derived from different human ESC lines exhibit distinctive cellular properties due to the fact that human ESC lines were established under diverse conditions and from embryos with different genetic backgrounds. Comparison of neurons derived from HSF1 and HSF6 ESC human lines has revealed that the HSF1 line produces forebrain neurons with GABAergic and dopaminergic neurotransmitter phenotypes, while HSF6-derived neurons produce midbrain/hindbrain neurons bearing dopaminergic, cholinergic, serotonergic, non-forebrain GABAergic, and glutamatergic phenotypes [116]. Significant differences in the miRNA expression profile was noted between these 2 human ESC lines [116], suggesting that miRNA expression patterns might dictate in defining various neuronal subtypes arisen from ESCs.

5. Conclusions

Epigenetic mechanisms are regulatory processes that control gene expression via changes in chromatin structure without alterations in the DNA sequence. Changes in chromatin structure alter the accessibility of transcription factors and RNA polymerase to genes packed into chromatin, thereby modulating the efficiency of gene transcription. Epigenetic mechanisms act to control this accessibility through histone modifications, DNA methylation, chromatin remodeling, and non-coding RNAs. Each of these epigenetic events interacts with intrinsic (ex. transcription factors) and/or extrinsic factors (ex. developmental cues such as morphogens and cytokines). Studies so far have suggested that, during sequential transitions from pluripotent ESCs to terminally differentiated neurons, epigenetic mechanisms play critical roles in not only maintaining self-renewal capacity and pluripotency of ESCs, but also restricting cell lineage choices. Further investigation will therefore help clarifying the mechanisms that control pluripotency and neuronal/glial fate specification. Furthermore, the knowledge will be used in harnessing ESCs safely and effectively for clinical applications.

Ackknowledgments

The authors wish to thank the financial support of JSPS KAKENHI Grant Number 24592567 (to A. S.) and NIH RC1 DC010706 (to E.H.).

Author details

Atsushi Shimomura[1] and Eri Hashino[2*]

*Address all correspondence to: ehashino@iupui.edu

1 Department of Anatomy I, Fujita Health University School of Medicine, Toyoake, Aichi, Japan

2 Department of Otolaryngology-Head and Neck Surgery, Stark Neurosciences Research Institute, Indiana University School of Medicine, Indianapolis, IN, USA

References

[1] Evans MJ, Kaufman MH. Establishment in culture of pluripotential cells from mouse embryos. Nature 1981;292(5819) 154-156.

[2] Spivakov M, Fisher AG. Epigenetic signatures of stem-cell identity. Nat Rev Genet 2007;8(4) 263-271.

[3] Chen L, Daley GQ. Molecular basis of pluripotency. Hum Mol Genet 2008;17(R1) R23-27.

[4] Temple S. The development of neural stem cells. Nature 2001;414(6859) 112-117.

[5] Temple S. Division and differentiation of isolated CNS blast cells in microculture. Nature 1989;340(6233) 471-473.

[6] Kilpatrick TJ, Bartlett PF. Cloning and growth of multipotential neural precursors: requirements for proliferation and differentiation. Neuron 1993;10(2) 255-265.

[7] Hirabayashi Y, Gotoh Y. Stage-dependent fate determination of neural precursor cells in mouse forebrain. Neurosci Res 2005;51(4) 331-336.

[8] Hirabayashi Y, Gotoh Y. Epigenetic control of neural precursor cell fate during development. Nat Rev Neurosci 2010;11(6) 377-388.

[9] Loh YH, Wu Q, Chew JL, Vega VB, Zhang W, Chen X, Bourque G, George J, Leong B, Liu J, Wong KY, Sung KW, Lee CW, Zhao XD, Chiu KP, Lipovich L, Kuznetsov VA, Robson P, Stanton LW, Wei CL, Ruan Y, Lim B, Ng HH. The Oct4 and Nanog transcription network regulates pluripotency in mouse embryonic stem cells. Nat Genet 2006;38(4) 431-440.

[10] Zhou Q, Chipperfield H, Melton DA, Wong WH. A gene regulatory network in mouse embryonic stem cells. Proc Natl Acad Sci U S A 2007;104(42) 16438-16443.

[11] Walker E, Ohishi M, Davey RE, Zhang W, Cassar PA, Tanaka TS, Der SD, Morris Q, Hughes TR, Zandstra PW, Stanford WL. Prediction and testing of novel transcriptional networks regulating embryonic stem cell self-renewal and commitment. Cell Stem Cell 2007;1(1) 71-86.

[12] Young RA. Control of the embryonic stem cell state. Cell 2011;144(6) 940-954.

[13] Heo J, Lee JS, Chu IS, Takahama Y, Thorgeirsson SS. Spontaneous differentiation of mouse embryonic stem cells *in vitro*: characterization by global gene expression profiles. Biochem Biophys Res Commun 2005;332(4) 1061-1069.

[14] Loring JF, Porter JG, Seilhammer J, Kaser MR, Wesselschmidt R. A gene expression profile of embryonic stem cells and embryonic stem cell-derived neurons. Restor Neurol Neurosci 2001;18(2-3) 81-88.

[15] Bhattacharya B, Puri S, Puri RK. A review of gene expression profiling of human embryonic stem cell lines and their differentiated progeny. Curr Stem Cell Res Ther 2009;4(2) 98-106.

[16] Stein GS, Stein JL, Van Wijnen AJ, Lian JB, Montecino M, Croce CM, Choi JY, Ali SA, Pande S, Hassan MQ, Zaidi SK, Young DW. Transcription factor-mediated epigenetic regulation of cell growth and phenotype for biological control and cancer. Adv Enzyme Regul 2010;50(1) 160-167.

[17] Lunyak VV, Rosenfeld MG. Epigenetic regulation of stem cell fate. Hum Mol Genet 2008;17(R1) R28-36.

[18] Luger K, Mader AW, Richmond RK, Sargent DF, Richmond TJ. Crystal structure of the nucleosome core particle at 2.8 A resolution. Nature 1997;389(6648) 251-260.

[19] Yuan GC, Liu YJ, Dion MF, Slack MD, Wu LF, Altschuler SJ, Rando OJ. Genome-scale identification of nucleosome positions in S. cerevisiae. Science 2005;309(5734) 626-630.

[20] Muthurajan UM, Bao Y, Forsberg LJ, Edayathumangalam RS, Dyer PN, White CL, Luger K. Crystal structures of histone Sin mutant nucleosomes reveal altered protein-DNA interactions. EMBO J 2004;23(2) 260-271.

[21] Lieb JD, Clarke ND. Control of transcription through intragenic patterns of nucleosome composition. Cell 2005;123(7) 1187-1190.

[22] Bell O, Tiwari VK, Thoma NH, Schubeler D. Determinants and dynamics of genome accessibility. Nat Rev Genet 2011;12(8) 554-564.

[23] Bai L, Morozov AV. Gene regulation by nucleosome positioning. Trends Genet 2010;26(11) 476-483.

[24] Anderson JD, Lowary PT, Widom J. Effects of histone acetylation on the equilibrium accessibility of nucleosomal DNA target sites. J Mol Biol 2001;307(4) 977-985.

[25] Strahl BD, Allis CD. The language of covalent histone modifications. Nature 2000;403(6765) 41-45.

[26] Lewis BP, Burge CB, Bartel DP. Conserved seed pairing, often flanked by adenosines, indicates that thousands of human genes are microRNA targets. Cell 2005;120(1) 15-20.

[27] Kouzarides T. Chromatin modifications and their function. Cell 2007;128(4) 693-705.

[28] Zhang Y, Reinberg D. Transcription regulation by histone methylation: interplay between different covalent modifications of the core histone tails. Genes Dev 2001;15(18) 2343-2360.

[29] Peterson CL, Laniel MA. Histones and histone modifications. Curr Biol 2004;14(14) R546-551.

[30] Nishioka K, Rice JC, Sarma K, Erdjument-Bromage H, Werner J, Wang Y, Chuikov S, Valenzuela P, Tempst P, Steward R, Lis JT, Allis CD, Reinberg D. PR-Set7 is a nucleosome-specific methyltransferase that modifies lysine 20 of histone H4 and is associated with silent chromatin. Mol Cell 2002;9(6) 1201-1213.

[31] Schotta G, Lachner M, Sarma K, Ebert A, Sengupta R, Reuter G, Reinberg D, Jenuwein T. A silencing pathway to induce H3-K9 and H4-K20 trimethylation at constitutive heterochromatin. Genes Dev 2004;18(11) 1251-1262.

[32] Kouzarides T. Histone methylation in transcriptional control. Curr Opin Genet Dev 2002;12(2) 198-209.

[33] Martin C, Zhang Y. The diverse functions of histone lysine methylation. Nat Rev Mol Cell Biol 2005;6(11) 838-849.

[34] Wang Y, Jia S. Degrees make all the difference: the multifunctionality of histone H4 lysine 20 methylation. Epigenetics 2009;4(5) 273-276.

[35] Suzuki MM, Bird A. DNA methylation landscapes: provocative insights from epigenomics. Nat Rev Genet 2008;9(6) 465-476.

[36] Eden S, Cedar H. Role of DNA methylation in the regulation of transcription. Curr Opin Genet Dev 1994;4(2) 255-259.

[37] Law JA, Jacobsen SE. Establishing, maintaining and modifying DNA methylation patterns in plants and animals. Nat Rev Genet 2010;11(3) 204-220.

[38] Ballestar E, Wolffe AP. Methyl-CpG-binding proteins. Targeting specific gene repression. Eur J Biochem 2001;268(1) 1-6.

[39] Wade PA. Methyl CpG-binding proteins and transcriptional repression. Bioessays 2001;23(12) 1131-1137.

[40] Jones PL, Veenstra GJ, Wade PA, Vermaak D, Kass SU, Landsberger N, Strouboulis J, Wolffe AP. Methylated DNA and MeCP2 recruit histone deacetylase to repress transcription. Nat Genet 1998;19(2) 187-191.

[41] Nan X, Ng HH, Johnson CA, Laherty CD, Turner BM, Eisenman RN, Bird A. Transcriptional repression by the methyl-CpG-binding protein MeCP2 involves a histone deacetylase complex. Nature 1998;393(6683) 386-389.

[42] Cairns BR. Chromatin remodeling: insights and intrigue from single-molecule studies. Nat Struct Mol Biol 2007;14(11) 989-996.

[43] Hargreaves DC, Crabtree GR. ATP-dependent chromatin remodeling: genetics, genomics and mechanisms. Cell Res 2011;21(3) 396-420.

[44] Smith CL, Peterson CL. ATP-dependent chromatin remodeling. Curr Top Dev Biol 2005;65 115-148.

[45] Varga-Weisz PD, Blank TA, Becker PB. Energy-dependent chromatin accessibility and nucleosome mobility in a cell-free system. EMBO J 1995;14(10) 2209-2216.

[46] Ito T, Bulger M, Pazin MJ, Kobayashi R, Kadonaga JT. ACF, an ISWI-containing and ATP-utilizing chromatin assembly and remodeling factor. Cell 1997;90(1) 145-155.

[47] Zhang Y, Ng HH, Erdjument-Bromage H, Tempst P, Bird A, Reinberg D. Analysis of the NuRD subunits reveals a histone deacetylase core complex and a connection with DNA methylation. Genes Dev 1999;13(15) 1924-1935.

[48] Xie W, Ling T, Zhou Y, Feng W, Zhu Q, Stunnenberg HG, Grummt I, Tao W. The chromatin remodeling complex NuRD establishes the poised state of rRNA genes characterized by bivalent histone modifications and altered nucleosome positions. Proc Natl Acad Sci U S A 2012;109(21) 8161-8166.

[49] Brosnan CA, Voinnet O. The long and the short of noncoding RNAs. Curr Opin Cell Biol 2009;21(3) 416-425.

[50] Cannell IG, Kong YW, Bushell M. How do microRNAs regulate gene expression? Biochem Soc Trans 2008;36(Pt 6) 1224-1231.

[51] Lagos-Quintana M, Rauhut R, Lendeckel W, Tuschl T. Identification of novel genes coding for small expressed RNAs. Science 2001;294(5543) 853-858.

[52] Lee Y, Jeon K, Lee JT, Kim S, Kim VN. MicroRNA maturation: stepwise processing and subcellular localization. EMBO J 2002;21(17) 4663-4670.

[53] He L, Thomson JM, Hemann MT, Hernando-Monge E, Mu D, Goodson S, Powers S, Cordon-Cardo C, Lowe SW, Hannon GJ, Hammond SM. A microRNA polycistron as a potential human oncogene. Nature 2005;435(7043) 828-833.

[54] Azuara V, Perry P, Sauer S, Spivakov M, Jorgensen HF, John RM, Gouti M, Casanova M, Warnes G, Merkenschlager M, Fisher AG. Chromatin signatures of pluripotent cell lines. Nat Cell Biol 2006;8(5) 532-538.

[55] Bernstein BE, Mikkelsen TS, Xie X, Kamal M, Huebert DJ, Cuff J, Fry B, Meissner A, Wernig M, Plath K, Jaenisch R, Wagschal A, Feil R, Schreiber SL, Lander ES. A bivalent chromatin structure marks key developmental genes in embryonic stem cells. Cell 2006;125(2) 315-326.

[56] Mikkelsen TS, Ku M, Jaffe DB, Issac B, Lieberman E, Giannoukos G, Alvarez P, Brockman W, Kim TK, Koche RP, Lee W, Mendenhall E, O'Donovan A, Presser A, Russ C, Xie X, Meissner A, Wernig M, Jaenisch R, Nusbaum C, Lander ES, Bernstein BE. Genome-wide maps of chromatin state in pluripotent and lineage-committed cells. Nature 2007;448(7153) 553-560.

[57] Ringrose L, Paro R. Epigenetic regulation of cellular memory by the Polycomb and Trithorax group proteins. Annu Rev Genet 2004;38 413-443.

[58] Lee TI, Jenner RG, Boyer LA, Guenther MG, Levine SS, Kumar RM, Chevalier B, Johnstone SE, Cole MF, Isono K, Koseki H, Fuchikami T, Abe K, Murray HL, Zucker JP, Yuan B, Bell GW, Herbolsheimer E, Hannett NM, Sun K, Odom DT, Otte AP, Volkert TL, Bartel DP, Melton DA, Gifford DK, Jaenisch R, Young RA. Control of developmental regulators by Polycomb in human embryonic stem cells. Cell 2006;125(2) 301-313.

[59] Boyer LA, Plath K, Zeitlinger J, Brambrink T, Medeiros LA, Lee TI, Levine SS, Wernig M, Tajonar A, Ray MK, Bell GW, Otte AP, Vidal M, Gifford DK, Young RA, Jaenisch R. Polycomb complexes repress developmental regulators in murine embryonic stem cells. Nature 2006;441(7091) 349-353.

[60] Cao R, Zhang Y. The functions of E(Z)/EZH2-mediated methylation of lysine 27 in histone H3. Curr Opin Genet Dev 2004;14(2) 155-164.

[61] Cao R, Wang L, Wang H, Xia L, Erdjument-Bromage H, Tempst P, Jones RS, Zhang Y. Role of histone H3 lysine 27 methylation in Polycomb-group silencing. Science 2002;298(5595) 1039-1043.

[62] Schwartz YB, Pirrotta V. Polycomb silencing mechanisms and the management of genomic programmes. Nat Rev Genet 2007;8(1) 9-22.

[63] Jiang H, Shukla A, Wang X, Chen WY, Bernstein BE, Roeder RG. Role for Dpy-30 in ES cell-fate specification by regulation of H3K4 methylation within bivalent domains. Cell 2011;144(4) 513-525.

[64] Burgold T, Spreafico F, De Santa F, Totaro MG, Prosperini E, Natoli G, Testa G. The histone H3 lysine 27-specific demethylase Jmjd3 is required for neural commitment. PLoS One 2008;3(8) e3034.

[65] Schmitz SU, Albert M, Malatesta M, Morey L, Johansen JV, Bak M, Tommerup N, Abarrategui I, Helin K. Jarid1b targets genes regulating development and is involved in neural differentiation. EMBO J 2011;30(22) 4586-4600.

[66] Meshorer E, Yellajoshula D, George E, Scambler PJ, Brown DT, Misteli T. Hyperdynamic plasticity of chromatin proteins in pluripotent embryonic stem cells. Dev Cell 2006;10(1) 105-116.

[67] Song MR, Ghosh A. FGF2-induced chromatin remodeling regulates CNTF-mediated gene expression and astrocyte differentiation. Nat Neurosci 2004;7(3) 229-235.

[68] Meshorer E, Misteli T. Chromatin in pluripotent embryonic stem cells and differentiation. Nat Rev Mol Cell Biol 2006;7(7) 540-546.

[69] Hayakawa T, Nakayama J. Physiological roles of class I HDAC complex and histone demethylase. J Biomed Biotechnol 2011;2011 129383.

[70] Sapountzi V, Logan IR, Robson CN. Cellular functions of TIP60. Int J Biochem Cell Biol 2006;38(9) 1496-1509.

[71] Fazzio TG, Huff JT, Panning B. An RNAi screen of chromatin proteins identifies Tip60-p400 as a regulator of embryonic stem cell identity. Cell 2008;134(1) 162-174.

[72] Meissner A, Mikkelsen TS, Gu H, Wernig M, Hanna J, Sivachenko A, Zhang X, Bernstein BE, Nusbaum C, Jaffe DB, Gnirke A, Jaenisch R, Lander ES. Genome-scale DNA methylation maps of pluripotent and differentiated cells. Nature 2008;454(7205) 766-770.

[73] Isagawa T, Nagae G, Shiraki N, Fujita T, Sato N, Ishikawa S, Kume S, Aburatani H. DNA methylation profiling of embryonic stem cell differentiation into the three germ layers. PLoS One;6(10) e26052.

[74] Mohn F, Weber M, Rebhan M, Roloff TC, Richter J, Stadler MB, Bibel M, Schubeler D. Lineage-specific polycomb targets and *de novo* DNA methylation define restriction and potential of neuronal progenitors. Mol Cell 2008;30(6) 755-766.

[75] Fouse SD, Shen Y, Pellegrini M, Cole S, Meissner A, Van Neste L, Jaenisch R, Fan G. Promoter CpG methylation contributes to ES cell gene regulation in parallel with Oct4/Nanog, PcG complex, and histone H3 K4/K27 trimethylation. Cell Stem Cell 2008;2(2) 160-169.

[76] Brinkman AB, Gu H, Bartels SJ, Zhang Y, Matarese F, Simmer F, Marks H, Bock C, Gnirke A, Meissner A, Stunnenberg HG. Sequential ChIP-bisulfite sequencing enables direct genome-scale investigation of chromatin and DNA methylation cross-talk. Genome Res 2012;22(6) 1128-1138.

[77] Kaji K, Caballero IM, MacLeod R, Nichols J, Wilson VA, Hendrich B. The NuRD component Mbd3 is required for pluripotency of embryonic stem cells. Nat Cell Biol 2006;8(3) 285-292.

[78] Kaji K, Nichols J, Hendrich B. Mbd3, a component of the NuRD co-repressor complex, is required for development of pluripotent cells. Development 2007;134(6) 1123-1132.

[79] Ho L, Ronan JL, Wu J, Staahl BT, Chen L, Kuo A, Lessard J, Nesvizhskii AI, Ranish J, Crabtree GR. An embryonic stem cell chromatin remodeling complex, esBAF, is essential for embryonic stem cell self-renewal and pluripotency. Proc Natl Acad Sci U S A 2009;106(13) 5181-5186.

[80] Lessard J, Wu JI, Ranish JA, Wan M, Winslow MM, Staahl BT, Wu H, Aebersold R, Graef IA, Crabtree GR. An essential switch in subunit composition of a chromatin remodeling complex during neural development. Neuron 2007;55(2) 201-215.

[81] Marson A, Levine SS, Cole MF, Frampton GM, Brambrink T, Johnstone S, Guenther MG, Johnston WK, Wernig M, Newman J, Calabrese JM, Dennis LM, Volkert TL, Gupta S, Love J, Hannett N, Sharp PA, Bartel DP, Jaenisch R, Young RA. Connecting microRNA genes to the core transcriptional regulatory circuitry of embryonic stem cells. Cell 2008;134(3) 521-533.

[82] Wang Y, Baskerville S, Shenoy A, Babiarz JE, Baehner L, Blelloch R. Embryonic stem cell-specific microRNAs regulate the G1-S transition and promote rapid proliferation. Nat Genet 2008;40(12) 1478-1483.

[83] Sinkkonen L, Hugenschmidt T, Berninger P, Gaidatzis D, Mohn F, Artus-Revel CG, Zavolan M, Svoboda P, Filipowicz W. MicroRNAs control *de novo* DNA methylation through regulation of transcriptional repressors in mouse embryonic stem cells. Nat Struct Mol Biol 2008;15(3) 259-267.

[84] Delaloy C, Liu L, Lee JA, Su H, Shen F, Yang GY, Young WL, Ivey KN, Gao FB. MicroRNA-9 coordinates proliferation and migration of human embryonic stem cell-derived neural progenitors. Cell Stem Cell 2010;6(4) 323-335.

[85] Krichevsky AM, Sonntag KC, Isacson O, Kosik KS. Specific microRNAs modulate embryonic stem cell-derived neurogenesis. Stem Cells 2006;24(4) 857-864.

[86] Gao FB. Context-dependent functions of specific microRNAs in neuronal development. Neural Dev 2010;5 25.

[87] Hirabayashi Y, Itoh Y, Tabata H, Nakajima K, Akiyama T, Masuyama N, Gotoh Y. The Wnt/beta-catenin pathway directs neuronal differentiation of cortical neural precursor cells. Development 2004;131(12) 2791-2801.

[88] Hirabayashi Y, Suzki N, Tsuboi M, Endo TA, Toyoda T, Shinga J, Koseki H, Vidal M, Gotoh Y. Polycomb limits the neurogenic competence of neural precursor cells to promote astrogenic fate transition. Neuron 2009;63(5) 600-613.

[89] Lee S, Lee B, Lee JW, Lee SK. Retinoid signaling and neurogenin2 function are coupled for the specification of spinal motor neurons through a chromatin modifier CBP. Neuron 2009;62(5) 641-654.

[90] Marin-Husstege M, Muggironi M, Liu A, Casaccia-Bonnefil P. Histone deacetylase activity is necessary for oligodendrocyte lineage progression. J Neurosci 2002;22(23) 10333-10345.

[91] Balasubramaniyan V, Boddeke E, Bakels R, Kust B, Kooistra S, Veneman A, Copray S. Effects of histone deacetylation inhibition on neuronal differentiation of embryonic mouse neural stem cells. Neuroscience 2006;143(4) 939-951.

[92] Hsieh J, Nakashima K, Kuwabara T, Mejia E, Gage FH. Histone deacetylase inhibition-mediated neuronal differentiation of multipotent adult neural progenitor cells. Proc Natl Acad Sci U S A 2004;101(47) 16659-16664.

[93] Rossler R, Boddeke E, Copray S. Differentiation of non-mesencephalic neural stem cells towards dopaminergic neurons. Neuroscience 2010;170(2) 417-428.

[94] Humphrey GW, Wang YH, Hirai T, Padmanabhan R, Panchision DM, Newell LF, McKay RD, Howard BH. Complementary roles for histone deacetylases 1, 2, and 3 in differentiation of pluripotent stem cells. Differentiation 2008;76(4) 348-356.

[95] Chong JA, Tapia-Ramirez J, Kim S, Toledo-Aral JJ, Zheng Y, Boutros MC, Altshuller YM, Frohman MA, Kraner SD, Mandel G. REST: a mammalian silencer protein that restricts sodium channel gene expression to neurons. Cell 1995;80(6) 949-957.

[96] choenherr CJ, Paquette AJ, Anderson DJ. Identification of potential target genes for the neuron-restrictive silencer factor. Proc Natl Acad Sci U S A 1996;93(18) 9881-9886.

[97] Ballas N, Mandel G. The many faces of REST oversee epigenetic programming of neuronal genes. Curr Opin Neurobiol 2005;15(5) 500-506.

[98] Sun YM, Greenway DJ, Johnson R, Street M, Belyaev ND, Deuchars J, Bee T, Wilde S, Buckley NJ. Distinct profiles of REST interactions with its target genes at different stages of neuronal development. Mol Biol Cell 2005;16(12) 5630-5638.

[99] Abrajano JJ, Qureshi IA, Gokhan S, Zheng D, Bergman A, Mehler MF. REST and CoREST modulate neuronal subtype specification, maturation and maintenance.

PLoS One 2009;4(12) e7936. http://www.plosone.org/article/info%3Adoi%2F10.1371%2Fjournal.pone.0007936 (accessed 7 December 2009)

[100] Takizawa T, Nakashima K, Namihira M, Ochiai W, Uemura A, Yanagisawa M, Fujita N, Nakao M, Taga T. DNA methylation is a critical cell-intrinsic determinant of astrocyte differentiation in the fetal brain. Dev Cell 2001;1(6) 749-758.

[101] Fan G, Martinowich K, Chin MH, He F, Fouse SD, Hutnick L, Hattori D, Ge W, Shen Y, Wu H, ten Hoeve J, Shuai K, Sun YE. DNA methylation controls the timing of astrogliogenesis through regulation of JAK-STAT signaling. Development 2005;132(15) 3345-3356.

[102] Martins-Taylor K, Schroeder DI, Lasalle JM, Lalande M, Xu RH. Role of DNMT3B in the regulation of early neural and neural crest specifiers. Epigenetics 2012;7(1) 71-82.

[103] Yoo AS, Crabtree GR. ATP-dependent chromatin remodeling in neural development. Curr Opin Neurobiol 2009;19(2) 120-126.

[104] Wu JI, Lessard J, Olave IA, Qiu Z, Ghosh A, Graef IA, Crabtree GR. Regulation of dendritic development by neuron-specific chromatin remodeling complexes. Neuron 2007;56(1) 94-108.

[105] Wang W, Chi T, Xue Y, Zhou S, Kuo A, Crabtree GR. Architectural DNA binding by a high-mobility-group/kinesin-like subunit in mammalian SWI/SNF-related complexes. Proc Natl Acad Sci U S A 1998;95(2) 492-498.

[106] Yun M, Wu J, Workman JL, Li B. Readers of histone modifications. Cell Res 2011;21(4) 564-578.

[107] Deo M, Yu JY, Chung KH, Tippens M, Turner DL. Detection of mammalian microRNA expression by in situ hybridization with RNA oligonucleotides. Dev Dyn 2006;235(9) 2538-2548.

[108] Kapsimali M, Kloosterman WP, de Bruijn E, Rosa F, Plasterk RH, Wilson SW. MicroRNAs show a wide diversity of expression profiles in the developing and mature central nervous system. Genome Biol 2007;8(8) R173.

[109] Shi Y, Chichung Lie D, Taupin P, Nakashima K, Ray J, Yu RT, Gage FH, Evans RM. Expression and function of orphan nuclear receptor TLX in adult neural stem cells. Nature 2004;427(6969) 78-83.

[110] Li W, Sun G, Yang S, Qu Q, Nakashima K, Shi Y. Nuclear receptor TLX regulates cell cycle progression in neural stem cells of the developing brain. Mol Endocrinol 2008;22(1) 56-64.

[111] Zhao C, Sun G, Li S, Shi Y. A feedback regulatory loop involving microRNA-9 and nuclear receptor TLX in neural stem cell fate determination. Nat Struct Mol Biol 2009;16(4) 365-371.

[112] Yoo AS, Staahl BT, Chen L, Crabtree GR. MicroRNA-mediated switching of chromatin-remodelling complexes in neural development. Nature 2009;460(7255) 642-646.

[113] Smirnova L, Grafe A, Seiler A, Schumacher S, Nitsch R, Wulczyn FG. Regulation of miRNA expression during neural cell specification. Eur J Neurosci 2005;21(6) 1469-1477.

[114] Conaco C, Otto S, Han JJ, Mandel G. Reciprocal actions of REST and a microRNA promote neuronal identity. Proc Natl Acad Sci U S A 2006;103(7) 2422-2427.

[115] Yeo M, Lee SK, Lee B, Ruiz EC, Pfaff SL, Gill GN. Small CTD phosphatases function in silencing neuronal gene expression. Science 2005;307(5709) 596-600.

[116] Wu H, Xu J, Pang ZP, Ge W, Kim KJ, Blanchi B, Chen C, Sudhof TC, Sun YE. Integrative genomic and functional analyses reveal neuronal subtype differentiation bias in human embryonic stem cell lines. Proc Natl Acad Sci U S A 2007;104(34) 13821-13826.

Chapter 13

Neural Fate of Mesenchymal Stem Cells and Neural Crest Stem Cells: Which Ways to Get Neurons for Cell Therapy Purpose?

Virginie Neirinckx, Cécile Coste,
Bernard Rogister and Sabine Wislet-Gendebien

Additional information is available at the end of the chapter

1. Introduction

The treatment of neurological disorders represents a critical issue in clinical research, since no complete recovery of patients can be achieved with actual therapeutic means, despite symptomatic improvements. Indeed, whereas restricted brain areas still house cells competent to generate newborn neurons in adulthood, those neural stem cells are present in restricted amounts. Moreover, this limited neurogenesis does not seem to be sufficient to enable neuronal regeneration in cases of traumatic, ischemic or degenerative lesions of the central nervous system. Therefore, other sources of neural cells have to be considered in a cell therapy objective.

Stem cells are characterized as cells endowed with continuous self-renewal ability and pluri- or multipotentiality, and could consequently give rise to a wide panel of cell types. Non-germinal stem cells are classified into different categories: (1) Embryonic stem cells (ES) are found in the inner cell mass of blastocyst and are pluripotent stem cells that can generate any mature cell of each of the three germ layers; (2) Induced pluripotent stem cells (iPS) are adult somatic cells that are reprogrammed into pluripotent cells with ES-like abilities; (3) Somatic stem cells are tissue-specific and more restricted than ES cells in terms of differentiation capabilities. They can be isolated from various fetal and adult tissues, which make them an attractive supply of material for cell therapy. Indeed, while neurons have already been successfully generated from ES cells [1] or iPS cells [2, 3], the use of adult somatic stem cells definitely remain of significant interest regarding technical, ethical and immunological issues concerning cell transplantation for brain diseases. In this regard, mesenchymal stem cells (MSCs) and neural crest-derived stem cells (NCSCs) that can be found in various locations of the adult organism (and even in perinatal tissues) represent an important source of easily-accessible multipotent cells to use in a cell therapy purpose.

In this chapter, we will describe the major features of MSCs and NCSCs isolated from five different tissues, which constitute the main exploited and accessible sources for cell isolation in an objective of cell therapy protocols for neurological disorders (Figure 1). Moreover, we will detail the multiple ways they can generate neuron-like cells *in vitro*. Indeed, numerous culture conditions and differentiation protocols do exist and are demonstrated as efficient, supporting the fact that neural differentiation can occur through different cellular signaling mechanisms. Therefore, we will review the various signaling pathways that could trigger the neural fate adoption of MSCs and NCSCs, and the related cell-based therapy experiments that have been done downstream.

2. Different types of mesenchymal stem cells

Mesenchymal stem cells (MSCs) are plastic-adherent, fibroblast-like cells, which are conventionally able to self-renew and differentiate into tissues of the mesodermic lineage, such as bone, adipose tissue and cartilage. Whereas those cells have traditionally been isolated from bone marrow stroma, many reports have now described the presence of MSCs in a variety of fetal, perinatal and adult tissues, including peripheral blood, umbilical cord Wharton's Jelly and blood, fetal liver and lungs, adipose tissue, skeletal muscles, amniotic fluid, synovium and circulatory system, where they work as supportive cells and maintain tissue homeostasis.

2.1. Bone marrow mesenchymal stem cells

The initial study of non-hematopoietic bone marrow (BM) cells was performed by Friedenstein et al. in the late 80's [4, 5]. After establishing single cell suspensions of BM, they showed that those cells were able to generate colonies of adherent fibroblast-shaped cells when cultured *in vitro*. They demonstrated that these colony-forming unit - fibroblasts (CFU-F) presented the ability to undergo osteogenic differentiation [5, 6]. These bone marrow mesenchymal stem cells (BM-MSCs) were then demonstrated as multipotent progenitors that were able to self-renew [7] and could differentiate into any cell of the mesodermic lineage, like osteoblasts, chondrocytes, or adipocytes [8, 9]. More interestingly, it has been showed that BM-MSCs were able to "trans-differentiate" into cells with endodermal or ectodermal characteristics [10], and particularly into neuron-like cells [11-15]. These stem cells are therefore raising huge interest, since they represent a promising source of material for cell therapy protocols, such as mesenchymal tissue engineering or neurological disorder treatments as well.

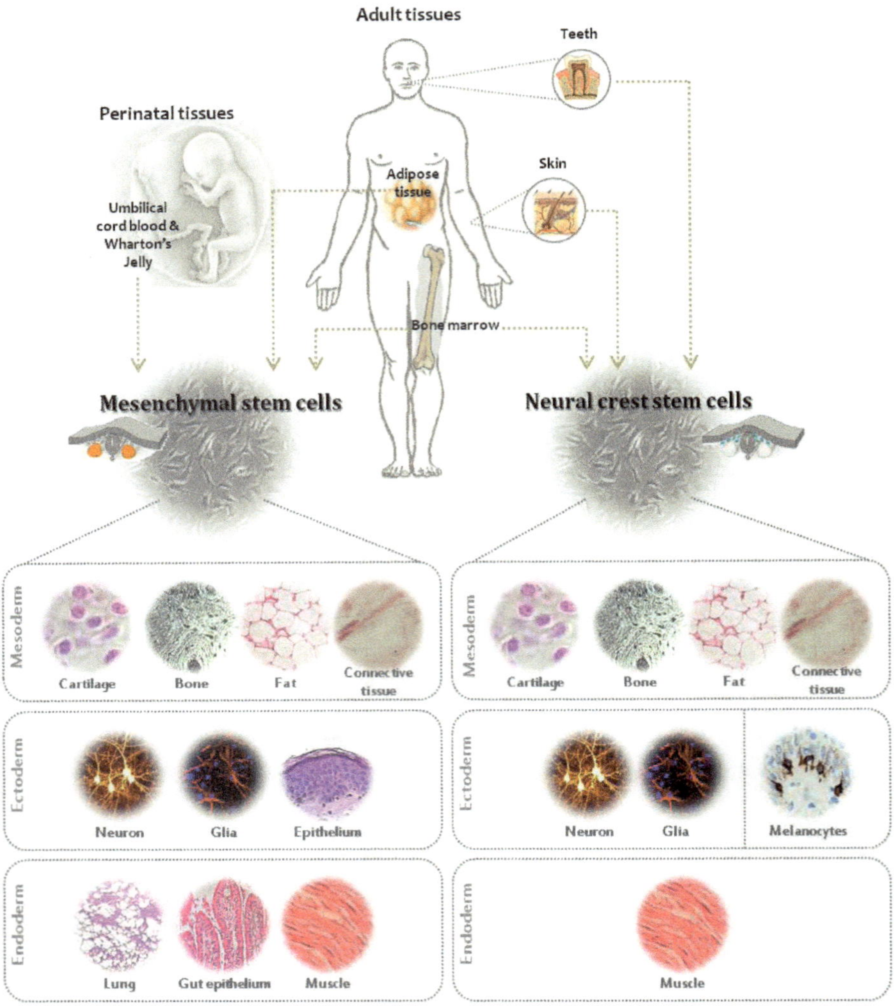

Figure 1. Mesenchymal and neural crest stem cells from different perinatal and adult tissues. The upper part describes the presence of mesenchymal and/or neural crest stem cells in various adult tissue. The lower part describes cell fate that have been demonstrated for each type of stem cells regarding the mesodermic, endodermic or ectodermic cell lineage.

The main debate concerning BM-MSCs resides in the lack of exact phenotypic characterization, due to the absence of specific membrane markers and non-standardized culture methods. Consequently, several groups described BM-MSCs with a wide variety of different phenotypes: Verfaillie's group described a rare population of cells in human BM stroma as mesodermal adult progenitor cells (MAPCs)[12, 16]; D'Ippolito and collaborators cultured cells in low oxygen tension and characterized marrow isolated adult multilineage inducible (MIAMI) cells [17, 18]; whereas a lot of other groups kept the mesenchymal stem cell concept as defined by Pittenger et al. [9].

In addition to the phenotypic differences of BM-MSCs which are inherent to culture settings, it has been demonstrated that BM stroma was a mixed population of cells arising from different embryonic lineages. Although adult BM-MSCs were commonly considered to be of mesodermal origin (bone marrow mesenchymal stem cells) [19], several studies have shown that some adult BM-MSCs derive from the embryonic neural crest [20-24] (see paragraph below). Hence, the different studies that are detailed below often describe BM-MSCs without distinguishing mesenchymal and neural-crest derived cells.

2.2. Adipose tissue stem cells

Similarly to the main part of BM stroma, adipose tissue derives from mesodermic lineage and contains stem cells able to differentiate into bone, cartilage, fat and muscle. Likewise, adipose tissue mesenchymal stem cells (AT-MSCs) can adopt a neural-like phenotype [25, 26], which makes them another potential source of cells to use in replacement therapy.

2.3. Umbilical cord blood and Wharton's jelly mesenchymal stem cells

Wharton's jelly constitutes the gelatinous matrix of umbilical cord. Mainly composed of collagen fibers, proteoglycans and stromal cells, this tissue has also been described to enclose mesenchymal cells endowed with stem cells properties (WJ-MSCs); They are easily cultured and expanded *in vitro,* and are able to differentiate into a wide range of cell types, including neural cells [27-29].

Whereas adult peripheral blood only contains a tiny number of MSCs, umbilical cord blood is a richer source and allows to culture adherent MSCs more efficiently. These umbilical cord blood MSCs (UCB-MSCs) are considered as a more primitive population, but can be largely expanded and maintained in long term culture [30], and were described to be an osteogenic, adipogenic, chondrogenic and even a neurogenic cell population [31-33]. Altogether, these data confirmed umbilical cord as a new source of cells for cellular therapeutics for stromal, bone, and, potentially, neural repair [34].

3. Different types of neural crest stem cells

During embryonic development of vertebrates, neural crest is specified at the border of the neural plate and the non-neural ectoderm after gastrulation. During neurulation, the neural folds both join at the dorsal midline to form the neural tube. Subsequently, neural crest cells (NCC) from the roof plate of the neural tube undergo an epithelial to mesenchymal transition (EMT), delaminating from the neuroectoderm. Those multipotent NCC then migrate towards different locations in the body where they differentiate into various cell types, including melanocytes, craniofacial cartilage and bone, smooth muscle, peripheral and enteric neuron, and glia.

In the past few years, multipotent and self renewing neural crest stem cells (NCSCs) have been described to persist in the adult organism. Those post-migratory NCSCs were found in the gut [35], the skin [36-38], the cornea [39], the heart [40], the teeth [41, 42], the dorsal root ganglion and the bone marrow [21, 22, 43]. As the skin, the teeth and the bone marrow constitute the most easily-accessible and available sources of NCSCs to use in therapy protocols, we will describe those three tissues more precisely.

3.1. Bone marrow neural crest stem cells

Regarding the striking similarities of bone marrow stromal cells and embryonic NCSCs concerning their neural differentiation potential, the question of the presence of a neural crest-derived cell subpopulation in bone marrow was raised. Indeed, the mesodermal origin of bone marrow stromal cells was definitely queried since a study of Takashima et al. demonstrated that a first wave of mesenchymal stem cells in the embryo derives from the Sox1-positive neuroepithelium through a neural crest stage [20].

Lately, convincing evidence for the subsistence of NCSCs in bone marrow emerged from a study by Nagoshi et al. They isolated neural crest-derived cells from the bone marrow using Wnt1-Cre/FloxedEGFP mice for *in vivo* fate mapping. Those cells could be propagated in sphere cultures for a couple of passages. A bit more than 3% of these isolated $EGFP^+$ cells had the capacity to differentiate into neurons, glia, and smooth muscle cells (this proportion was sustainably increased by collagenase treatment, suggesting their tight contact with bone surface) [21, 22]. The same group used another transgenic mouse (P0-Cre/FloxedEGFP) to isolate NCSCs among the bone marrow stromal cells, and demonstrated their ability to differentiate into neural crest lineages but also into mesenchymal lineages such as adipocytes, chondrocytes and osteocytes [22]. Using a Wnt1-Cre/FloxedLacZ transgenic mouse, the group of Wislet-Gendebien generated neural-crest derived clones of passage 5 bone marrow stromal cells, and compared them with mesenchymal clones. They showed that the two types of populations were surprisingly similar at the transcriptomic level and in terms of differentiation abilities, and that both of them could give rise to neurons [43]. Altogether, the different results about bone marrow NCSCs make those cells as exciting as their MSCs neighbors in a context of therapy. Moreover, their neural crest origin may confer them particular additional properties in a perspective of nervous system repair.

3.2. Skin-derived neural crest stem cells

Using the same type of Wnt1-Cre reporter mice, the groups of Sieber-Blum and Toma identified neural crest-derived stem cells in the facial skin of adult mice and humans [36, 37, 44, 45]. Those skin-derived precursors (SKPs) are located in the dermal papillae and in the hair follicle, and are able to differentiate *in vitro* into neurons, smooth muscle cells, Schwann cells and melanocytes.

Other skin-derived NCSCs, termed epidermal NCSCs (EPI-NCSCs) were isolated from the bulge region of whisker follicles. Similarly to SKPs, EPI-NCSCs can give rise to neurons, smooth muscle cells, Schwann cells and melanocytes [37, 44, 46]. As an easy-accessible autologous source of highly multipotent stem cells, the skin and its SKPs and EPI-NCSCs are of significant interest in cell therapy.

3.3. Dental neural crest stem cells

The dental pulp is the connective tissue that forms the inner part of the teeth, and contains ondotoblasts which are responsible of dentin formation. Few years ago, a population of stem cells has been identified in dental pulp, and is thought to arise from the embryonic cranial neural crest [47, 48]. These dental pulp stem cells (DP-SCs) are endowed with high proliferative potential, self-renewal ability and multi-lineage differentiation [42, 49], making them an attractive tool for stem cell therapeutic strategies. Whereas the DP-SCs are isolated from the adult teeth, the same type of stem cells can be found in the human exfoliated deciduous teeth (SHED cells), identified as immature DP-SCs.

The properties of self-renewal and multi-lineage differentiation ability of all described stem cells make them truly attractive candidates for cell therapy. Furthermore, they offer the non-negligible advantage of being easily obtained without invasive method. Indeed, whereas umbilical cord is usually intended to trash after birth and can rather be preserved in order to collect cells, bone marrow aspiration, lipo-aspiration, or teeth extraction are non-heavy procedures that are commonly performed in clinical context. Those procedures could even be performed in patients when needed, allowing autologous grafts and avoiding immunological rejects. Additionally, the use of MSCs/NCSCs, from either adult origin or isolated from umbilical cord, get round the ethical problems related to fetal cells use. Moreover, those cells are supposed to be safer than embryonic stem cells or induced pluripotent stem cells in terms of tumorigenicity and genomic modifications [24, 50].

4. Signaling pathways involved in neural differentiation of MSCs and NCSCs

As already mentioned, a wide range of culture settings for MSCs/NCSCs neural differentiation were commonly experienced, with some of them giving rise to substantial results. Hence, it can be inferred that MSCs/NCSCs can give rise to neuronal cells through the activation/deactivation of many intracellular signaling pathways. In this chapter, we will focus on the analysis of several differentiating protocols that highlighted specific signaling pathways in neuronal fate decision. We will dissect those pathways from the ligand molecules to the different cellular and molecular effectors that are involved within, up to the gene expression modulation. We will then describe the different downstream effects experimentally observed after activation of those pathways, in the context of neural fate adoption by different type of MSCs/NCSCs and summarized in Figure 2 and Table 1.

4.1. Cyclic-adenosine-monophosphate and PKA signaling pathway

Cyclic-adenosine-monophosphate (cAMP) is a well-known intracellular messenger, which is physiologically synthesized from adenosine-triphosphate by a membrane-anchored adenylyl cyclase, when this last is induced by an active G protein-coupled receptor. In the cytoplasm, cAMP essentially activates the protein kinase A (PKA), which then reach the nucleus where it supports the phosphorylation of a transcription factor (cAMP responsive element binding protein, or CREB protein). Once phosphorylated, CREB protein binds CREB-binding protein (CREBB protein or CBP), and with the support of different co-factors, join specific DNA sequences and regulate the expression of different genes (coding for c-fos, brain derived neurotrophic factor (BDNF)[51], or tyrosine hydroxylase (TH)[52]). The destruction of intracellular cAMP is mediated by phosphodiesterases (PDE), which convert cAMP into AMP, then regulating cAMP cytoplasmic concentrations. This cAMP-dependent pathway has been demonstrated to be fundamental in embryonic development, neural cells survival and other processes like long term memory and neuronal plasticity [53-55].

cAMP is frequently used in culture media to induce MSCs/NCSCs into neural lineage, as well as other molecules which raise the intracellular cAMP levels. For example, forskolin activates adenylyl-cyclase, dibutyryl-cAMP (db-cAMP) and 3-isobutyl-1-methylxanthine (IBMX) both act as inhibitors of phosphodiesterases, and 8-bromo-cAMP activates PKA and is long-acting because of its resistance to degradation by phosphodiesterases.

The main cytoplasmic target of cAMP, which is the PKA, has effectively been demonstrated to mediate neural differentiation. Wang et al. studied the impact of PKA activation on neurite outgrowth and on neural markers glial acidic fibrillary protein (GFAP) and neurofilament (NF) expression. They observed that the complete inactivation of this kinase led to a total absence of neural differentiation in UCB-MSCs, while the level of phosphorylated CREB was upregulated in forskolin-treated cells (this effect was inhibited in presence of PKA inhibitor) [56]. The involvement of PKA in the neural differentiation of MSCs was also confirmed by several others studies [57,58].

According to Lepski et al., neuronal differentiation of human BM-MSCs resulted from a specific mechanism dependent upon the PKA pathway. Indeed, they demonstrated that the presence of a PKA inhibitor in the induction medium impaired the differentiation process (induced by IBMX, coupled with brain-derived neurotrophic factor (BDNF), see paragraph 3.4.), and that CREB was phosphorylated in differentiated MSCs [59]. Moreover, MSC-derived cells showed significant voltage-dependent ionic currents (Na^+, K^+ and Ca^{2+} currents).

Besides, UCB-MSCs were induced to neural outcome with db-cAMP and IBMX treatment, which was demonstrated to be necessary and sufficient for neurite-like outgrowth and for nuclear receptor related 1 protein (Nurr1) expression. Nurr1 is known to play a key role in dopaminergic system maintenance. In addition, those data showed evidence for cAMP-pathway control on differential phosphorylation of TH isoforms [60].

Lin et al. studied the ability of granulocyte-macrophage colony-stimulating-factor (GM-CSF) to promote neural differentiation in BM-MSCs through the phosphorylation of CREB [61]. Indeed, GM-CSF-treated BM-MSCs expressed higher levels of neuron specific enolase (NSE) over time, whereas transiently increased nestin expression. In parallel, a substantial increase of phosphorylated-CREB level was observed in the GM-CSF-treated BM-MSCs compared with control (CREB levels were not different between the two groups), and that the kinetics of this increase was consistent with the progress in neural differentiation.

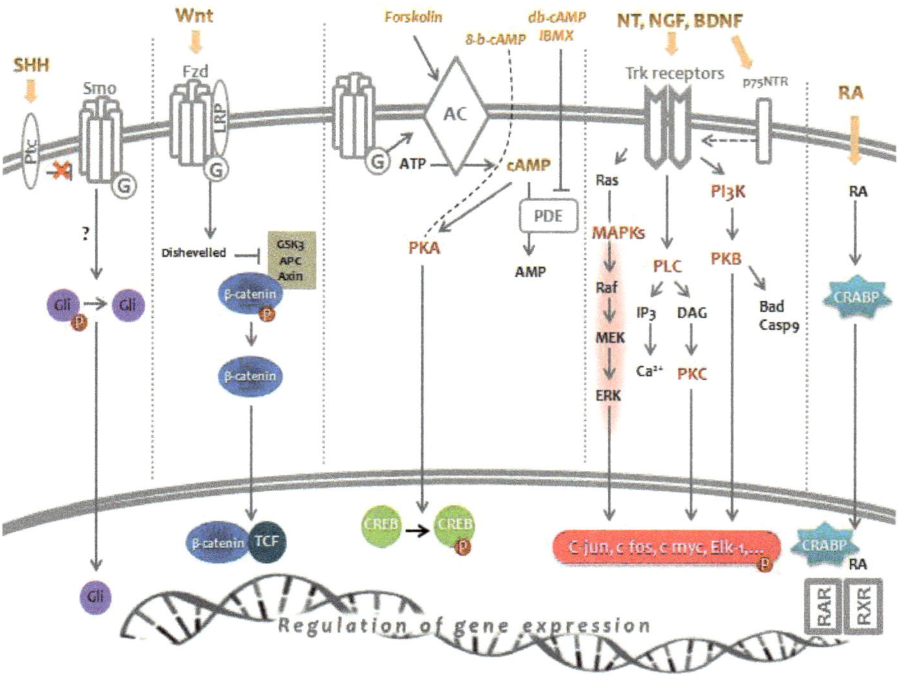

Figure 2. Different signaling pathways are involved in neural differentiation of MSCs and NCSCs.Each pathway and modulating substances are described in the text.

While cAMP pathway is supposed to be involved in neural differentiation of MSCs, its precise role in this differentiation process still needs to be defined. Zhang et al. showed evidence for the involvement of cAMP in two differentially-regulated processes, which are early transient neuron-like morphology changes, like cytoskeleton rearrangement, and later neural markers expression associated with neuronal function, but demonstrated that cAMP-treated BM-MSCs did not achieve complete differentiation [62]. Another hypothesis was made by Rooney et al., who examined the effect of intracellular cAMP elevation on BM-MSCs' fate [63]. They demonstrated that forskolin and 8-bromo-cAMP induced a transient increase in βIII-tubulin expression and changes in cell morphology, but no expression of growth associated protein 43 (GAP-43) [64] was seen in the neural-like BM-MSCs, excluding authentic neurite formation. They therefore concluded that this effect was mostly due to a modification of culture conditions rather than in a differentiation process.

	Cell type	Passage	Pathways	Induction protocol	Protocol length	Neural phenotype	Electro-physiological profile	Inhibitor	Reference
1	**UCB-MSCs**	ns	cAMP-PKA-CREB	Forskolin	1 to 7 days	NF, GFAP	No	H89, U0126	[56]
2	**BM-MSCs**	P12-P24	cAMP-PKA-CREB, NT	1) EGF, bFGF. 2) cAMP, IBMX, BDNF	1) 1 week. 2) 12 hours	NF-200, NFM, NeuroD, MAP2, NeuN, GABA	Inward Na+ currents and outward K+ currents	PKAi fragment 6–22 amide	[59]
3	**BM-MSCs**	P3-P6	cAMP-PKA-CREB	GM-CSF	6 to 96 hours	Nestin, NSE, GFAP	No	No	[61]
4	**BM-MSCs**	P0?	cAMP-PKA	Forskolin, IBMX	1 hour to 2 days	βIII-tubulin, GFAP, NSE	No	H89	[62]
5	**BM-MSCs**	ns	cAMP	Forskolin / 8-bromo-cAMP	6 and 24 hours / 1 and 4 days	βIII-tubulin	No	No	[63]
6	**BM-MSCs**	ns	NT, SHH	SHH, FGF8, bFGF (+ BDNF)	12 days	NeuN, TH, βIII-tubulin, DAT	Inward Na+ currents and outward K+ currents	No	[65, 66]
7	**BM-MSCs**	P3-P8	cAMP, RA, SHH	Forskolin, SHH and/or RA	2 days	Nestin, Sox2, NSE, GFAP, synapsin, ACh	Neuronal resting potential	No	[67]
8	**BM-MSCs**	P3-P5	cAMP, NT, RA, SHH	1) bFGF, Forskolin. 2) Forskolin, IBMX, RA, SHH, BDNF	7 days	GATA3, Sox10, GluR4, Irx2, calretinin, MAP2, NeuN, βIII-tubulin	No	No	[68]
9	**MIAMI cells**	P3-P9	cAMP, NT, RA, SHH	1) bFGF. 2) NT-3, SHH, RA, FGF8. 3) Forskolin, NT-3, BDNF, NGF, GDNF.	1) 24h. 2- 2 days. 3) 3-7 days	NSE, GFAP, βIII-tubulin, NF-L, NF-M, Nurr1, TH	Inward Na+ currents and outward K+ currents	No	[69]
10	**AT-MSCs**	ns	cAMP, NT, RA, SHH	bFGF, IBMX. 2) SHH,RA. 3) BDNF, GNDF	6 hours. 2) 1 week. 3) ns	βIII-tubulin, ChAT, Nkx2.2, Pax6, Hb9, Olig2	No	No	[70]
11	**UCB-MSCs**	P5-P8	cAMP-PKA, NT, RA	RA, IBMX, NGF, bFGF	8 hours to 7 days	GFAP, NF-L, NF-M, NF-H, NSE, Nurr-1, TH, Tau	No	H89	[60]
12	**BM-MSCs**	P4	cAMP, PKC, RA	Forskolin, IBMX, TPA / RA	Up to 48 hours / 7 days	βIII-tubulin, GFAP, NSE, NF-M	No	No	[71]

	Cell type	Passage	Pathways	Induction protocol	Protocol length	Neural phenotype	Electro-physiological profile	Inhibitor	Reference
13	**BM-MSCs**	P3-P4	cAMP, RA (RARβ)	1) RA. 2) Forskolin	1) 24 hours. 2) ns	Nestin, NSE, MAP2	Neuronal resting potential	No	[72]
14	**DP-SCs**	P0?	RA	1) EGF, bFGF. 2) bFGF. 3) bFGF, RA	1) 7 days. 2) 7 days. 3) 7 days.	Nestin, βIII-tubulin, NF-M, NFH, PSA-NCAM	Inward Na+ currents	No	[41]
15	**MIAMI cells**	P5-P9	cAMP, NT	1) EGF, bFGF. 2) bFGF. 3) bFGF, NT-3. 4) 3) Forskolin, NT-3, BDNF, NGF.	1) 10 days. 2) 24 hours. 3) 2 days. 4) 3 days	βIII-tubulin, NF-M, NF-H, NF-L, GalC	No	No	[73]
16	**MIAMI cells**	ns	NT (TrkC)-Rac1-Mek1/2-Erk1/2	1) bFGF. 2) NT-3.	1) 24 hours. 2) 48 hours	βIII-tubulin, NF-M, NF-H, NF-L, Nestin	No	U0126, K252a, NSC23766	[74]
17	**SKPs**	P3-P9	NT	1) bFGF, EGF. 2) NT-3, NGF, BDNF	1) 2-3 weeks. 2) 2-3 weeks.	NF-M, GAP43, βIII-tubulin, MAP2	No	No	[37]
18	**BM-NCSCs**	P5 clones	MAPKs	Co-culture with CGN	5 days	βIII-tubulin	Inward Na+ currents and outward K+ currents (PA for BM-MSCs clones)	PD98059	[43]
19	**SKPs**	ns	NT	1) bFGF, EGF. 2) NGF	ns	NF-M, βIII-tubulin, GFAP	No	No	[75]
20	**UCB-MSCs**	ns	NT-Raf1-MAPK/ERK, RA	bFGF, RA, BDNF	7 days	βIII-tubulin, NeuN, GFAP, MBP	No	LY294002, PD98059	[76]
21	**UCB-MSCs**	ns	NT (TrkB)-Raf1-MAPK-ERK, B-catenin	BDNF gene transfection		βIII-tubulin, NeuN, GFAP, MBP	No	K252A	[77]
22	**WJ-MSCs**	P3	NT	BDNF / HCNP / rDHE	14 days	MAP2, AChT	No	No	[78]

	Cell type	Passage	Pathways	Induction protocol	Protocol length	Neural phenotype	Electro-physiological profile	Inhibitor	Reference
23	**AT-MSCs**	ns	cAMP-NT	1) bFGF, EGF, BDNF. 2) IBMX	1) 3 days. 2) 48 hours	βIII-tubulin, GFAP	No	No	[79]
24	**BM-MSCs & DP-SCs**	P3	cAMP-NT	bFGF, EGF, BDNF, IBMX	3-5 days.	GFAP, c-fos, NF, HNK1, enolase-2, βIII-tubulin, MAP2, Sox2, Tenascin-C, Connexin-43 and nestin	No	No	[80]
25	**DP-SCs**	P1-P4	cAMP, PKC, RA	1) bFGF, 5-azacytidine. 2) bFGF, IBMX, TPA, db-cAMP, Forskolin, NT-3, NGF. 3) db-cAMP, NT-3.	1) 48 hours. 2) 3 days. 3) 3-7 days.	βIII-tubulin, NF-M, GFAP, NeuN, NSE	Inward Na+ currents and outward K+ currents	No	[81]
26	**SKPs**	P3	NT, RA	1) RA. 2) NT-3	1) 7 days. 2) 7 days.	βIII-tubulin, GFAP, MAP-2, NeuN	No	K252a, Pep5	[82]
27	**SKPs**	ns	cAMP, NT, RA	1) RA, NT-3, BDNF, NGF, db-cAMP	2 weeks to 1 month	PGP9.5, NF, FMI-43, NMDAR	No	No	[83]
29	**BM-MSCs**	P3-P4	cAMP-MAPK-MEK-ERK-Raf	Forskolin	48 hours	βIII-tubulin, NF200, NSE	No	PD98059	[58]
30	**BM-MSCs**	ns	cAMP-PKA, PKC, MAPK-MEK-ERK	1) bFGF. 2) Forskolin.	1) Overnight. 2) Up to 7 days	NF	No	K252a, KT5720, AG879, KN-62, LY294002, PD98059	[57]
31	**BM-MSCs**	P0?	cAMP-Wnt	bFGF, IBMX, Forskolin, Wnt1	3 to 7 days	Ngn1, Brn3a, NeuroD, P2X3, GluR2, GluR4	No	No	[84]

("ns" indicates that the passage or the incubation length are not specified. "No" indicates that no electrophysiological results are described in the study or that no inhibitor has been tested to confirm the pathway). **Hedgehog signaling pathway**

Table 1. In vitro protocols for neural differentiation of different types of MSCs/NCSCs and detailed results.

The hedgehog-mediated signalization is involved in the embryonic development, and its main ligand, Sonic Hedgehog (SHH) plays a role of morphogenic factor, defining which fate has to be applied to cells at each place of the embryo: its role in the nervous system organization is crucial and depends on precise concentration gradients which are essential for a correct patterning of the embryo. Indeed, SHH signaling is the chief actor in the definition of the dorsoventral axis of the nervous system. This signalization mostly takes place in cell cilia, and implies two different receptors that, once activated, generate a tricky reorganization of cytoplasmic protein complexes. SHH binds its receptor Patched1 (Ptc), relieving Ptc-mediated inhibition of a second receptor Smoothened (Smo): Ptc leaves the cilium where Smo then accumulates and induces the activation of Gli family of transcription factors (Gli1, Gli2, and Gli3) [85, 86].

SHH was used to induce dopaminergic differentiation of human BM-MSCs, as demonstrated by Trzaska et al. After a 12-days incubation with SHH, coupled with fibroblast growth factor 8 (FGF8) and basic fibroblast growth factor (bFGF), a great number of cells turned into putative dopaminergic neurons, as showed by tyrosine hydroxylase (TH) expression and electrophysiological features. Those cells showed higher expression of neuronal markers, and downregulated genes which are involved in cell cycle regulation, like cyclin-dependent kinase 2 (CDK2) and proliferating cell nuclear antigen (PCNA), indicating that they entered a post-mitotic fate [65, 66].

Qi and al. analyzed the abilities of rhesus monkey BM-MSCs to differentiate into cholinergic neural cells. While SHH alone in the culture medium did not trigger any modification of resting potential, they demonstrated that BM-MSCs exhibited neuronal resting membrane potential when retinoic acid (RA) was present in the culture medium, and under the combination of both SHH and RA. Moreover, cells from the SHH+RA inducing group expressed higher levels of synapsin and acetylcholine (ACh), indicating that the combination of both signals was the best way to obtain cholinergic neurons [67].

Many other studies demonstrated a synergic role of SHH and RA in neural induction of BM-MSCs. Kondo et al. identified those two signals as sensory factors, showing that SHH+RA application leaded to the expression of glutamatergic sensory neuron markers (including GATA3, Sox10 or GluR4) by treated BM-MSCs [68]. On the other hand, the combination of SHH+RA added to FGF8 (before neurotrophin incubation) was showed to promote dopaminergic fate in MIAMI cells [69], which expressed TH and other molecules involved in dopaminergic differenciation, like Nurr1.

Human AT-MSCs were induced to neural differentiation through the action of SHH and RA. After induction, immunochemical labeling showed βIII-tubulin, choline acetyltransferase (ChAT), and NSE expression. The differentiated cells were then characterized by RT-PCR and results showed that those cells were restricted to a ventral spinal fate (Nkx2.2, Pax6, Hb9, and Olig2), suggesting that those cells could be good candidates for motoneurons generation, in the context of spinal cord injuries therapy [70].

4.2. Retinoic acid signaling pathway

Retinoic acid (RA) is physiologically metabolized from retinol, thanks to the sequential action of cellular retinol-binding protein (CRBP), retinol dehydrogenase (RoDH) and retinaldehyde dehydrogenases (RALDHs). Once in the cytoplasm, RA is bound by cellular RA-binding protein (CRABP) and enters the nucleus to bind its specific receptors (RARs) and the retinoid X receptors (RXRs), which themselves heterodimerize and bind to DNA sequences known as the RAREs (RA-response elements). This activates transcription of target genes (Hox genes, Oct4,...) [87]. This RA signalization is involved in brain development and more particularly in the definition of the anterio-posterior axis of the nervous system, by regulating the expression of Hox genes in defined localized domains of the embryo [88].

Whereas SHH was often coupled with RA in cell culture differentiation medium, the implication of RA signaling in neuronal differentiation was also studied without a combination with SHH. RA was demonstrated to act on the up-regulation of NF-L expression in UCB-MSCs, while applied with IBMX, db-cAMP, nerve growth factor (NGF) and bFGF [60]. This study also highlighted the role of RA and cAMP/PKA pathways in the differential phosphorylation of TH during differentiation. Indeed, neurally differentiated cells express neuronal markers as Tau or NSE, whereas TH and Nurr-1 expression assessed their dopaminergic profile.

In the study of Scintu et al., two different protocols were used to differentiate BM-MSCs into neuronal cells. The first one was carried out by activating the cAMP and PKC pathway (with forskolin, TPA and IBMX), whereas the second one consisted in RA treatment. Both protocols leaded to NSE, βIII-tubulin, GFAP and NF positive cells [71].

Similarly, pre-treatment with RA before incubation with forskolin leaded BM-MSCs to express higher levels of nestin, NSE, and microtubule associated protein 2 (MAP2) and exhibit neural-like resting membrane potential and increased intracellular calcium concentration [72]. They also demonstrated that only RA specific receptors RARa and RARc were expressed in native BM-MSCs. Conversely, the expression of RARb was significantly increased in differentiated neurons, suggesting its major role in neural differentiation.

Arthur et al. performed RA treatment of human DP-SCs, which subsequently showed neural morphology and expression of βIII-tubulin, NF-M and NF-H, and more interestingly exhibited electrophysiological activity characteristic of sodium voltage-gated channels, assessing for their potential ability to give rise to functional neurons [41].

4.3. Neurotrophic factors and downstream signaling pathways

Neurotrophins are secreted growth factors that are involved in the development of neurons in the nervous system, as well as in their survival and functionality. This family of proteins is constituted by the "prototypical" nerve growth factor (NGF), brain-derived growth factor (BDNF), and the neurotrophins (NT-) 3, 4/5 and 6. Those members promote neural cells to survive, grow, differentiate and function through the activation of high-affinity tyrosine-kinase (tropomyosin-related) receptors (TrkA, TrkB and TrkC are respectively bound by NGF/NT-6, BDNF/NT-4, and NT-3), and through the activation of a common low-affinity receptor, the $p75^{LNR}$, which has no intrinsic kinase property. While $p75^{LNR}$ activation is sufficient to induce events like neurite formation, its role seems to facilitate the binding of neurotrophins to Trk receptors. After trans-phosphorylation, Trk receptors function as activators of three main signaling pathways, respectively mitogen-activated protein kinases (MAPKs), phospholipase C (PLC) and phosphatidyl-inositol-3-kinase (PI3K) [89,90].

Briefly, the MAPKs pathway consists in a set of sequentially-activated kinase proteins grouped in three main connected cascades, involving regulators of alpha-foetoproteins (Raf), extracellular-regulated kinases (ERK), p38 or jun-kinase 1/2/3, resulting in the phosphorylation of transcription factors and then regulating gene expression. MAPKs are abundantly expressed in the central nervous system (CNS), and ERKs are known to be involved in different processes, including neuronal maturation, survival, and synaptic functions.

The PLC signalization pathway mostly induces intracellular calcium mobilization, but furthermore stimulates protein kinase C (PKC) via the production of diacylglycerol (DAG). The PKC can also be directly activated by 12-*O*-tetradecanoylphorbol-13-acetate (TPA), and is also able to activate MAPKs pathway.

Finally, PI3K controls another downstream kinase called Akt (also named protein kinase B or PKB) that is a crucial player in cell survival through the regulation of apoptosis among other roles.

Several additional neurotrophic factors are regrouped in a second family, the GDNF family of ligands (GFL). Briefly, the glial neurotrophic factor (GDNF) is a protein that has been shown to promote the survival and differentiation of dopaminergic neurons and motoneurons, and constitutes then an important potential actor in the management of neurological diseases such as Parkinson's disease [91, 92], amyotrophic lateral sclerosis or spinal cord injuries. Neurturin, artemin and persephin are similar ligands that also play a role in cell survival, neurite outgrowth, and cell differentiation migration. Those four members act by the activation of a tyrosine kinase receptor RET, which in association with a co-receptor (GFRα), triggers auto-transphosphorylation and downstream signaling processes.

A cocktail of the three main neurotrophins (BDNF, NGF and NT-3) was used to direct neural differentiation of MIAMI cells, which began to develop a complex neuritic arborization and to express neuronal markers, e.g. NF-L or NeuN [69]. Moreover, those differentiated cells showed inward Na^+ and outward K^+ currents. This study also highlighted the importance of NT-3 in the neural commitment and differentiation step, through the demonstration of a dramatic decrease in viability, βIII-tubulin expression, neuron-like morphology and branching of differentiated cells without NT-3 treatment. Those results were then further detailed and showed the enhanced neural specification from MIAMI cells thanks to epidermal growth factor (EGF) and bFGF pre-treatment [73]; the implication of Rho-GTPase Rac1, which was thought to regulate Mek1/2-Erk1/2 phosphorylation, mediating transcription of genes involved in neural differentiation versus proliferation during NT-3-induced neuronal commitment [74].

The first assessment of the ability of SKPs to generate neural cells was achieved by the group of Toma, who first described that about 9,4% of SKPs were NF-M, GAP43, βIII-tubulin and MAP2 positive after being treated with NGF, BDNF and NT-3 [37].

When co-cultivated with immature cerebellar granules, nestin-positive BM-MSCs are able to differentiate into functional neuronal cells [93], as showed by βIII-tubulin expression and action potentials firings. After characterizing two subpopulations of BM-MSCs which were respectively derived and non-derived from the embryonic neural crest (after generating clonal cultures), Wislet-Gendebien and collaborators demonstrated that the neural differentiation of BM-NCSCs in co-culture conditions was abolished in the presence of a MAPKs inhibitor. Those results confirmed the importance of MAPKs pathway in neural differentiation of adult BM-NCSCs [43].

After adding NGF in the culture medium of human SKPs, Bakthiari et al. obtained NF-M, βIII-tubulin, S100 and GFAP positive cells, and that after different conditions of cryopreservation [75].

Lim et al. demonstrated the important role of BDNF in neural differentiation of human UCB-MSCs, and provided a deeper study of the different involved pathways. Addition of BDNF in the induction medium leaded to the phosphorylation of Raf-1 and ERK, then to the downstream up-regulation of p35 expression, which was not observed when ERK was blocked with a specific inhibitor. p35 is known as an anti-apoptotic factor able to block procaspase maturation and to protect neurons from cell death [94, 95].

They also analyzed the contribution of BDNF to cell viability, and demonstrated an up-regulation of the anti-apoptotic gene Bcl2, which was mediated by the activity of PI3K and Akt phosphorylation [76]. Few years later, after genetically modifying UCB-MSCs through transfection with a BDNF-expressing plasmid, they showed the expression of βIII-tubulin, NeuN, GFAP and myelin basic protein (MBP) in differentiated cells, associated with an up-regulated phosphorylation level of TrkB, Raf-1 and ERKs [77].

BDNF was also used to induce bi-multipolar morphology and MAP2 expression in WJ-MSCs. When used in combination with hippocampal cholinergic neurostimulating peptide (HCNP) and/or denervated hippocampal extract (rDHE), WJ-MSCs turned into Choline-acetyltransferase (ChAT) positive cells [96].

Coupled with IBMX, BDNF was able to induce GFAP and βIII-tubulin expression in AT-MSCs, as demonstrated by Ying et al. [79]. The same combination of IBMX and BDNF was used to differentiate DP-SCs into GFAP, c-fos, NF, HNK1, enolase-2, βIII-tubulin, MAP2, Sox2, Tenascin-C, Connexin-43 and nestin positive cells [80].

Neural induction of DP-SCs was achieved by Kiraly et al. through the activation of both cAMP and PKC signaling pathways. After reprogramming by 5-azacytidine treatment, cells where treated with IBMX, db-cAMP, forskolin, TPA, NGF and NT-3, and showed an increase in neurogenin-2, βIII-tubulin, NSE, NF-M and GFAP expression, while electrophysiological recordings revealed voltage dependent sodium channels activity [81].

The study of Zhang et al. demonstrated that RA induced SKPs to neural differentiation through the up-regulation of the transcription factor NeuroD and the cell-cycle regulatory protein p21 [82]. In the meantime, RA also induced $p75^{NTR}$ up-regulation that leaded to apoptotic cell death. They showed that when treated with NT-3 after RA induction, the survival and neural differentiation of SKPs were improved significantly, and cell apoptosis induced by RA was decreased. These effects were reversible as confirmed by the way of a $p75^{NTR}$ inhibitor Pep5 instead of Trk receptor inhibitor K252a.

The three pathways of RA, cAMP and NT were recruited together to differentiate SKPs into neuronal cells. After adding RA, db-cAMP, NGF, BDNF and NT-3 to the culture medium, Lebonvallet et al. identified NF and PGP9.5 positive cells, which were also able to incorporate FMI-43 staining, indicating the presence of synaptic vesicles. Furthermore, they showed an overexpression of neuron-related genes in differentiated SKPs [83].

Kim et al. studied the involvement of non-neurotrophin-activated MAPKs pathway. They showed that cAMP and PKA (resulting of forskolin treatment) promoted the phosphorylation/activation of B-Raf, MEK and ERK [58]. Confirmation was specified with the use of an inhibitor of MAPKs pathway that induced a significant decrease in neural features of forskolin-treated BM-MSCs. The same observation was carried out by Jori et al., confirming that neural-like BM-MSCs reverted to uncommitted cells when cultured with a MEK-ERK inhibitor [57].

4.4. Wnt signaling pathway

The Wnt signaling pathway is constituted by a network of proteins that are involved in the regulation of multiple developmental events during embryogenesis, but also in adulthood, in several physiological processes and tissue homeostasis through cell fate specification, differentiation, or proliferation..

Wnt proteins act on cells by binding Frizzled (Fzd)/low density lipoprotein (LDL) receptor-related protein (LRP) receptor complex. When Wnt signal is inactive, the levels of cytoplasmic transcription factor β-catenin are kept low through continuous proteasome-mediated degradation, which is regulated by a complex including glycogen synthase kinase-3β (GSK-3), Axin, and Adenomatous Polyposis Coli (APC). Once Wnt ligands activate Fzd/LRP, the degradation pathway is inhibited (through the activity of Dishevelled (Dsh)) and β-catenin accumulates in the cytoplasm. After nuclear translocation, it interacts with T-cell specific transcription factors (TCF) among others, which allows transcription regulation [97, 98].

Kondo et al. exposed that BM-MSCs induced to neural differentiation (with forskolin and IBMX) showed significant dose-dependent upregulation of sensory neurons markers Ngn1, NeuroD, Brn3a and P2X3 when the induction medium was supplemented with recombinant Wnt1 (whereas Wnt3a exhibited comparable but slighter effects)[84]. Glutamate receptors GluR2 and GluR4 were also up-regulated in those conditions.

5. Implications in cell therapy

With regards to their accessibility and their multipotentiality, adult and perinatal MSCs and NCSCs constitute ideal stem cells to use in cell therapy. As it has been shown that those cells could give rise to neuron-like cells via multiple ways of induction, we can infer that they could be of valuable interest in the treatment of neurological lesions. In this paragraph, we will collect the results of some studies that focused on cell therapy of Parkinson's disease and spinal cord injuries, using different types of MSCs/NCSCs and different ways to differentiate them into neurons before being transferred in animal models. Those results are summarized in the Table 2.

5.1. Dopaminergic neurons and Parkinson's disease

Parkinson's disease (PD) is the second most common neurodegenerative disorder after Alzheimer's disease, with a prevalence of 0,3% of the population in industrialized countries, reaching 1% after 60 years of age [110]. This pathology is characterized by typical clinical symptoms, like bradykinesia, rigidity, gait troubles and resting tremor, while the main pathological feature is the loss of dopaminergic neurons in the Substantia Nigra pars compacta (SNpc), associated with ubiquitinated protein aggregates called Lewy bodies in different locations of the brain [111, 112].

In the last 80's, clinical trials have been started, using fetal mesencephalic dopaminergic neurons to transplant in PD patients [113, 114]. Despite the demonstration of several benefits in terms of clinical symptoms and pathology, few problems remain. Fetal tissue heterogeneity, influence of harvesting methods on the graft efficiency, need of too much fetuses for only one patient, altogether coupled with ethical concerns, left no option but finding other ways to proceed. One of the main goals in this field relies in the replacement of lost dopaminergic neurons in the nigrostriatal system, which could be achieved through the use of different types of stem cells. As explained earlier, MSCs/NCSCs are interesting candidates in this objective [115].

In this paragraph, we will review the results of some studies aiming to differentiate diverse types of MSCs and NCSCs in dopaminergic neurons before grafting those cells *in vivo*, using animal models mimicking the symptoms of PD (which are required to study the putative usefulness of stem cells in regenerative therapy).

After *in vitro* differentiation of WJ-MSCs in dopaminergic neural cells using a SHH and FGF8 treatment (in combination with brain-conditioned medium), Fu et al transplanted those differentiated cells inside the striatum of hemiparkinsonian rats, previously treated with 6-hydroxydopamine (6-OHDA). 20 days after transplantation, TH positive cells were found around the implantation site, and those cells were shown to be grafted WJ-MSCs. Moreover, the number of amphetamine-induced rotations (giving idea of motor performances of hemiparkinsonian rats) was decreased, and this decrease was gradual over time, showing an important improvement in the nigrostriatal pathway function [99].

Cell type	Differentiation protocol	Animal model	Histology	Behavioral aspects	Ref.
Dopaminergic neurons - Parkinson's Disease					
WJ-MSCs	SHH, FGF8 (+ brain-conditioned medium)	6-OHDA rat	Survival after 20 days TH positive grafted cells.	Decrease of amphetamine-induced rotations over time.	[99]
BM-MSCs	SHH, FGF8, GDNF	6-OHDA rat	Transient survival No differentiation	No	[100]
DP-SCs / SHED	Nothing	6-OHDA rat	TH-positive grafted cells	Decrease of apomorphine-induced rotations over time.	[101]
	Forskolin, SHH, FGF8, GDNF	(in vitro)	In vitro expression of βIII-tubulin, MAP2, and TH	No	
BM-MSCs	Forskolin, IBMX, db-cAMP and TPA	6-OHDA rat	<4 weeks survival Few TH expression Many GABA positive cells	No	[102]
Motoneurons - Spinal Cord Injuries					
BM-MSCs	8-bromo-AMP and Rolipram	Rat with contused SC	A2B5, NCAM and B3T positive cells	Recovery of hind limb stepping and hind limb weight support	[103]
BM-MSCs	RA + NT-3 overexpression	Rat with transected SC	MAP2, NF and GFAP positive cells Reduction of cystic cavity size Rescue of surviving neurons	Improvement of hinclim locomotion	[104]
BM-MSCs	Hb9 and Olig2 overexpression + RA, forskolin, SHH	Injured organotypic SC slice	Integration in slice ChAT positive cells	No	[105]
BM-MSCs	RA, db-cAMP, forskolin, IBMX	Rat with contused SC	In vitro expression of MAP2, NSE, nestin, βIII-tubulin Reduced cystic cavity	Improvement in motor performances	[106]
UCB-MSCs	Nothing	Rat with hemisection SC injury	Accumulation near the lesion Reduction of lesion size Enhanced axon regrowth	Enhancement of functional locomotor abilities	[107]

Cell type	Differentiation protocol	Animal model	Histology	Behavioral aspects	Ref.
SKPs	Nothing	Rat with contused SC	Survival rate of Reduced cavity size Myelination of endogenous axons Recruitment of endogenous Schwann cells	Heightened sensory responses	[108]
	Forskolin (+ neuregulin-1β)	Rat with contused SC	Survival rate of Reduced cavity size Myelination of endogenous axons Recruitment of endogenous Schwann cells Bypass of the lesion Reduced gliosis Axonal growth	Increased BBB score and Basso locomotor subscore Decease in the number of hind limb errors No impact of sensitivity to sensory stimuli	
EPI-NCSCs	Nothing	Rat with contused SC	No migration, no proliferation Close contact with host neuritis βIII-tubulin, GAD67, RIP and MBP positive cells. No GFAP	No	[109]

("No" indicates that no behavioral testing is described in the study. Protocols describing *in vitro* differentiation in the meantime than *in vivo* studies are also included in the table, as well as some *in vivo* studies using non-differentiated cells).

Table 2. Different results obtained in cell-based therapy experiments using MSCs and NCSCs.

On the other hand, Khoo et al showed that neuronal-primed human BM-MSCs (with SHH, FGF8, GDNF and other growth factors) did survive transiently in the brain of 6-OHDA-treated rats, but no further differentiation in functional dopaminergic neurons was observed, even when a co-transplantation with olfactory ensheating cells (OECs) was performed to enhance to graft efficiency [100].

The same cocktail was used by Wang et al. to differentiate SHED cells (DP-SCs) into dopaminergic neurons, this time supplemented with forskolin. Differentiated cells were βIII-tubulin, MAP2 and TH positive *in vitro*. They further characterized naïve SHED cells by transplanting them into the striatum of a hemiparkinsonian rat. While some TH-positive cell bodies were found in the graft zone, a significant decrease in apomorphine-induced rotations was observed, attesting of a beneficial effect of the cell transplantation [101].

cAMP pathway was recruited to differentiate BM-MSCs (after EGF/bFGF-induced sphere formation) in dopaminergic neurons, using forskolin, IBMX and db-cAMP (coupled with the PKC activator TPA) [102]. Differentiated cells showed *in vitro* expression of βIII-tubulin, neurofilament, Nurr-1, TH, AADC and GIRK2. After transplantation into the striatum of 6-OHDA rats, few cells were βIII-tubulin and TH positive, whereas a higher number of grafted cells became GABA-positive (maybe due to the striatal environment mainly composed of GABA neurons). Unfortunately, no behavioral observation was described by Suon et al.

5.2. Motoneurons and spinal cord injuries

Whereas peripheral nerves are able to regenerate when a lesion occurs, the motoneurons and nervous fibers in the spinal cord can't be replaced in case of spinal cord injury (SCI). Indeed, traumatic spinal cord injury results in a wide panel of pathophysiological events counteracting any possibility of neural regeneration, and those events are generally grouped in two phases. The primary injury phase can be due to either contusion or compression, and is characterized by section of axons, necrosis, degeneration, oligodendrocytes apoptosis, gliosis and macrophage infiltration. Altogether, those events lead to secondary lesions like ischemia, inflammation, alteration of ion balance, insult of the blood-brain-barrier, lipid peroxidation and glutamate-induced excitotoxicity. Despite a slight spontaneous recovery, all those events collectively constitute an environment that hampers axonal regeneration [116]. Since the clinical consequences of such lesions are dramatic and rarely reversible (para-, hemi-, tetraplegy, respiratory problems, loss of sphincters control, all leading to important socio-economic issues), it's crucial to find out efficient therapies to improve the recuperation of motor function.

Stem cell grafting has been suggested as a therapeutic strategy for spinal cord repair, hence the obtainment of mature motoneurons is critical.

Human BM-MSCs were induced to differentiate into neural cells through the activation of cAMP signaling pathway, via the addition of 8-bromo-cAMP and Rolipram (inhibitor of phosphodiesterases) in the culture medium. Those neurally-induced BM-MSCs were then transplanted into a segment of the spinal cord of rats, previously wounded by contusion. After confirming neural nature of differentiated cells by immunostaining of A2B5, NCAM, B3T, *in vitro* as well as *in vivo* after transplantation, behavioral testing of rats revealed that the motor recovery (assessed by hind limb stepping and weight support) was significantly different at 2 to 12 weeks post-recovery in the group that was transplanted with neurally-induced BM-MSCs when compared with the control groups that received non differentiated BM-MSCs and saline solution [103].

Another protocol was tested by Zhang et al., who treated BM-MSCs with RA before genetically modifying them to overexpress the gene coding for the neurotrophin 3 (NT-3) [104]. Once they've showed that RA pretreatment enhanced NT-3 expression and secretion by MSCs after genetic engineering, they transplanted cells into the transected spinal cord of rats. Some transplanted cells were positive for MAP2, NF and GFAP labeling. Moreover, cell transplantation leaded to the reduction of cystic cavity, improvement of local environment, rescue of surviving neurons from retrograde atrophy, and improvement of hind limb locomotion.

Liqing et al. induced AT-MSCs to neural fate through the action of SHH and RA, and showed that those cells expressed the transcription factors Nkx2.2, Pax6, Hb9, and Olig2, suggesting those cells as attractive nominees to become mature motoneurons [70]. While no *in vivo* testing has been performed in this study, another experiment focusing on ventral spinal-specific transcription factors was carried out by Park and al., who genetically modified human BM-MSCs to express Hb9 and Olig2, just before treating them with neural induction medium consisting in sequential incubation with RA, forskolin, SHH and FGF. *In vitro,* those cells were excitable and were able to connect muscle fibers; while after transplantation into an injured organotypic spinal cord slice culture, they survive and integrate the slice, while expressing motoneurons-specific markers, e.g. ChAT [105].

Pedram et al. performed comparative study of the potencies of BM-MSCs to take part in the repair of spinal cord damages, either when neurally-differentiated than when used in their native state [106]. BM-MSCs were cultured following a multi-step protocol, in presence of RA and bFGF, db-cAMP, forskolin and IBMX. After assessing the neural nature of differentiated cells (expression of MAP2, NSE, nestin, and βIII-tubulin), they transplanted cells into the lesion cavity of contused rat spinal cords. Either undifferentiated BM-MSCs or neurally-induced BM-MSCs transplantation leaded to a reduced cavity, but a significant improvement in motor performances was observed in rats that received neurally-differentiated BM-MSCs (compared to control group and native BM-MSCs-transplanted group).

Obtaining myelinating glial cells is another way to manage spinal cord injuries. In that purpose, Biernaskie et al. studied the effect of SKPs on spinal cord lesions, when transplanted in their naïve state or when pre-differentiated into Schwann cells (using forskolin and neuregulin-1β) [108]. They showed that a graft of both the naïve SKPs and SKPs-derived Schwann cells leaded to a reduced cystic cavity size, and that the cells myelinated host axons and recruited host Schwann cells. Still, the SKPs-derived Schwann cells were the only ones to generate a bridge across the lesion and to induce a growth-permissive environment, while a substantial improvement was observed at the behavioral level (Increased BBB score and Basso locomotor subscore and decrease in the number of hind limb errors).

Significant enhancement of functional locomotor abilities was observed by Schira et al. after transplantation of unrestricted UCB-MSCs into the surrounding area of a hemisection injury, accompanied by cell accumulation near the lesion, reduction in its size and enhanced axon regrowth [107]. This study gives an example of what can be observed using naïve stem cells in cell therapy, without any pre-differentiation. In the same way, Sieber-Blum et al. transplanted EPI-NCSCs in the core of a spinal cord lesion, and observed βIII-tubulin, GAD67, RIP and MBP positive cells among the grafted cells. Those cells were tightly close to endogenous neuritis, but did not show any sign of proliferation nor migration in the tissue [109].

6. Conclusions

Mesenchymal stem cells (MSCs) and neural crest stem cells (NCSCs) are multipotent cells that are able to generate a wide range of cell types, including neural cells, which makes them incredibly interesting in restorative therapies for patients suffering from neurological diseases. A lot of induction protocols indicate that many signaling pathways may be involved in the neural fate of MSCs and NCSCs. Indeed, the signalization pathways of cAMP, Retinoic acid, Hedgehog, Wnt and the neurotrophins-activated pathways have been implicated into the maturation of adult MSCs/NCSCs into neural-like cells. After an induction process consisting in various activators, lengths and conditions of culture, treated cells adopt a neural morphology express markers (at the transcriptome level as well as at the protein level) that are usually described to characterize neurons at different developmental stages [117, 118] in MSCs as well as in NCSCs. Despite the expression of those specific neural markers, only a tiny number of *in vitro* protocols were able to provide convincing evidence for a neuron-specific electrophysiological signature of the differentiated cells.

During neural development, immature neural cells undergo a differentiation process towards functional neurons through different stages that are accurately defined by specific electrophysiological features. Briefly, the first currents that occur in the cell consist in voltage-dependent outward potassium currents. As maturation proceeds, voltage-dependent inward calcium and sodium currents arise sequentially. The ultimate step is finally characterized by the elicitation of action potential through the activity of several mature voltage-gated sodium channels: an important depolarization triggers intracellular modifications, proteins activation, and vesicular trafficking that are required for proper synaptic chemical and electrical function/transmission [119-121]. As clearly observed in Table 1, even if a few data attest of electrophysiological activity in MSCs/NCSCs-derived neuron-like cells (as showed by sodium and potassium currents), there is no sufficient evidence for action potential firings and for an appropriate neuronal function.

As showed by the diagram on the figure 3, most of the collected studies describe the cAMP signaling pathway to play a key role in the neural differentiation of MSCs/NCSCs. On the other hand, neurotrophins are often used for neural differentiation, whereas MAPKs have been shown to be involved too. RA represents the third most used signaling molecule. We can see that the most part of studies showing significant electrophysiological recordings use RA treatment for differentiation, suggesting its noteworthy role in this process (16,1 % of the total number of studies (5/31) and 62,5 % of the number of studies showing significant electrophysiological recordings (5/8)). Additionally, a major number of protocols were performed in association with cAMP pathway activation. On the other hand, 40% of the differentiation protocols using SHH signalization (2/5 studies) were able to induce changes in electrical activity (see Table 1). That presumably raises the question of a role for RA and SHH in the last stages of maturation of MSCs/NCSCs into neural-like cells.

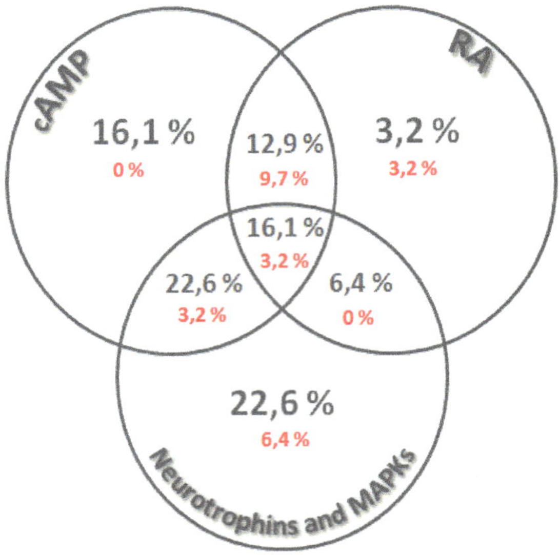

Figure 3. Percentages of differentiation protocols involving cAMP, RA or neurotrophins/MAPKs signaling pathways among the 31 detailed studies. Percentages are expressed in regard to the total number of studies. Numbers in red indicate the percentages of studies describing significant electrophysiological recordings.

Overall, we tend to conclude that although the cells express neural-specific proteins and exhibit a preliminary electrical activity [122, 123], MSCs and NCSCs do not seem to be able to fully differentiate and generate functional neurons in order to reach the objective of cell-based therapy in human neurological treatments.

However, several *in vivo* studies based on MSCs/NCSCs-derived neural cells demonstrate a significant improvement of symptoms and lesions in animal models of neurological disorders, such as Parkinson's disease or spinal cord injury [24]. In these studies, the transplantation of differentiated MSCs/NCSCs leads to the limitation of the lesions and the recovering of motor functions. Regarding other successful cell therapy experiments based on the transplantation of non-differentiated MSCs/NCSCs, we can infer that the experimental enhancement is more likely to be due to the intrinsic properties of the grafted cells, and not to a genuine differentiation process nor to an authentic neuronal electrical activity. Indeed, even if their ability to generate neurons is present but quite limited, they still display important immunomodulatory and anti-inflammatory properties, they secrete a lot of growth and neurotrophic factors, they modulate apoptosis processes, and promote endogenous precursors recruitment [124-128]

In conclusion, those observations confirmed the significance of MSCs and NCSCs use in cell therapy procedures to treat several neurological disorders, sustaining their high capacity to protect or restore neural tissue through many proceedings that are probably more owed to intrinsic abilities than to neuronal differentiation.

Author details

Virginie Neirinckx[1], Cécile Coste[1], Bernard Rogister[1,2,3] and Sabine Wislet-Gendebien[1*]

*Address all correspondence to: s.wislet@ulg.ac.be

1 GIGA Neurosciences, University of Liège, Belgium

2 GIGA Development, Stem Cells and Regenerative Medicine, University of Liège, Belgium

3 Neurology Department, University of Liège, Belgium

References

[1] Patani, R., et al., Retinoid-independent motor neurogenesis from human embryonic stem cells reveals a medial columnar ground state. Nat Commun, 2011. 2: p. 214.

[2] Swistowski, A., et al., Efficient generation of functional dopaminergic neurons from human induced pluripotent stem cells under defined conditions. Stem Cells, 2010. 28(10): p. 1893-904.

[3] Malgrange, B., et al., Using human pluripotent stem cells to untangle neurodegenerative disease mechanisms. Cell Mol Life Sci, 2011. 68(4): p. 635-49.

[4] Friedenstein, A.J., et al., Precursors for fibroblasts in different populations of hematopoietic cells as detected by the in vitro colony assay method. Exp Hematol, 1974. 2(2): p. 83-92.

[5] Friedenstein, A.J., et al., Stromal cells responsible for transferring the microenvironment of the hemopoietic tissues. Cloning in vitro and retransplantation in vivo. Transplantation, 1974. 17(4): p. 331-40.

[6] Friedenstein, A.J., Stromal mechanisms of bone marrow: cloning in vitro and retransplantation in vivo. Haematol Blood Transfus, 1980. 25: p. 19-29.

[7] Prockop, D.J., Adult stem cells gradually come of age. Nat Biotechnol, 2002. 20(8): p. 791-2.

[8] Bianco, P., et al., Bone marrow stromal stem cells: nature, biology, and potential applications. Stem Cells, 2001. 19(3): p. 180-92.

[9] Pittenger, M.F., et al., Multilineage potential of adult human mesenchymal stem cells. Science, 1999. 284(5411): p. 143-7.

[10] Uccelli, A., L. Moretta, and V. Pistoia, Mesenchymal stem cells in health and disease. Nat Rev Immunol, 2008. 8(9): p. 726-36.

[11] Jiang, Y., et al., Pluripotency of mesenchymal stem cells derived from adult marrow. Nature, 2002. 418(6893): p. 41-9.

[12] Reyes, M. and C.M. Verfaillie, Characterization of multipotent adult progenitor cells, a subpopulation of mesenchymal stem cells. Ann N Y Acad Sci, 2001. 938: p. 231-3; discussion 233-5.

[13] Woodbury, D., et al., Adult rat and human bone marrow stromal cells differentiate into neurons. J Neurosci Res, 2000. 61(4): p. 364-70.

[14] Brazelton, T.R., et al., From marrow to brain: expression of neuronal phenotypes in adult mice. Science, 2000. 290(5497): p. 1775-9.

[15] Sanchez-Ramos, J., et al., Adult bone marrow stromal cells differentiate into neural cells in vitro. Exp Neurol, 2000. 164(2): p. 247-56.

[16] Verfaillie, C.M., Multipotent adult progenitor cells: an update. Novartis Found Symp, 2005. 265: p. 55-61; discussion 61-5, 92-7.

[17] D'Ippolito, G., et al., Marrow-isolated adult multilineage inducible (MIAMI) cells, a unique population of postnatal young and old human cells with extensive expansion and differentiation potential. J Cell Sci, 2004. 117(Pt 14): p. 2971-81.

[18] D'Ippolito, G., et al., Isolation and characterization of marrow-isolated adult multilineage inducible (MIAMI) cells. Exp Hematol, 2006. 34(11): p. 1608-10.

[19] Dennis, J.E. and P. Charbord, Origin and differentiation of human and murine stroma. Stem Cells, 2002. 20(3): p. 205-14.

[20] Takashima, Y., et al., Neuroepithelial cells supply an initial transient wave of MSC differentiation. Cell, 2007. 129(7): p. 1377-88.

[21] Nagoshi, N., et al., Ontogeny and multipotency of neural crest-derived stem cells in mouse bone marrow, dorsal root ganglia, and whisker pad. Cell Stem Cell, 2008. 2(4): p. 392-403.

[22] Morikawa, S., et al., Development of mesenchymal stem cells partially originate from the neural crest. Biochem Biophys Res Commun, 2009. 379(4): p. 1114-9.

[23] Glejzer, A., et al., Wnt1 and BMP2: two factors recruiting multipotent neural crest progenitors isolated from adult bone marrow. Cell Mol Life Sci, 2011. 68(12): p. 2101-14.

[24] Wislet-Gendebien, S., et al., Adult bone marrow: which stem cells for cellular therapy protocols in neurodegenerative disorders? J Biomed Biotechnol, 2012. 2012: p. 601560.

[25] Zuk, P.A., et al., Human adipose tissue is a source of multipotent stem cells. Mol Biol Cell, 2002. 13(12): p. 4279-95.

[26] Gimble, J. and F. Guilak, Adipose-derived adult stem cells: isolation, characterization, and differentiation potential. Cytotherapy, 2003. 5(5): p. 362-9.

[27] Mitchell, K.E., et al., Matrix cells from Wharton's jelly form neurons and glia. Stem Cells, 2003. 21(1): p. 50-60.

[28] Wang, H.S., et al., Mesenchymal stem cells in the Wharton's jelly of the human umbilical cord. Stem Cells, 2004. 22(7): p. 1330-7.

[29] Fu, Y.S., et al., Transformation of human umbilical mesenchymal cells into neurons in vitro. J Biomed Sci, 2004. 11(5): p. 652-60.

[30] Kern, S., et al., Comparative analysis of mesenchymal stem cells from bone marrow, umbilical cord blood, or adipose tissue. Stem Cells, 2006. 24(5): p. 1294-301.

[31] Lee, O.K., et al., Isolation of multipotent mesenchymal stem cells from umbilical cord blood. Blood, 2004. 103(5): p. 1669-75.

[32] Sanchez-Ramos, J.R., et al., Expression of neural markers in human umbilical cord blood. Exp Neurol, 2001. 171(1): p. 109-15.

[33] Goodwin, H.S., et al., Multilineage differentiation activity by cells isolated from umbilical cord blood: expression of bone, fat, and neural markers. Biol Blood Marrow Transplant, 2001. 7(11): p. 581-8.

[34] Baksh, D., R. Yao, and R.S. Tuan, Comparison of proliferative and multilineage differentiation potential of human mesenchymal stem cells derived from umbilical cord and bone marrow. Stem Cells, 2007. 25(6): p. 1384-92.

[35] Kruger, G.M., et al., Neural crest stem cells persist in the adult gut but undergo changes in self-renewal, neuronal subtype potential, and factor responsiveness. Neuron, 2002. 35(4): p. 657-69.

[36] Fernandes, K.J., et al., A dermal niche for multipotent adult skin-derived precursor cells. Nat Cell Biol, 2004. 6(11): p. 1082-93.

[37] Toma, J.G., et al., Isolation and characterization of multipotent skin-derived precursors from human skin. Stem Cells, 2005. 23(6): p. 727-37.

[38] Wong, C.E., et al., Neural crest-derived cells with stem cell features can be traced back to multiple lineages in the adult skin. J Cell Biol, 2006. 175(6): p. 1005-15.

[39] Yoshida, S., et al., Isolation of multipotent neural crest-derived stem cells from the adult mouse cornea. Stem Cells, 2006. 24(12): p. 2714-22.

[40] Tomita, Y., et al., Cardiac neural crest cells contribute to the dormant multipotent stem cell in the mammalian heart. J Cell Biol, 2005. 170(7): p. 1135-46.

[41] Arthur, A., et al., Adult human dental pulp stem cells differentiate toward functionally active neurons under appropriate environmental cues. Stem Cells, 2008. 26(7): p. 1787-95.

[42] Gronthos, S., et al., Stem cell properties of human dental pulp stem cells. J Dent Res, 2002. 81(8): p. 531-5.

[43] Wislet-Gendebien, S., et al., Mesenchymal stem cells and neural crest stem cells from adult bone marrow: characterization of their surprising similarities and differences. Cell Mol Life Sci, 2012.

[44] Toma, J.G., et al., Isolation of multipotent adult stem cells from the dermis of mammalian skin. Nat Cell Biol, 2001. 3(9): p. 778-84.

[45] Sieber-Blum, M., et al., Pluripotent neural crest stem cells in the adult hair follicle. Dev Dyn, 2004. 231(2): p. 258-69.

[46] Sieber-Blum, M. and Y. Hu, Epidermal neural crest stem cells (EPI-NCSC) and pluripotency. Stem Cell Rev, 2008. 4(4): p. 256-60.

[47] Peters, H. and R. Balling, Teeth. Where and how to make them. Trends Genet, 1999. 15(2): p. 59-65.

[48] Thesleff, I. and T. Aberg, Molecular regulation of tooth development. Bone, 1999. 25(1): p. 123-5.

[49] Gronthos, S., et al., Postnatal human dental pulp stem cells (DPSCs) in vitro and in vivo. Proc Natl Acad Sci U S A, 2000. 97(25): p. 13625-30.

[50] Mizuno, H., M. Tobita, and A.C. Uysal, Concise review: adipose-derived stem cells as a novel tool for future regenerative medicine. Stem Cells, 2012. 30(5): p. 804-10.

[51] Suzuki, A., et al., Upregulation of CREB-mediated transcription enhances both short- and long-term memory. J Neurosci, 2011. 31(24): p. 8786-802.

[52] Lim, J., et al., Regulation of tyrosine hydroxylase gene transcription by the cAMP-signaling pathway: involvement of multiple transcription factors. Mol Cell Biochem, 2000. 212(1-2): p. 51-60.

[53] Bourtchuladze, R., et al., Deficient long-term memory in mice with a targeted mutation of the cAMP-responsive element-binding protein. Cell, 1994. 79(1): p. 59-68.

[54] Dworkin, S., et al., CREB activity modulates neural cell proliferation, midbrain-hindbrain organization and patterning in zebrafish. Dev Biol, 2007. 307(1): p. 127-41.

[55] Mantamadiotis, T., et al., Disruption of CREB function in brain leads to neurodegeneration. Nat Genet, 2002. 31(1): p. 47-54.

[56] Wang, T.T., et al., Neural differentiation of mesenchymal-like stem cells from cord blood is mediated by PKA. Biochem Biophys Res Commun, 2007. 357(4): p. 1021-7.

[57] Jori, F.P., et al., Molecular pathways involved in neural in vitro differentiation of marrow stromal stem cells. J Cell Biochem, 2005. 94(4): p. 645-55.

[58] Kim, S.S., et al., cAMP induces neuronal differentiation of mesenchymal stem cells via activation of extracellular signal-regulated kinase/MAPK. Neuroreport, 2005. 16(12): p. 1357-61.

[59] Lepski, G., et al., Limited Ca2+ and PKA-pathway dependent neurogenic differentiation of human adult mesenchymal stem cells as compared to fetal neuronal stem cells. Exp Cell Res, 2010. 316(2): p. 216-31.

[60] Tio, M., et al., Roles of db-cAMP, IBMX and RA in aspects of neural differentiation of cord blood derived mesenchymal-like stem cells. PLoS One, 2010. 5(2): p. e9398.

[61] Lin, X., et al., GM-CSF enhances neural differentiation of bone marrow stromal cells. Neuroreport, 2007. 18(11): p. 1113-7.

[62] Zhang, L., et al., cAMP initiates early phase neuron-like morphology changes and late phase neural differentiation in mesenchymal stem cells. Cell Mol Life Sci, 2011. 68(5): p. 863-76.

[63] Rooney, G.E., et al., Elevation of cAMP in mesenchymal stem cells transiently upregulates neural markers rather than inducing neural differentiation. Stem Cells Dev, 2009. 18(3): p. 387-98.

[64] Zhao, C.P., et al., Signals in pathological CNS extracts of ALS mice promote hMSCs neurogenic differentiation in vitro. Cell Biol Int, 2007. 31(11): p. 1428-35.

[65] Trzaska, K.A., E.V. Kuzhikandathil, and P. Rameshwar, Specification of a dopaminergic phenotype from adult human mesenchymal stem cells. Stem Cells, 2007. 25(11): p. 2797-808.

[66] Trzaska, K.A. and P. Rameshwar, Dopaminergic neuronal differentiation protocol for human mesenchymal stem cells. Methods Mol Biol, 2011. 698: p. 295-303.

[67] Qi, Y., et al., Cholinergic neuronal differentiation of bone marrow mesenchymal stem cells in rhesus monkeys. Sci China Life Sci, 2010. 53(5): p. 573-80.

[68] Kondo, T., et al., Sonic hedgehog and retinoic acid synergistically promote sensory fate specification from bone marrow-derived pluripotent stem cells. Proc Natl Acad Sci U S A, 2005. 102(13): p. 4789-94.

[69] Tatard, V.M., et al., Neurotrophin-directed differentiation of human adult marrow stromal cells to dopaminergic-like neurons. Bone, 2007. 40(2): p. 360-73.

[70] Liqing, Y., et al., Directed differentiation of motor neuron cell-like cells from human adipose-derived stem cells in vitro. Neuroreport, 2011. 22(8): p. 370-3.

[71] Scintu, F., et al., Differentiation of human bone marrow stem cells into cells with a neural phenotype: diverse effects of two specific treatments. BMC Neurosci, 2006. 7: p. 14.

[72] Bi, Y., et al., Pre-activation of retinoid signaling facilitates neuronal differentiation of mesenchymal stem cells. Dev Growth Differ, 2010. 52(5): p. 419-31.

[73] Delcroix, G.J., et al., EGF and bFGF pre-treatment enhances neural specification and the response to neuronal commitment of MIAMI cells. Differentiation, 2010. 80(4-5): p. 213-27.

[74] Curtis, K.M., L.A. Gomez, and P.C. Schiller, Rac1b regulates NT3-stimulated Mek-Erk signaling, directing marrow-isolated adult multilineage inducible (MIAMI) cells toward an early neuronal phenotype. Mol Cell Neurosci, 2012. 49(2): p. 138-48.

[75] Bakhtiari, M., et al., Proliferation and differentiation potential of cryopreserved human skin-derived precursors. Cell Prolif, 2012. 45(2): p. 148-57.

[76] Lim, J.Y., et al., Brain-derived neurotrophic factor stimulates the neural differentiation of human umbilical cord blood-derived mesenchymal stem cells and survival of differentiated cells through MAPK/ERK and PI3K/Akt-dependent signaling pathways. J Neurosci Res, 2008. 86(10): p. 2168-78.

[77] Lim, J.Y., et al., Neural Differentiation of Brain-derived Neurotrophic Factor-expressing Human Umbilical Cord Blood-derived Mesenchymal Stem Cells in Culture via TrkB-mediated ERK and beta-catenin Phosphorylation and following Transplantation into the Developing Brain. Cell Transplant, 2011.

[78] Zhang, Y.Q., et al., Neurotrophin-3 Gene-Modified Schwann Cells Promote TrkC Gene-Modified Mesenchymal Stem Cells to Differentiate into Neuron-Like Cells in Poly(Lactic-Acid-Co-Glycolic Acid) Multiple-Channel Conduit. Cells Tissues Organs, 2012. 195(4): p. 313-22.

[79] Ying, C., et al., Neural Differentiation of Rat Adipose-Derived Stem Cells in Vitro. Cell Mol Neurobiol, 2012.

[80] Karaoz, E., et al., Human dental pulp stem cells demonstrate better neural and epithelial stem cell properties than bone marrow-derived mesenchymal stem cells. Histochem Cell Biol, 2011. 136(4): p. 455-73.

[81] Kiraly, M., et al., Simultaneous PKC and cAMP activation induces differentiation of human dental pulp stem cells into functionally active neurons. Neurochem Int, 2009. 55(5): p. 323-32.

[82] Zhang, W., et al., Neurotrophin-3 improves retinoic acid-induced neural differentiation of skin-derived precursors through a p75NTR-dependent signaling pathway. Neurosci Res, 2009. 64(2): p. 170-6.

[83] Lebonvallet, N., et al., Characterization of neurons from adult human skin-derived precursors in serum-free medium : a PCR array and immunocytological analysis. Exp Dermatol, 2012. 21(3): p. 195-200.

[84] Kondo, T., et al., Wnt signaling promotes neuronal differentiation from mesenchymal stem cells through activation of Tlx3. Stem Cells, 2011. 29(5): p. 836-46.

[85] Litingtung, Y. and C. Chiang, Specification of ventral neuron types is mediated by an antagonistic interaction between Shh and Gli3. Nat Neurosci, 2000. 3(10): p. 979-85.

[86] Litingtung, Y. and C. Chiang, Control of Shh activity and signaling in the neural tube. Dev Dyn, 2000. 219(2): p. 143-54.

[87] Gudas, L.J. and J.A. Wagner, Retinoids regulate stem cell differentiation. J Cell Physiol, 2011. 226(2): p. 322-30.

[88] Maden, M., Retinoid signalling in the development of the central nervous system. Nat Rev Neurosci, 2002. 3(11): p. 843-53.

[89] Reichardt, L.F., Neurotrophin-regulated signalling pathways. Philos Trans R Soc Lond B Biol Sci, 2006. 361(1473): p. 1545-64.

[90] Huang, E.J. and L.F. Reichardt, Trk receptors: roles in neuronal signal transduction. Annu Rev Biochem, 2003. 72: p. 609-42.

[91] Gill, S.S., et al., Direct brain infusion of glial cell line-derived neurotrophic factor in Parkinson disease. Nat Med, 2003. 9(5): p. 589-95.

[92] Slevin, J.T., et al., Improvement of bilateral motor functions in patients with Parkinson disease through the unilateral intraputaminal infusion of glial cell line-derived neurotrophic factor. J Neurosurg, 2005. 102(2): p. 216-22.

[93] Wislet-Gendebien, S., et al., Plasticity of cultured mesenchymal stem cells: switch from nestin-positive to excitable neuron-like phenotype. Stem Cells, 2005. 23(3): p. 392-402.

[94] Martinou, I., et al., Viral proteins E1B19K and p35 protect sympathetic neurons from cell death induced by NGF deprivation. J Cell Biol, 1995. 128(1-2): p. 201-8.

[95] Sung, J.H., et al., Viral caspase inhibitor p35, but not crmA, is neuroprotective in the ischemic penumbra following experimental stroke. Neuroscience, 2007. 149(4): p. 804-12.

[96] Zhang, L., et al., In vitro differentiation of human umbilical cord mesenchymal stem cells (hUCMSCs), derived from Wharton's jelly, into choline acetyltransferase (ChAT)-positive cells. Int J Dev Neurosci, 2012.

[97] Logan, C.Y. and R. Nusse, The Wnt signaling pathway in development and disease. Annu Rev Cell Dev Biol, 2004. 20: p. 781-810.

[98] Toledo, E.M., M. Colombres, and N.C. Inestrosa, Wnt signaling in neuroprotection and stem cell differentiation. Prog Neurobiol, 2008. 86(3): p. 281-96.

[99] Fu, Y.S., et al., Conversion of human umbilical cord mesenchymal stem cells in Wharton's jelly to dopaminergic neurons in vitro: potential therapeutic application for Parkinsonism. Stem Cells, 2006. 24(1): p. 115-24.

[100] Khoo, M.L., et al., Transplantation of neuronal-primed human bone marrow mesenchymal stem cells in hemiparkinsonian rodents. PLoS One, 2011. 6(5): p. e19025.

[101] Wang, J., et al., Stem cells from human-exfoliated deciduous teeth can differentiate into dopaminergic neuron-like cells. Stem Cells Dev, 2010. 19(9): p. 1375-83.

[102] Suon, S., M. Yang, and L. Iacovitti, Adult human bone marrow stromal spheres express neuronal traits in vitro and in a rat model of Parkinson's disease. Brain Res, 2006. 1106(1): p. 46-51.

[103] Alexanian, A.R., et al., Transplanted neurally modified bone marrow-derived mesenchymal stem cells promote tissue protection and locomotor recovery in spinal cord injured rats. Neurorehabil Neural Repair, 2011. 25(9): p. 873-80.

[104] Zhang, W., et al., Implantation of adult bone marrow-derived mesenchymal stem cells transfected with the neurotrophin-3 gene and pretreated with retinoic acid in completely transected spinal cord. Brain Res, 2010. 1359: p. 256-71.

[105] Park, H.W., et al., Directed induction of functional motor neuron-like cells from genetically engineered human mesenchymal stem cells. PLoS One, 2012. 7(4): p. e35244.

[106] Pedram, M.S., et al., Transplantation of a combination of autologous neural differentiated and undifferentiated mesenchymal stem cells into injured spinal cord of rats. Spinal Cord, 2010. 48(6): p. 457-63.

[107] Schira, J., et al., Significant clinical, neuropathological and behavioural recovery from acute spinal cord trauma by transplantation of a well-defined somatic stem cell from human umbilical cord blood. Brain, 2012. 135(Pt 2): p. 431-46.

[108] Biernaskie, J., et al., Skin-derived precursors generate myelinating Schwann cells that promote remyelination and functional recovery after contusion spinal cord injury. J Neurosci, 2007. 27(36): p. 9545-59.

[109] Sieber-Blum, M., et al., Characterization of epidermal neural crest stem cell (EPI-NCSC) grafts in the lesioned spinal cord. Mol Cell Neurosci, 2006. 32(1-2): p. 67-81.

[110] de Lau, L.M. and M.M. Breteler, Epidemiology of Parkinson's disease. Lancet Neurol, 2006. 5(6): p. 525-35.

[111] Nussbaum, R.L. and C.E. Ellis, Alzheimer's disease and Parkinson's disease. N Engl J Med, 2003. 348(14): p. 1356-64.

[112] Hornykiewicz, O., Biochemical aspects of Parkinson's disease. Neurology, 1998. 51(2 Suppl 2): p. S2-9.

[113] Lindvall, O., et al., Grafts of fetal dopamine neurons survive and improve motor function in Parkinson's disease. Science, 1990. 247(4942): p. 574-7.

[114] Kordower, J.H., et al., Dopaminergic transplants in patients with Parkinson's disease: neuroanatomical correlates of clinical recovery. Exp Neurol, 1997. 144(1): p. 41-6.

[115] Wakeman, D.R., H.B. Dodiya, and J.H. Kordower, Cell transplantation and gene therapy in Parkinson's disease. Mt Sinai J Med, 2011. 78(1): p. 126-58.

[116] Ronaghi, M., et al., Challenges of stem cell therapy for spinal cord injury: human embryonic stem cells, endogenous neural stem cells, or induced pluripotent stem cells? Stem Cells, 2010. 28(1): p. 93-9.

[117] Diez del Corral, R. and K.G. Storey, Markers in vertebrate neurogenesis. Nat Rev Neurosci, 2001. 2(11): p. 835-9.

[118] von Bohlen Und Halbach, O., Immunohistological markers for staging neurogenesis in adult hippocampus. Cell Tissue Res, 2007. 329(3): p. 409-20.

[119] Baines, R.A. and M. Bate, Electrophysiological development of central neurons in the Drosophila embryo. J Neurosci, 1998. 18(12): p. 4673-83.

[120] Wislet-Gendebien, S., et al., Astrocytic and neuronal fate of mesenchymal stem cells expressing nestin. Brain Res Bull, 2005. 68(1-2): p. 95-102.

[121] Carleton, A., et al., Becoming a new neuron in the adult olfactory bulb. Nat Neurosci, 2003. 6(5): p. 507-18.

[122] Foudah D., S.A., Redondo J., Tredici G., Miloso M., Evaluation of neural markers expression in human mesenchymal stem cells after mesengenic differentiation. Italian Journal of Anatomy and Embryology, 2011. 16(1).

[123] Liu, J., et al., Electrophysiological properties and synaptic function of mesenchymal stem cells during neurogenic differentiation - a mini-review. Int J Artif Organs, 2012. 35(5): p. 323-37.

[124] Lin, Y.T., et al., Human mesenchymal stem cells prolong survival and ameliorate motor deficit through trophic support in Huntington's disease mouse models. PLoS One, 2011. 6(8): p. e22924.

[125] Park, H.J., et al., Neuroprotective effect of human mesenchymal stem cells in an animal model of double toxin-induced multiple system atrophy parkinsonism. Cell Transplant, 2011. 20(6): p. 827-35.

[126] Snyder, B.R., et al., Human multipotent stromal cells (MSCs) increase neurogenesis and decrease atrophy of the striatum in a transgenic mouse model for Huntington's disease. PLoS One, 2010. 5(2): p. e9347.

[127] Quertainmont, R., et al., Mesenchymal Stem Cell Graft Improves Recovery after Spinal Cord Injury in Adult Rats through Neurotrophic and Pro-Angiogenic Actions. PLoS One, 2012. 7(6): p. e39500.

[128] Prockop, D.J. and J.Y. Oh, Medical therapies with adult stem/progenitor cells (MSCs): a backward journey from dramatic results in vivo to the cellular and molecular explanations. J Cell Biochem, 2012. 113(5): p. 1460-9.

Permissions

The contributors of this book come from diverse backgrounds, making this book a truly international effort. This book will bring forth new frontiers with its revolutionizing research information and detailed analysis of the nascent developments around the world.

We would like to thank Sabine Wislet-Gendebien, PhD, for lending her expertise to make the book truly unique. She has played a crucial role in the development of this book. Without her invaluable contribution this book wouldn't have been possible. She has made vital efforts to compile up to date information on the varied aspects of this subject to make this book a valuable addition to the collection of many professionals and students.

This book was conceptualized with the vision of imparting up-to-date information and advanced data in this field. To ensure the same, a matchless editorial board was set up. Every individual on the board went through rigorous rounds of assessment to prove their worth. After which they invested a large part of their time researching and compiling the most relevant data for our readers. Conferences and sessions were held from time to time between the editorial board and the contributing authors to present the data in the most comprehensible form. The editorial team has worked tirelessly to provide valuable and valid information to help people across the globe.

Every chapter published in this book has been scrutinized by our experts. Their significance has been extensively debated. The topics covered herein carry significant findings which will fuel the growth of the discipline. They may even be implemented as practical applications or may be referred to as a beginning point for another development. Chapters in this book were first published by InTech; hereby published with permission under the Creative Commons Attribution License or equivalent.

The editorial board has been involved in producing this book since its inception. They have spent rigorous hours researching and exploring the diverse topics which have resulted in the successful publishing of this book. They have passed on their knowledge of decades through this book. To expedite this challenging task, the publisher supported the team at every step. A small team of assistant editors was also appointed to further simplify the editing procedure and attain best results for the readers.

Our editorial team has been hand-picked from every corner of the world. Their multi-ethnicity adds dynamic inputs to the discussions which result in innovative outcomes. These outcomes are then further discussed with the researchers and contributors who give their valuable feedback and opinion regarding the same. The feedback is then collaborated with the researches and they are edited in a comprehensive manner to aid the understanding of the subject.

Apart from the editorial board, the designing team has also invested a significant amount of their time in understanding the subject and creating the most relevant covers. They scrutinized every image to scout for the most suitable representation of the subject and create an appropriate cover for the book.

The publishing team has been involved in this book since its early stages. They were actively engaged in every process, be it collecting the data, connecting with the contributors or procuring relevant information. The team has been an ardent support to the editorial, designing and production team. Their endless efforts to recruit the best for this project, has resulted in the accomplishment of this book. They are a veteran in the field of academics and their pool of knowledge is as vast as their experience in printing. Their expertise and guidance has proved useful at every step. Their uncompromising quality standards have made this book an exceptional effort. Their encouragement from time to time has been an inspiration for everyone.

The publisher and the editorial board hope that this book will prove to be a valuable piece of knowledge for researchers, students, practitioners and scholars across the globe.

List of Contributors

Tanja Vogel
Dept. of Molecular Embryology, Institute for Anatomy and Cell Biology, Albert-Ludwigs-University Freiburg, Germany

Sonia Villapol, Trevor T. Logan and Aviva J. Symes
Department of Pharmacology and Center for Neuroscience and Regenerative Medicine, Uniformed Services University of the Health Sciences, Bethesda, MD, USA

Uwe Ueberham and Thomas Arendt
Department for Molecular and Cellular Mechanisms of Neurodegeneration, Paul Flechsig Institute for Brain Research, University Leipzig, Leipzig, Germany

Nibaldo C. Inestrosa and Lorena Varela-Nallar
Center for Aging and Regeneration (CARE), Department of Cell and Molecular Biology, Faculty of Biological Sciences, Pontifical Catholic University of Chile, Santiago, Chile

Adam R. Cole
Neurosignalling Group, Garvan Institute of Medical Research, Darlinghurst, Sydney, Australia

Liang-Wei Chen
Institute of Neurosciences, The Fourth Military Medical University, Xi'an, China

Jenny Wong
Illawarra Health and Medical Research Institute, University of Wollongong, Wollongong, NSW, 2522, Australia
School of Biological Sciences, University of Wollongong, Wollongong, NSW, 2522, Australia

Yonggang Zhang and Wenhui Hu
Department of Neuroscience, Temple University School of Medicine, Philadelphia, USA

Harleen S. Basrai, Kimberly J. Christie and Ann M. Turnley
Centre for Neuroscience Research, Department of Anatomy and Neuroscience, The University of Melbourne, Victoria, Australia

Roxana Nat, Galina Apostolova and Georg Dechant
Institute for Neuroscience, Innsbruck Medical University, Innsbruck, Austria

Ryan Salewski and Hamideh Emrani
Toronto Western Research Institute, University Health Network, Toronto Western Hospital, Canada

Michael G. Fehlings
Division of Neurosurgery and Spinal Program University of Toronto, Krembil Neuroscience Centre, UHN, Toronto Western Hospital, Canada

Atsushi Shimomura
Department of Anatomy I, Fujita Health University School of Medicine, Toyoake, Aichi, Japan

Eri Hashino
Department of Otolaryngology-Head and Neck Surgery, Stark Neurosciences Research Institute, Indiana University School of Medicine, Indianapolis, IN, USA

Bernard Rogister
GIGA Neurosciences, University of Liège, Belgium
GIGA Development, Stem Cells and Regenerative Medicine, University of Liège, Belgium
Neurology Department, University of Liège, Belgium

Virginie Neirinckx, Cécile Coste, and Sabine Wislet-Gendebien
GIGA Neurosciences, University of Liège, Belgium